E. Deltz A. Thiede H. Hamelmann (Eds.)

Small-Bowel Transplantation

Experimental and Clinical Fundamentals

With 78 Figures

Springer-Verlag Berlin Heidelberg New York
London Paris Tokyo

Priv.-Doz. Dr. Eberhard Deltz
Professor Dr. Arnulf Thiede
Professor Dr. Horst Hamelmann

Abtl. Allgemeine Chirurgie an der
Christian-Albrechts-Universität Kiel
Arnold-Heller Straße 7, D-2300 Kiel

ISBN-13:978-3-642-71089-6 e-ISBN-13:978-3-642-71087-2
DOI: 10.1007/978-3-642-71087-2

Library of Congress Cataloging-in-Publication Data.
Small-Bowel Transplantation. Experimental and Clinical Fundamentals. Based on a meeting held in Kiel, West Germany, in Oct. 1985. Includes index. 1. Intestine, Small–Transplantation–Congresses. 2. Transplantation immunology–Congresses. 3. Surgery, Experimental–Congresses. I. Deltz, Eberhard. II. Thiede, Arnulf. III. Hamelmann, H. [DNLM: 1. Intestine, Small–transplantation–congresses. WI 500 E96 1985]
RD540.7.E97 1986 617'.5541 86-20356
ISBN-13:978-3-642-71089-6 (U.S.)

Softcover reprint of the hardcover 1st edition 1986

2123/3145-543210

Preface

In contrast to the continuously increasing success in kidney, liver, heart, and pancreas transplantation, small-bowel transplantation has not shown similarly impressive progress until recently.

The few clinical attempts at small-intestinal transplantation in the late 1960s and early 1970s were unsuccessful. In spite of these initial failures, a few groups of surgeons continued to investigate the problems of small-bowel transplantation from the technical, functional, and immunologic point of view. Now, about 15 years later, conditions have changed. Total parenteral nutrition has made tremendous progress, thus maintaining patients with short-bowel syndrome who are potential recipients of small-bowel grafts in an acceptable physical condition. Immunologists and clinicians have furthermore been able to expand our knowledge of basic immunologic reactions induced by transplanted organs. In addition, within the last 8 years, new immunosuppressive drugs and regimens have been introduced which have proved to be extremely effective.

Taking all these aspects into account, we regarded it as an extremely worthwhile and effective undertaking to invite scientists from all over the world who are working in the field of small-bowel transplantation to participate in a symposium on this topic. This meeting, the first to deal exclusively with small-bowel transplantation, was held in Kiel, West Germany, in October 1985. Its aims were twofold:

1.) To stimulate direct communication between basic scientists and clinicians
2.) To articulate the problems in this new field of transplantation research which remain to be solved through experimental research and clinical investigations

This volume compiles all the contributions made at the workshop and covers ten main topics of importance in small-bowel transplantation: experimental animal models (Sess. 1, 2), the absorptive and adaptive capacity of the transplanted small-bowel (Sess. 3), immunology and immunosuppression (Sess. 4, 5) surgical techniques (Sess. 6), clinical considerations relating to recipient evaluation and donor procurement (Sess. 7, 8), and post-transplantation monitoring and indications for small-bowel transplantation (Sess. 9, 10). In addition summaries of the discussions on each topic appear at the end of each section.

We hope that this book will, in addition to contributing toward the fulfillment of the two aims stated above, stimulate further successful experimental work in this fascinating field of transplantation research and, above all, provide a basis for initial clinical trials of intestinal transplantation in the very near future.

Kiel, October 1986

E. DELTZ
A. THIEDE
H. HAMELMANN

Table of Contents

List of Contributors

ARNAUD-BATTANDIER, F., Dr.
Departement de Pédiatrie, Service de Gastroentérologie, Pédiatrique et de Nutrition, Hôpital des Enfants-Malades,
149 Rue de Sèvres 75730 Paris Cedex 15, France

COHEN, Z., M.D., F.R.C.S. (C)
F.A.C.S., Toronto General Hospital, 101 College Street,
Eaton Bldg., 9–211, Toronto, Ontario, M5G 1L7, Canada

COLLIN, J., Dr.
University of Oxford, Nuffield Department of Surgery
John Radcliffe Hospital, Headington, Oxford OX 3 9DU, U.K.

DELTZ, E., Priv.-Doz. Dr. med.
Chirurg. Universitätsklinik, Arnold-Heller Str. 7, D-2300 Kiel,
West Germany

FERGUSON, A., PhD FRCP FRCPath
Gastro-Intestinal Unit, Western General Hospital, Crewe Road,
Edinburgh EH 4 2 XU, Scotland, U.K.

GEBHARDT, J. H.
Chirurg. Universitätsklinik, Arnold-Heller Str. 7, D-2300 Kiel,
West Germany

GUNDLACH, M.
Chirurg. Universitätsklinik, Arnold-Heller Str. 7, D-2300 Kiel,
West Germany

HARDY, M. A., M.D.
College of Physicians and Surgeons of Columbia University, Department of Surgery, Transplant Service, 630 West 168th Street, New York,
N.Y. 10032, USA

KIRKMAN, R. L., M.D.
Transplant and General Surgery, Brigham and Women's Hospital,
75 Francis Street, Boston, Massachusetts 02115, USA

Lee, K. K. W., Dr.
The University of Chicago, Department of Surgery
950 East Fifty-Ninth-Street, Chicago, Illinois 60637, USA

Leimenstoll, G., Dr. med.
I. Medizinische Universitätsklinik, Abteilung Spezielle Nephrologie und Dialyse, Schittenhelmstr. 12, D-2300 Kiel, West Germany

Liedgens, P.
Chirurgische Universitätsklinik, Arnold-Heller Str. 7, D-2300 Kiel, West Germany

Lünstedt, B., Dr. med.
Chirurgische Universitätsklinik, Arnold-Heller Str. 7, D-2300 Kiel, West Germany

Marks, W. H., M.D., Ph.D.
Department of Surgery, Loyola University Stritch School of Medicine, 2160 South First Avenue, Maywood, Illinois 60153, USA

Mengel, W., Prof. Dr. med.
Chirurgische Universitätsklinik, Arnold-Heller Str. 7, D-2300 Kiel, West Germany

Müller, J. M., Prof. Dr.
Chirurgische Universitätsklinik Köln-Lindenthal
Joseph-Stelzmann-Str. 9, D-5000 Köln 41, West Germany

Müller-Hermelink, H. K., Prof. Dr. med.
Pathologisches Institut der Universität Luitpoldkrankenhaus, D-8700 Würzburg, West Germany

Nordgren, S., M.D.
University of Göteborg, Department of Surgery II, Sahlgrenska sjukhuset, S-413 45 Göteborg, Sweden

Preissner, W. Ch., Dr. rer. nat. Dr. med.
Chirurgische Universitätsklinik, Arnold-Heller Str. 7, D-2300 Kiel, West Germany

Revillon, Y., Dr.
Department de Pediatrie, Service de Gastroenterologie, Pediatrique et de Nutrition, Hôpital des Enfants-Malades, 149 Rue de Sèvres
75730 Paris Cedex 15, France

Ricour, C., Pr AG
Department de Pediatrie, Service de Gastroenterologie, Pediatrique et de

Nutrition, Hôpital des Enfants-Malades, 149 Rue de Sèvres
75730 Paris Cedex 15, France

ROTMAN, N., Dr.
Service de Générale, Hôpital Henri Mondor, 94010 Créteil 207-51-41, Poste 2410, France

SANDFORTH, F., Dr.
Klinikum Steglitz, Innere Medizin, Abt. Gastroenterologie
Hindenburgdamm 30, D-1000 Berlin 45, West Germany

SCHRAUT, W. H., M.D.
The University of Chicago, Department of Surgery
5841 S. Maryland Avenue, Chicago, Illinois 60637, USA

SCHROEDER, P., Dr. med.
Chirurgische Universitätsklinik, Arnold-Heller Str. 7, D-2300 Kiel, West Germany

SEIFERT, J., Prof. Dr. med.
Chirurgische Universitätsklinik, Arnold-Heller Str. 7, D-2300 Kiel, West Germany

STAUFFER, U. G., Prof. Dr. med.
Universitäts-Kinderklinik Zürich, Steinwiesstr. 75, CH-8032 Zürich, Switzerland

TANNENBAUM, G., Dr.
Department of Surgery, Transplant Service, College of Physicians and Surgeons of Columbia University, 630 West 168th Street, New York N.Y. 10032, USA

VESTWEBER, K.-H., Dr. med.
Chirurgische Klinik Köln-Merheim, Ostmerheimer Str. 200
D-5000 Köln 91, West Germany

WALTER, M., Dr. med.
Chirurg. Universitätsklinik Köln, Joseph-Stelzmann-Str. 9
D-5000 Köln 41, West Germany

WESTPHAL, E., Dr. med.
Hygiene-Institut, Abt. Immunologie, Brunswiker Str. 2–6, D-2300 Kiel, West-Germany

WOLMAN, S. L., M.D., F.R.C.P. (C)
Toronto General Hospital, Gastroenterologie, Nutrition Room 220, 9th Floor, Eaton Wing, Toronto, Ontario M5G1L7, Canada

Session 1

Evaluation of Experimental Models of Small-Bowel Transplantation in the Rat

Microsurgical Techniques of Heterotopic and Orthotopic Small-Bowel Transplantation in the Rat

W. CH. PREISSNER, P. SCHROEDER, M. GUNDLACH, P. LIEDGENS, E. SCHRÖDER, and E. DELTZ

Introduction

Within the last 10 years, clinical kidney transplantation has reached the stage where it can be considered a routine procedure. Transplantation of the liver and heart is being performed with considerable success at several surgical centers. However, the history of human small-bowel grafting has so far been characterized largely by setbacks. To date, small-bowel transplantation has been performed in a few cases only (HARDY et al. 1985), with a maximum survival time of 79 days (FORTNER et al. 1972).

Major obstacles, both technical and immunologic, have prevented any recent clinical attempts in small-bowel transplantation.

The immunologic response in small-bowel transplantation includes not only rejection but also a graft-versus-host reaction, which are mediated by the epithelial and mesenchymal elements in the intestinal wall and the mesentery (MONCHIK and RUSSELL 1971; STAUFFER 1977; THIEDE and DELTZ 1978) respectively. The latter include in particular immunocompetent cells in the Peyer's patches, the lymph follicles of the intestinal wall, and the mesenteric lymph nodes. When these cells pass into the recipient, a graft-versus-host reaction directed against the recipient occurs. On the other hand a rejection reaction, the host-versus-graft reaction, also takes place. Complex immunologic reactions can be expected by the interaction of these two reactions. For analysis of these complicated immunologic reactions, experiments with defined constant immunogenetic conditions, with known histoincompatibility antigens of the major histoincompatibility complex (MHC) are necessary. MHC-typed rats are available that permit microsurgical procedures to be carried out in numbers large enough for a statistical evaluation of experimental results. For this reason, microsurgical models in the rat are best suited for experimental organ grafting and for solving the complicated problems related to transplantation surgery (MÜLLER-RUCHHOLTZ 1985).

Among microsurgical techniques for small-bowel transplantation, it is important to distinguish between two different types of experimental designs:

1) Heterotopic transplantation, in which the small intestine of the recipient is not removed and the transplant is grafted alongside the recipient's organ.
2) Orthotopic transplantation, in which the small bowel of the recipient is removed and the transplanted organ replaces it in orthotopic position.

Heterotopic Small-Bowel Transplantation

Heterotopic small-bowel transplantation is possible by three different methods. The various models of heterotopic small-bowel transplantation (DELTZ and THIEDE 1984; 1985) differ in their manner of handling the oral and aboral ends of the graft. It is possible to place both ends of the graft as an ileostoma and duodenostoma in the abdominal wall of the recipient. The disadvantage of this model in rats is that the maintainance of the stomas can be extremly complicated, as the rats lose large amounts of fluid and electrolytes through the stomas.

Another possibility is to anastomose the aboral end of the gut to the terminal ileum of the recipient and to suture the other end to the abdominal wall as a duodenostoma. Finally, it is possible to anastomose the aboral end of the graft to the terminal ileum of the recipient and to close the oral end with a circular ligature (Fig. 1). This is the technique used by the microsurgical group in Kiel (DELTZ and THIEDE 1984; 1985).

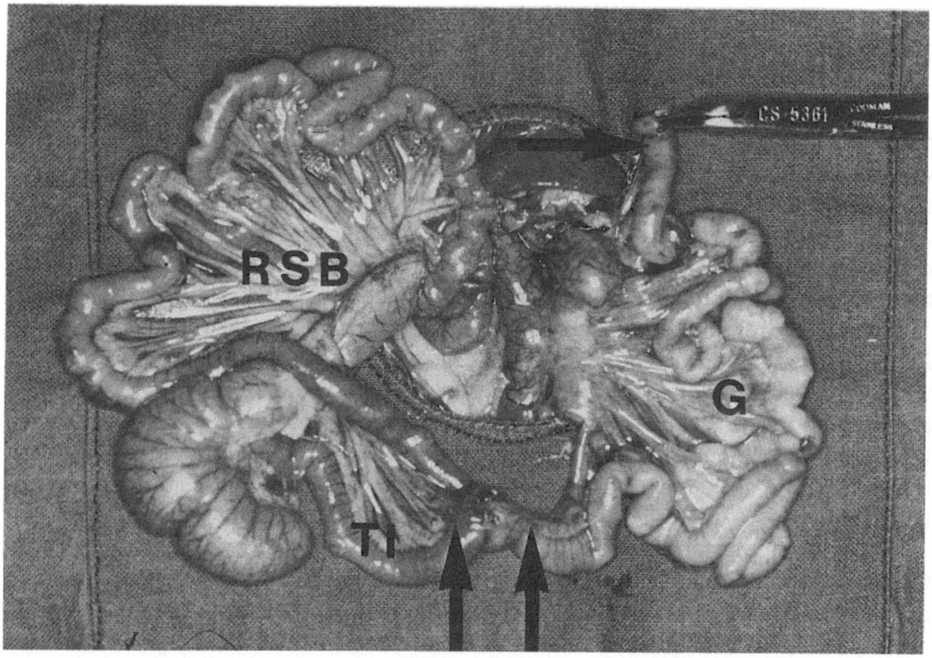

Fig. 1. Heterotopic small-bowel transplantation in the rat. →, oral end of the graft *(G)*; ⇉, ileoileal anastomosis of the graft and recipient's terminal ileum *(TI)*; *RSB*, recipient's small bowel

Operative Technique

Using ether anesthesia, the abdomen of the donor is opened by a midline incision. The operation starts with the separation of the small-bowel mesentery from the colon. First, the middle colic artery and its branches are ligated, and the mesocolon is divided. The portal vein and the superior mesenteric vein are divided after ligature of their tributaries and isolation from the pancreas.

After the retroperitoneum is entered and the celiac trunk is freed of surrounding tissue, the lienal artery and a lumbal artery are ligated and the lymph vessels divided. Then, the aorta is cross-clamped proximally and distally of the superior mesenteric artery, and the portal vein and the intestine are divided at the duodenojejunal flexure and at the terminal ileum. Following this step, the aortic cuff is punctured and the graft perfused with 0.9% NaCl solution at 4°C until the graft appears white and the effluent is clear. After this, the aorta is ligated distally, and the graft is removed by dissecting the aorta. Finally, the intestinal graft is perfused with 20 ml 0.9% NaCl solution beginning at the oral end of the graft to remove the intraluminal contents.

Transplantation

After opening the abdomen of the recipient by a midline incision, the small bowel of the recipient is retracted to the right to expose the abdominal aorta and the inferior vena cava. Both vessels are isolated along a stretch of 1 cm, clamped proximally and distally, and opened longitudinally. The vessels must be rinsed free of blood to reduce the chance of thrombosis.

After bringing the graft into position, an end-to-side anastomosis of the aortic cuff of the graft to the abdominal aorta of the recipient is performed using a running suture. The posterior suture is performed from the lumen, the anterior suture from the exterior of the vessel. The next step is the end-to-side anastomosis of the portal vein to the inferior vena cava of the recipient. The anastomoses are sutured with 8-0 nonabsorbable material (Ethilon, Ethicon, Hamburg). In the vein-to-vein anastomosis, care must be taken to avoid stenosis, which would lead to stasis in the graft. The clamps are removed and the blood stream released. As a substitute for blood loss, 2 ml hydroxyethyl starch is injected into the tail vein. The oral end of the graft is closed with a circular ligature. The aboral end of the graft is anastomosed by an end-to-side anastomosis to the terminal ileum of the recipient by a continuous one-layer suture with nonabsorbable material. Finally, the intestine of the recipient and the graft are returned to the abdomen, and the abdominal wall is closed with a continuous two-layer suture.

The whole operation takes about 120 min, and the cold ischemic time is 30–40 min. Complications are venous thrombosis in the region of the anastomosis and bleeding from the arterial anastomosis. Both complications lead to a shock situation resulting in the death of the recipient within 24 h.

With sufficient microsurgical practice and experience, the postoperative long-term survival rate is more than 90%.

Orthotopic Small-Bowel Transplantation

In our laboratory, orthotopic small-bowel transplantation is achieved by the so-called two-step operative technique. The first operative step is the heterotopic auxiliary transplantation, as described above.

After 3 weeks, the lymph vessels between graft and recipient are regenerated (REZNICK et al. 1982). At this time, the second operative step is performed. The abdomen of the recipient is opened by a midline incision, the graft small bowel is retracted to the right, that of the recipient is retracted to the left side. The second operative step consists of resection of the recipient's small bowell by ligatures of the mesenteric vessels. Then, anastomosis of the oral end of the graft to the duodenum of the recipient is accomplished by end-to-end anastomosis using a continuous one-layer suture with nonabsorbable material (Fig. 2). The intestine is returned to the abdomen, and the abdominal wall ist closed with a continuous one-layer suture.

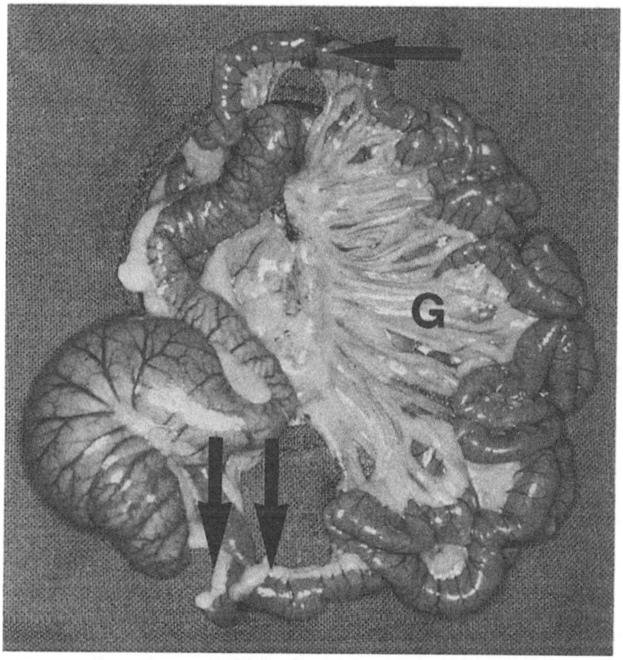

Fig. 2. Orthotopic small-bowel transplantation. →, oral duodenojejunal anastomosis; ⇉, ileoileal anastomosis; graft *(G)* in orthotopic position

By this method, orthotopic small-bowel transplantation with portosystemic blood drainage is achieved. The duration of the second operative step ist about 40 min. After the second operative step, the animals receive a liquid synthetic oligopeptide diet (Peptisorb, Pfrimmer, Erlangen, Federal Republic of Germany) for the first 5 days, after which they receive a normal diet with water ad libidum. Heparin and antibiotics are unnecessary. With sufficient microsurgical practice and experience, the long-term survival rate of syngeneic transplantation is more than 85%, with a survival time of more than 180 days.

Discussion of Microsurgical Models

Of the two different types of small-bowel transplantation, heterotopic and orthotopic transplantation, the heterotopic model represents a bypass model with a simple technique and a very high survival rate. In comparison, orthotopic transplantation of small bowel is much more complicated. There are two types of orthotopic transplantation: the two-step operative technique described above that we are using and the single-step technique described by Kort (1984). In our laboratory, we use the two-step operative technique because, compared with the single-step technique, surgical mortality is lower.

Heterotopic models are better suited for investigations of immunologic reactions such as rejection reaction and graft-versus-host reaction because the recipient survives even when the graft sustains extensive damage that in the orthotopic graft would lead to the early death of the recipient. In contrast, orthotopic models are more suited for preclinical studies, including studies of graft function and absorption capacity under physiologic conditions and in interaction with immunologic reactions.

References

Deltz E, Thiede A (1984) Experimental transplantation of small-intestine: Microsurgical techniques and their applicability in research. In: Olszewski WL (ed) Handbook of Microsurgery, vol 2. CRC Press, Boca Raton, Florida, pp 419–429

Deltz E, Thiede A (1985) Microsurgical technique for small-intestine transplantation. In: Thiede A, Deltz E, Engemann R, Hamelmann H (eds) Microsurgical models in rats for transplantation research. Springer, Berlin Heidelberg New York Tokyo, pp 51–55

Fortner JG, Sichuk G, Litwin SD, Beattie EH (1972) Immunological responses to an intestinal allograft with HL-identical donor-recipient. Transplantation 14:531–535

Hardy MA, Iga Ch, Lau H (1985) Intestinal transplantation: Laboratory experience of clinical consequences. In: Thiede A, Deltz E, Engemann R, Hamelmann H (eds) Microsurgical models in rats for transplantation research. Springer, Berlin Heidelberg New York Tokyo, pp 337–346

Kort WJ (1984) Orthotopic total small bowel transplantation in the rat. In: Olszewski W (ed) Handbook of microsurgery, vol 2. CRC Press, Boca Raton, Florida, pp 431–435

Monchick GJ, Russell PS (1971) Transplantation of small-bowel in the rat: Technical and immunological considerations. Surgery 70:693–702

Müller-Ruchholtz W (1985) Theoretical aspects of rat organ transplantation. In: Thiede A, Deltz E, Engemann R, Hamelmann H (eds) Microsurgical models in rats for transplantation research. Springer, Berlin Heidelberg New York Tokyo, pp 77–81

Reznick BK, Graddock GN, Langer B, Gilas T, Cullen JB (1982) Structure and function of small bowel allografts in the dog: Immunosuppression with cyclosporin A. Can J Surg 25:51–55

Stauffer U (1977) The present state of small bowel transplantation in animal research and in man. Z Kinderchir 22:241–248

Thiede A, Deltz E (1978) Morphological reaction in transplanted small-intestines using immunogenetically defined rat strain combinations. Langenbecks Arch Chir 346:119–127

Small-Bowel Transplantation in the Rat: Graft Survival with Heterotopic vs Orthotopic Position

K. K. W. Lee and W. H. Schraut

Introduction

Experimental studies on a variety of vascularized organ allografts have suggested that graft rejection may be delayed if venous outflow is directed into the portal rather than the systemic circulation (Fukuda et al. 1969; Sakai 1970). In studies of small-bowel transplantation, in which portal rather than caval venous drainage establishes an anatomically and physiologically normal state, the beneficial effects of portal drainage on the survival of both graft and recipient have been confirmed (Kort et al. 1973; Schraut et al. 1983). These studies, however, have been limited to the heterotopic model of intestinal transplantation in which the small-bowel allograft remains defunctionalized, i.e., it constitutes an accessory graft which is not in continuity with the recipient's gastrointestinal tract. In future clinical intestinal transplantation, the graft is likely to be placed orthotopically, in gastrointestinal continuity, either at the time of transplantation or later. In this position, the intestinal allograft is exposed to the fecal stream and is required to absorb enterally administered nutrients. Using the rat model of vascularized small-bowel transplantation, we studied the effect of venous drainage upon graft survival following both heterotopic and orthotopic transplantation.

Materials and Methods

Experimental Groups

Transplantation was performed in the Lewis x Brown Norway F_1 (LBN F_1) hybrid to Lewis (LEW) rat strain combination using males weighing between 200 and 250 g. We prepared four groups of animals which differed with respect to graft position (heterotopic or orthotopic) and route of venous drainage (systemic or portal):

I. Heterotopic, systemic venous drainage (H-SVD), $n = 25$
II. Heterotopic, portal venous drainage (H-PVD), $n = 14$
III. Orthotopic, systemic venous drainage (O-SVD), $n = 15$
IV. Orthotopic, portal venous drainage (O-PVD), $n = 10$

Operative Procedures

Small-bowel transplantation was performed using standard microsurgical techniques as described by Schraut et al. (1983). The donor small bowel was removed on a vascular pedicle, which consisted of the superior mesenteric artery and the portal vein, after intraluminal irrigation of the bowel with cold (4°C) neomycin-saline solution (0.05%) and intravascular flushing with cold heparinized saline (10000 units/liter). After end-to-side anastomosis of the superior mesenteric artery to the recipient's infrarenal aorta, the portal vein was anastomosed either to the inferior vena cava (groups I and III) or to the portal vein (groups II and IV). In groups I and II, heterotopic transplantation was completed by construction of two enterostomas at the animals' abdominal wall. In groups III and IV, orthotopic transplantation was completed by resection of the recipients' own smal bowel from the ligament of Treitz to the ileocecal valve and by placement of the revascularized graft into intestinal continuity through end-to-end intestinal anastomoses.

Animals surviving for fewer than 4 days after the operation were regarded as technical failures and were excluded from further analysis.

Postoperative Care

All animals were permitted a regular laboratory diet ad libitum beginning on the second postoperative day, and their general health and appearance were closely monitored. The enterostomas of animals in groups I and II were examined daily, and the exteriorized grafts were periodically cannulated and irrigated with saline.

Determination of Graft Rejection

In animals undergoing heterotopic transplantation, evidence of rejection consisted of graft necrosis or fibrosis and closure of the enterostomas. Stomal necrosis was invariably associated with the recipient's death, thus providing a well-defined clinical end point of rejection. Stomal fibrosis and obliteration of the lumen were not associated with recipient death and thus constituted a less well-defined end point of rejection. Graft rejection following orthotopic transplantation was invariably associated with the recipient's death and was thus well-defined.

Pathohistologic Studies

After graft rejection was ascertained, all surviving animals were killed. Postmortem examinations were performed on all animals. The small-bowel graft and the recipient's small bowel, lymph nodes, spleen, and liver were prepared for light microscopy using hematoxylin and eosin stains.

Results

In heterotopic transplantation and either type of venous anastomosis, the technical failure rate was approximately 20%. Thrombosis of a vascular anastomosis was the primary cause for technical failure; other causes included graft volvulus and stomal complications such as prolapse or obstruction which led to perforation. In orthotopic transplantation, the technical failure rate was 20%–30% irrespective of the type of venous drainage used. In orthotopic transplantation, intestinal obstruction occurring at the site of intestinal anastomosis or as a result of adhesions was a cause for technical failure in addition to the causes noted for heterotopic transplantation.

Clinical Course and Survival: Heterotopic Transplantation

Rejection of LBN F_1 intestinal allografts following heterotopic transplantation with systemic venous drainage (H-SVD, group I) followed a rapid course characterized by necrosis of the enterostomas in association with progressive deterioration and death of the LEW recipient (Fig. 1). The mean survival time for these animals was 11.4 ± 0.4 days. After heterotopic transplantation with portal venous drainage (H-PVD, group II), graft rejection was more indolent. In these animals, the enterostomas became fibrotic and closed, preventing cannulation and irrigation of the graft, and the graft coalesced into a firm nodular abdominal mass. The overall health of these recipients was generally unaffected by the ongoing rejection of the allografts. The average graft survival of 19.8 ± 6.2 days in these animals was significantly longer than that for the H-SVD animals.

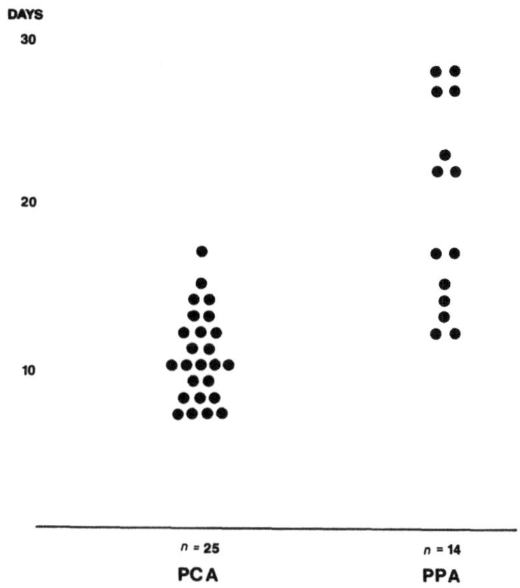

Fig. 1. Survival of intestinal allografts after heterotopic transplantation. In portocaval venous anastomosis *(PCA)*, recipient death constituted a well-defined end point of graft rejection; in portoportal venous anastomosis *(PPA)*, the end point of graft rejection was less well defined. The difference in graft survival is statistically significant

Clinical Course and Survival: Orthotopic Transplantation

The postoperative course and survival times following orthotopic transplantation were similar to those with systemic and portal venous drainage (Fig. 2). In the immediate postoperative period, all graft recipients lost weight because of perioperative fasting. With the resumption of a regular laboratory diet, the animals displayed normal appetites, with passage of normally formed feces and weight stabilization. Between 7 and 9 days after transplantation, the graft recipients developed diarrhea and lost weight. Both conditions became progressively severe and led to emaciation and death. In each group, one animal survived for 40 to 45 days; each of these animals had persistent diarrhea and appeared emaciated until it died. For the remaining animals in groups III (O-SVD) and IV (O-PVD), the mean survival times were 12.4 ± 1.7 and 13.1 ± 1.7 days respectively.

Histopathologic Findings: Heterotopic Transplantation

With rejection, H-SVD allografts (group I) became thin and friable, with patches of transmural necrosis and occasional perforations.

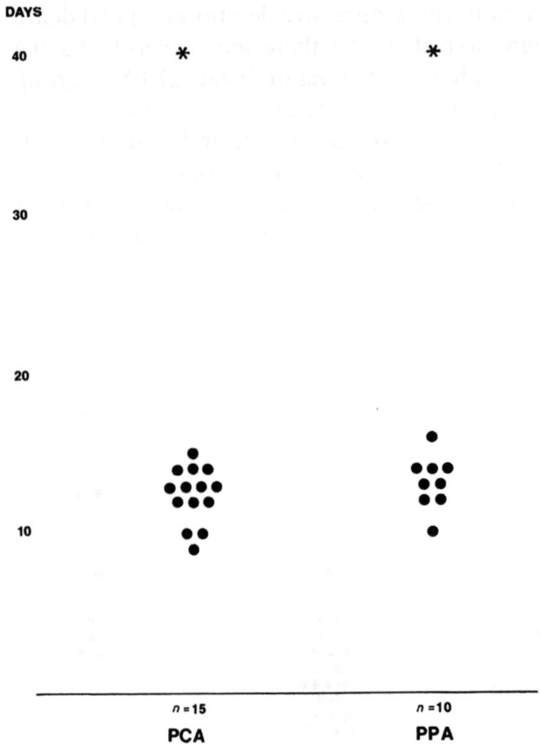

Fig. 2. Survival of intestinal allografts after orthotopic transplantation. For both portocaval anastomosis *(PCA)* and portoportal venous anastomosis *(PPA)*, recipient death provided a well-defined end point of graft rejection. Recipient survival is the same in both groups* longest survival time

When viewed microscopically, these grafts showed an intensive cellular infiltration of the mucosa and submucosa, widespread areas of mucosal destruction and sloughing, and peritonitis (Fig. 3a). After H-PVD (group II), the intestinal allograft became thickened and self-adherent, forming a firm, encapsulated nodular mass (Fig. 3b). The mucosa was absent, and the bowel wall was thickened, with granulation tissue and fibrosis of the submucosa and muscularis (Fig. 3c). Peritonitis was not detected in these animals.

Histopathologic Findings: Orthotopic Transplantation

With rejection, intestinal allografts in groups III (O-SVD) and IV (O-PVD) became thin and distended, with submucosal hemorrhage, while the graft mesentery became thickened. Microscopically, a prominent cellular infiltrate accompanied by extensive mucosal destruction and sloughing was seen (Fig. 4a, b). The allografts from each of the orthotopic graft recipients with the longest survival times showed destruction and denudation of the mucosa, with fibrosis and thickening of the remaining bowel wall (Fig. 4c).

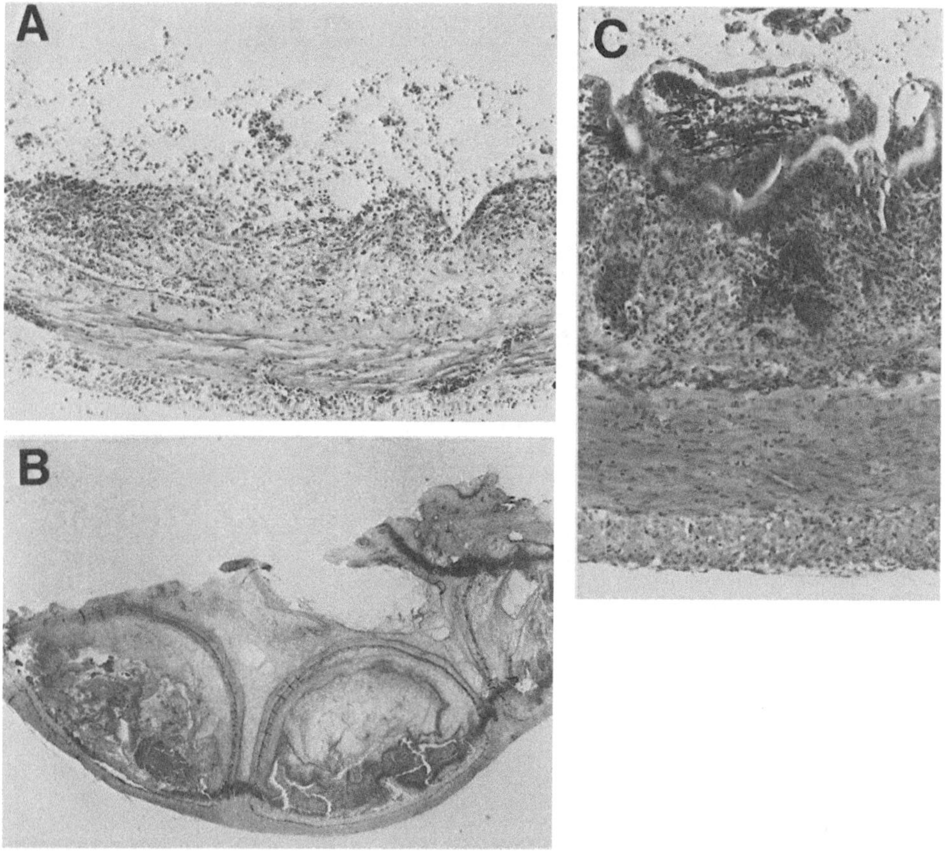

Fig. 3A–C. Pathohistologic changes in accessory intestinal allograft rejection. **A** Histologic appearance of a rejected heterotopic allograft with systemic drainage. There is complete mucosal destruction (× 100). **B** Whole-mount of a rejected heterotopic allograft with portal venous drainage. The intestinal loops are self-adherent and encapsulated (× 25). **C** Histologic appearance of a rejected heterotopic allograft with portal venous drainige. The bowel wall is thickened. The mucosa is still recognizable and heavily infiltrated (× 100). (Hematoxylin-eosin stain)

Discussion

These results demonstrate that, in small-bowel transplantation, the route of venous drainage may alter the course of allograft rejection. In the LBN $F_1 \rightarrow$ LEW strain combination, portal venous drainage of heterotopic intestinal transplants modifies rejection sufficiently to allow encapsulation and fibrosis of the graft, rather the perforation and transmural necrosis seen in systemic venous drainage. This leads to recipient survival despite rejection of the graft, rather than recipient death in concert with rejection of the graft. However, the time course for the histopathologic changes of rejection following portal venous drainage is delayed by only 1–3 days (Rosemurgy and Schraut 1986), suggesting that the beneficial effects of portal

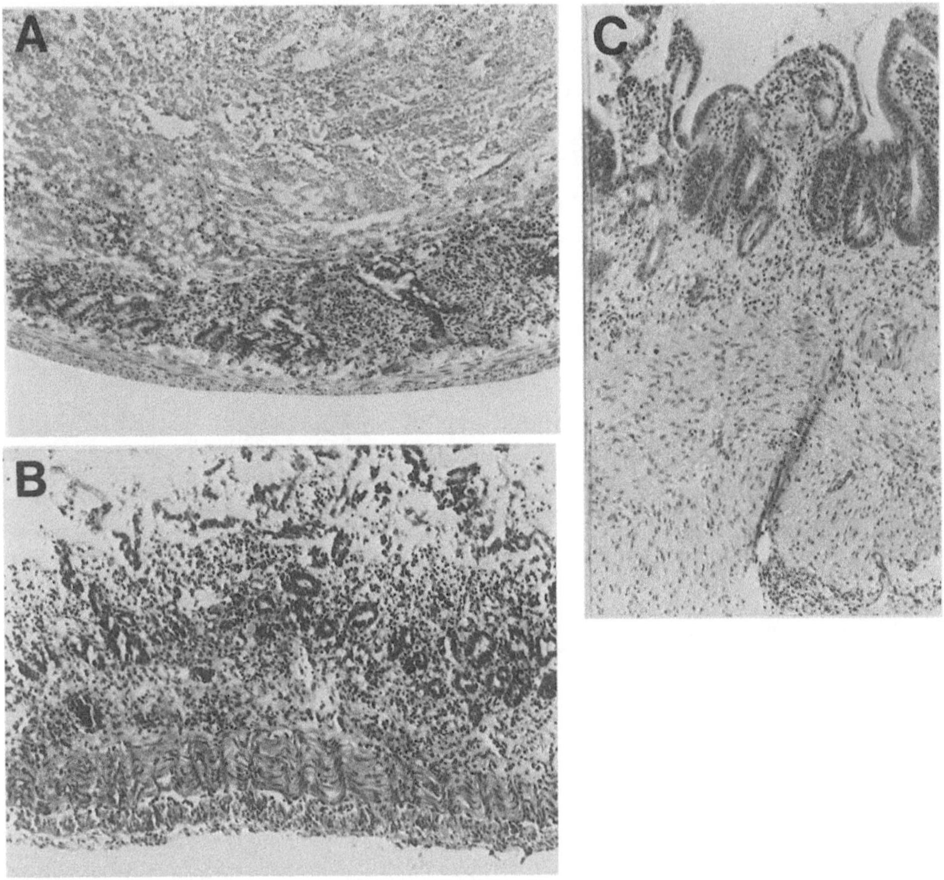

Fig. 4A–C. Pathohistologic changes in orthotopic intestinal allograft rejection. Acute graft rejection with systemic **(A)** and portal **(B)** venous drainage. Both grafts exhibit thinning of the bowel wall and mucosal destruction. **C** Histologic appearance of an orthotopic allograft from a long-term (42 days) surviving graft recipient. The mucosal layer is still present, although severely damaged. The bowel wall is thickened. (Hematoxylin-eosin stain; × 100)

venous drainage are relatively minor. Studies of functional graft survival using a maltose absorption test have also demonstrated only minor differences arising from portal venous drainage (Billiar et al. 1984).

With orthotopic graft placement, recipient survival depends on satisfactory preservation of graft function; i.e., a graft with markedly reduced functional (absorptive) capacity, even if it is otherwise intact, will lead to emaciation and death of the recipient. Loss of function due to rejection is paralleled by loss of the mucosal barrier function, an immediate and fatal effect of rejection for the recipient of an orthotopic graft. The transplanted bowel is constantly exposed to bacteria and other noxious substances in the lumen, which may interact synergistically with the rejection process and lead to rapid graft destruction. These events overshadow and prevent the minor beneficial effects of portal venous drainage from being expressed clinically.

Thus, compared with the heterotopic model of intestinal transplantation, the orthotopic model imposes more severe conditions for graft and recipient survival. Under these conditions, variations in graft rejection and recipient survival that arise from differences in the routes of venous outflow are not observed, further suggesting that this effect is minor, although real.

Successful clinical small-bowel transplantation in the future will entail orthotopic graft positioning, although heterotopic positioning may be employed as an initial step. The disparate findings in the heterotopic and the orthotopic models of small-bowel transplantation with respect to the types of venous drainage illustrate the potential hazards of extrapolating results obtained in the heterotopic model of the clinically more relevant orthotopic situation. They also point out the limitations of the heterotopic model as an investigational tool. The study of graft preservation and treatment of rejection, for example, should not rely on the use of the heterotopic model alone, but must also involve the orthotopic model, in which the existence of a degree of graft function sufficient to support the normal growth and nutrition of the recipient can be verified.

In the rat model of small-bowel transplantation, one-stage orthotopic transplantation requires slightly more operative time than does heterotopic transplantation. However, the incidence of technical failures is comparable and thus supports the use of orthotopic transplantation as an experimental model.

References

Billiar TR, Garberoglio C, Schraut WH (1984) Maltose absorption as an indicator of small-intestinal allograft rejection. J Surg Res 37:75–82

Fukuda A, Hanaoka T, Solowey AC, et al (1969) Inhibition of second-set renal allograft responses by portal vein drainage. Transplant Proc 1:602–604

Kort WJ, Westbroeck DL, MacDicken I, et al (1973) Orthotopic total small bowel transplantation in the rat. Eur Surg Res 5:81–89

Rosemurgy AS, Schraut WH (1986) Small-bowel allografts: Sequence of histologic changes in acute and chronic rejection. (To be published)

Sakai A (1970) Role of the liver in kidney allograft rejection in the rat. Transplantation 9:333–334

Schraut WH, Rosemurgy AS, Riddell RM (1983) Prolongation of intestinal allograft survival without immunosuppressive drug therapy: Transplantation of small bowel allografts. J Surg Res 34:597–607

Recent Results of Small-Bowel Transplantation in the Rat Model[1]

W. A. Koltun and R. L. Kirkman

Since its original description by Monchik and Russell (1971), the model of small-bowel transplantation in the rat has proved to be remarkably productive. The availability of inbred strains has allowed the phenomena of rejection and graft-vs-host disease (GvHD) to be studied separately in a controlled fashion that is not possible in large-animal models. Moreover, the advent of cyclosporine therapy has produced a flurry of new investigations employing the rat, as is evident from the contributions to this workshop.

Previous work from this la boratory has focused on the effect of cyclosporine on the immunology and function of small-bowel transplants in the rat (Kirkman et al., 1984; 1985). In our experimentation, cyclosporine has proved to be highly effective in the prevention of rejection. When the drug was given at a dose of 15 mg/kg per day for 7 days following transplantation, graft survival exceeded 100 days in the strain combination Lewis x Brown Norway F_1 hybrid (LBN) into Lewis and was significantly prolonged in the combination Lewis x Wistar Furth F_1 hybrid (LWF) into Lewis. Cyclosporine was less successful in preventing GvHD. When Lewis bowel was transplanted into either LBN or LWF recipients, host survival was prolonged by cyclosporine, but animals frequently succumbed to GvHD when cyclosporine was discontinued.

The histologic and functional correlates of rejection have also been carefully examined in our rat model (Madara and Kirkman 1985). Histologically, the earliest abnormalities in jejunal grafts occurred within 3 days post-transplantation and consisted of focal endothelial cell injury of the microvasculature and focal injury of crypt epithelial cells. Both alterations were associated with the infiltration of large lymphoid cells, and both progressed markedly over the ensuing 6 days. In contrast, the structure of the villus absorptive cells was not markedly altered until the 9th postoperative day. These structural abnormalities were largely paralleled by functional deficits in both passive and active ion transport, as determined in the Ussing chamber. These results have led to the hypothesis that the primary targets for rejection in small-bowel transplantation are the endothelial cells of the microvasculature and the crypt epithelial cells. Damage to the villus epithelium is most likely secondary and related to ischemia produced by microvascular injury and/or decreased epithelial regenerative ability which is secondary to crypt injury. Of importance, the histologic and functional abnormalities caused by rejection were markedly ameliorated by the use of cyclosporine in these short-term experiments.

[1] Supported by NIH Grants AM33040 and AM35929.

Recent laboratory investigations have turned to the longer-term consequences of small-bowel transplantation in the rat. This has required the development of techniques for placing the graft in continuity with the host gastrointestinal tract and has led to a significant increase in technical complications. Initial work has focused on the metabolic consequences of systemic, as opposed to portal, venous drainage. It seems likely that future clinical small-bowel transplants will employ systemic drainage for reasons of simplicity and safety. Nevertheless, the effects of a partial portacaval shunt on the nutrition and metabolism of the host have received little study. Aberrations in serum ammonia and amino acid levels have been observed following creation of an Eck's fistula in rats for studies of hepatic encephalopathy (Cummings et al. 1976; Hindfeldt et al. 1977; Hawkins et al. 1982). Whether this will be seen following small-bowel transplantation with systemic venous drainage remains unknown. The remainder of this paper will address this question. The data remain preliminary and are submitted in the spirit of a workshop contribution.

Materials and Methods

Animals

Adult male Lewis rats weighing between 150 and 250 g were obtained from Microbiological Associates, Walkersville, Maryland, USA, or from Charles River Laboratories, Kingston, New York, USA. Recipient and donor were always obtained from the same source.

Experimental Groups

Three groups of animals were studied:

1) Group I: (n = 6) unmanipulated controls
2) Group II: (n = 5) recipients of out-of-continuity small-bowel transplants, with both ends of the graft exteriorized as stomas
3) Group III: (n = 6) recipients of in-continuity small-bowel transplants, with near total resection of native jejunum and ileum

Venous drainage in both groups II and III was into the systemic circulation, and all transplants were isografts.

Operative Techniques

The technique for out-of-continuity small-bowel transplantation was modified from Monchik and Russell (1971) and has been previously described (Kirkman et al. 1984). For in-continuity grafts, the host intestine was resected from proximal jejunum to distal ileum, preserving the ileocecal valve.

Anastomoses between graft and host bowel were performed using a single layer of interrupted 7–0 silk, with the entire procedure performed as a single stage.

Postoperative Studies

All animals were weighed daily. Blood samples were obtained by cardiac puncture under light ether anesthesia. For ammonia levels, 1 ml heparinized blood was obtained 100–110 days after transplantation, iced, centrifuged, and the plasma assayed using the glutamate dehydrogenase technique (VAN ANKEN and SCHIPHORST 1974). Bilirubin, SGOT, alkaline phosphatase, total protein, and albumin were measured on serum samples obtained by separate puncture 1 week following ammonia determinations. Amino acid levels were obtained from heparinized blood 150–200 days following initiation of the study in groups I and III. The plasma was prepared by acid precipitation and stored at −20° C and analyzed on a Beckman amino acid analyzer (Model 6300) using the Ninhydrin technique.

Statistics
Groups were compared using the two-tailed *t* test.

Results

Growth curves for all three groups are illustrated in Fig. 1. Both transplanted groups weighed significantly less than the control group at 120 days ($P < 0.001$), but were not significantly different from each other.

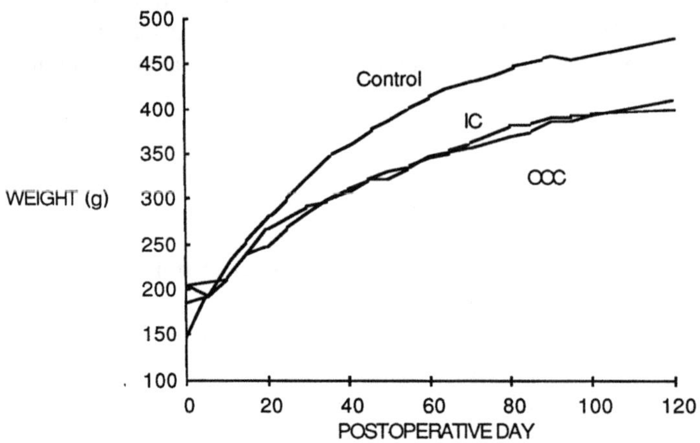

Fig. 1. Growth curves for control (n = 6), out-of-continuity *(OOC)* transplants (n = 5), and in-continuity *(IC)* transplants (n = 6). The difference between the controls and the other two groups is significant at 120 days ($P < 0.001$)

As seen in Fig. 2, chronic plasma ammonia levels were significantly greater in group III with in-continuity grafts (mean ± SE = 96 ± 9 µ*M*/liter) than in either group I (42.5 ± 1 µ*M*/liter) or group II (33.4 ± 5 µ*M*/liter) (both $P < 0.001$). The difference between groups I and II was not significant. Total protein, albumin, SGOT, alkaline phosphatase, and total bilirubin were not significantly different between any of the groups (data not shown).

Finally, five amino acids were identified which were significantly different in group III animals with in-continuity grafts when compared with the unmanipulated controls in group I. The five were glycine, serine, aspartate, histidine, and phenylalanine; significant changes in other amino acids were not detected. The percent age of change in these amino acids is shown in Fig. 3, with control values given in the legend.

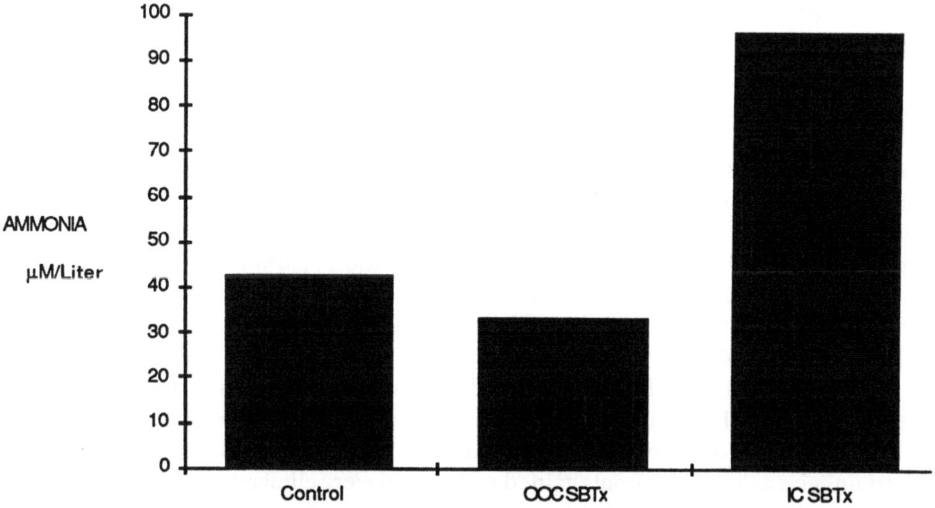

Fig. 2. Plasma ammonia levels in the three groups at 100–110 days after transplantation. The in-continuity *(ICSBT)* group is significantly different ($P < 0.001$) from the control and the out-of-continuity *(OOCSBT)* groups, which are not significantly different from each other

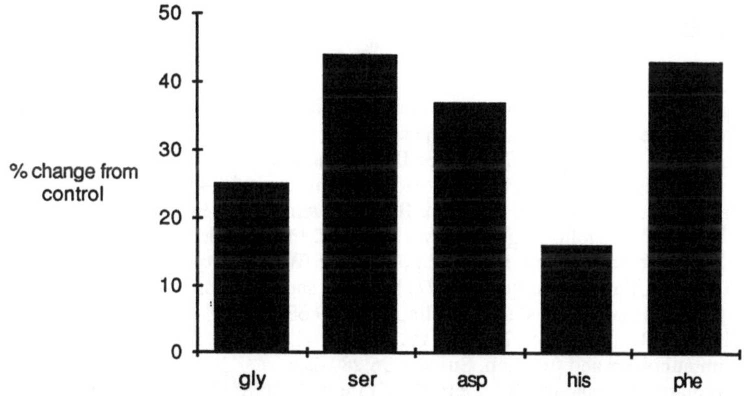

Fig. 3. Amino acid changes 150–200 days after transplantation in the in-continuity group (group III) expressed as percent age of change of control (group I) levels. Control levels were glycine *(gly)* 177 ± 8 n*M*/ml, serine *(ser)* 9 ± 2 n*M*/ml, aspartate *(asp)* 6 ± 1 n*M*/ml, histidine *(his)* 76 ± 2.5 n*M*/ml, and phenylalanine *(phe)* 63 ± 3 n*M*/ml. All changes were significant at the $P < 0.05$ level or better

Discussion

These preliminary results suggest that small-bowel transplantation with venous drainage into the systemic circulation will produce chronic abnormalities in ammonia and amino acid levels. Animals with total in-continuity small-bowel transplants displayed ammonia levels approximately twice those of unoperated controls. Since venous drainage from the colon continued to be into the portal circulation, the data suggest a role for the small bowel itself in the generation of ammonia. Furthermore, failure to observe the elevation in ammonia in animals whose transplants were not in-continuity indicates that food must be present in the bowel lumen for the production of ammonia. Abnormalities in ammonia levels could not be explained by liver dysfunction, as liver function tests remained normal in all groups.

The abnormalities in amino acid levels seen in these recipients of in-continuity small-bowel transplants are reminiscent of those reported in models of hepatic encephalopathy (Cummings et al. 1976; Aquirre et al. 1974). The pattern in those models includes elevations in the aromatic amino acids (phenylalanine, tyrosine, and tryptophan) as well as in aspartate, methionine, histidine, and glutamate. Decreased levels of the branched-chain amino acids leucine, isoleucine, and valine are also seen. These alterations have been correlated with changes in blood-brain barrier transport and the synthesis of false neurotransmitters such as octopamine (Smith et al. 1977; Hawkins et al. 1982). Failure to demonstrate all of these changes in our recipients of small-bowel transplants may reflect the incomplete nature of the portacaval shunt.

The significance of the observed abnormalities in ammonia and amino acid levels is uncertain, given that the animals gained weight and were clinically healthy. Nevertheless, these early data suggest that further study is required to determine the best route of venous drainage for clinical small-bowel transplants.

References

Aguirre A, Yoshimura N, Westman T, Fischer JE (1974) Plasma amino acids in dogs with two experimental forms of liver damage. J Surg Res 16:339–345

Cummings MG, Soeters PB, Janes JH, Keene JM, Fischer JE (1976) Regional brain indoleamine metabolism following chronic portocaval anastomosis in the rat. J Neurochem 27:501–509

Hawkins RA, Mans AM, Biebuyck JF (1982) Alterations in amino acid transport across blood brain barrier in rats following portacaval shunting. In: Blackburn GL, Grant JP, Young VR (ed) Amino acids: metabolism and medical applications. Wright, Boston, p 239

Hindfelt B, Plum F, Duffy TE (1977) Effect of acute ammonia intoxication on cerebral metabolism in rats with portacaval shunts. J Clin Invest 59:386–396

Kirkman RL, Lear PA, Madara JL, Tilney NL (1984) Small intestine transplantation in the rat-immunology and function. Surgery 96:280–286

Kirkman RL, Madara JL, Lear PA, Ythier A (1985) The utility of cyclosporin in small bowel transplantation. Transplant Proc 17:1401–1402

Madara JL, Kirkman RL (1985) Structural and functional evolution of jejunal allograft rejection in rats and the ameliorating effects of cyclosporine. J Clin Invest 75:502–512

Monchik GL, Russell PS (1971) Transplantation of small bowel in the rat, technical and immunological considerations. Surgery 70:693–702

Smith AR, Rossi-Fanelli F, Ziparo V, Janes JH, Perelle BA, Fischer JE (1977) Alterations in plasma and CSF amino acids, amines and metabolites in hepatic coma. Ann Surg 187:343–350

Van Anken HC, Schiphorst ME (1974) A kinetic determination of ammonia in plasma. Clin Chem Acta 56:151–157

Metabolic Effects of Systemic Venous Drainage in Small-Bowel Transplantation

K. K. W. LEE and W. H. SCHRAUT

Introduction

In vascularized transplants of the small bowel, venous outflow from the intestinal graft may be conveyed into either the portal or the systemic venous circulation. Studies on a variety of organ allografts (SAKAI 1970; BOECKX et al. 1975), including small-bowel allografts (KORT et al. 1973; SCHRAUT et al. 1983), have suggested that portal venous drainage confers immunologic benefits which favor prolonged allograft survival. These benefits appear to be minor, however, and may not be sufficient to justify the use of portal drainage in preference to systemic venous drainage in intestinal transplantation (SCHRAUT et al. 1985). Portal drainage, however, re-establishes the physiologic route of venous outflow, whereas systemic drainage creates a partial mesocaval shunt, the metabolic consequences of which have not been studied in detail. Therefore, using the rat model in orthotopic small-bowel transplantation, we compared the metabolic changes following transplantation with portal and with systemic venous drainage. Changes in body weight, blood ammonia levels, serum triglycerides, protein and albumin, maltose absorption, and liver weight were the parameters studied.

Materials and Methods

Experimental Groups

Male Lewis (LEW) rats weighing between 180 and 250 g were used in all experiments. Four groups of animals were studied:

1) LEW rats undergoing LEW syngeneic orthotopic small-bowel transplantation with end-to-side, portoportal venous anastomosis (PPA; $n = 7$)
2) LEW rats undergoing LEW syngeneic orthotopic small-bowel transplantation with end-to-side, portocaval venous anastomosis (PCA; $n = 8$)
3) LEW rats receiving a central end-to-side, portocaval shunt (PC shunt; $n = 15$)
4) Age-matched normal LEW rats (NL; $n = 6$)

Operative Procedures

Small-bowel transplantation was performed using a modification of the technique which we described previously (SCHRAUT et al. 1983). Briefly, the entire donor small bowel was harvested on a vascular pedicle consisting of the superior mesenteric artery and the portal vein. After end-to-side anastomosis of the superior mesenteric artery to the recipient's infrarenal aorta, the portal vein was anastomosed in end-to-side fashion to the recipient's portal vein (group 1) between the coronary vein and the confluence of the splenic and superior mesenteric veins or to the recipient's infrarenal inferior vena cava (group 2). The recipient's small bowel was resected from the ligament of Treitz to the ileocecal valve, and the revascularized intestinal graft was placed into gastrointestinal continuity by completion of two end-to-end intestinal anastomoses. Central end-to-side portocaval shunts were created in group 3 animals by dividing the portal vein at the hilum of the liver, ligating the central stump, and anastomosing the distal stump to the inferior vena cava in end-to-side fashion. Each type of venous anastomosis was completed in 10–15 min. The incidence of early venous thrombosis was approximately 15% in each group.

Postoperative Care

All animals were allowed a regular laboratory diet throughout the study period of 6 months. Total body weight and serum ammonia, protein, albumin, and triglyceride levels were measured periodically according to standard laboratory methods. Maltose absorption in the small-bowel grafts of groups 1 and 2 was also determined. At the end of the study period, the animals were killed and examined for patency of all anastomoses and for evidence of portal hypertension. Total body weight and relative liver weight were also recorded.

Results

The patterns of venous circulation resulting from the transplant procedures are illustrated in Fig. 1.

Animals undergoing transplantation with either portal or systemic venous drainage (groups 1 and 2) initially gained weight at rates slower than those for the age-matched normal rats (group 4), but by the end of the study period the total weight gain was comparable in all three groups (Table 1). Throughout this period, animals that had

Table 1. Influence of venous drainage on metabolic changes following orthotopic small-bowel transplantation in the rat

	Group	Weight change (%)	NH_3 (μg/dl)	Triglycerides (mg/dl) Early	Late	Relative liver weight (%)
PPA	1	45 ± 13	83 ± 10	47 ± 3*	70 ± 21	2.8 ± 0.2
PCA	2	39 ± 11	140 ± 22*	66 ± 20*	81 ± 26	2.6 ± 0.3
PC shunt	3	(−15 ± 10)*	560 ± 148*	40 ± 10*	51 ± 12*	2.0 ± 0.2*
Normal	4	39 ± 5	84 ± 15		94 ± 21	2.7 ± 0.2

* $P < 0.05$

undergone central portocaval shunting (group 3) suffered significant weight loss, and six of the 15 animals died of emaciation within 4 weeks after surgery.

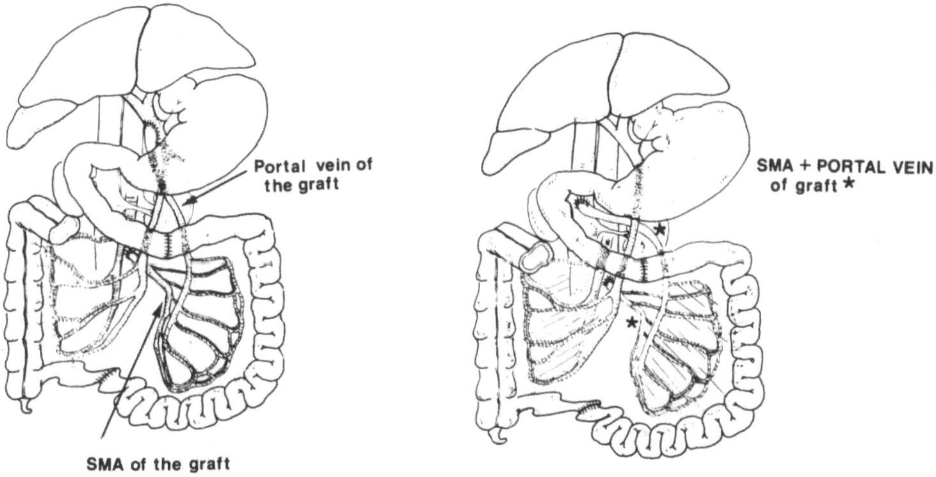

Fig. 1. Anatomic arrangement after transplantation of the entire small bowel of the rat with PPA *(left)* and with PCA *(right)*. The recipient's own small intestine has been resected, and the graft has been placed in intestinal continuity. (SMA, superior mesenteric artery)

Serum ammonia levels in animals undergoing transplantation with portal venous outflow (group 1) did not differ significantly from levels in normal animals, but in animals with systemically drained grafts (group 2), they were significantly elevated in comparison with levels in both group 1 and normal rats. Levels in group 3 animals (with central portocaval shunts) were markedly elevated in comparison with all three other groups.

In the early postoperative period, serum triglyceride levels were significantly decreased in animals undergoing small-bowel transplantation or central shunting when compared with levels in normal animals. By the end of the study period, levels no longer differed significantly from normal in transplanted animals (PPA and PCA), but remained significantly decreased in shunted animals.

Maltose absorption in transplanted grafts in groups 1 and 2 did not vary significantly from normal values. Serum protein electrophoresis in both groups of transplanted animals also gave normal results.

At the time of death, all venous anastomoses were patent, and there was no evidence of portal hypertension. The relative liver weight (liver weight/body weight) of group 1 rats was equal to the relative liver weight of normal animals. The relative liver weight of transplant recipients with PCA was somewhat lower than the weights for those with PPA and normal rats, but this difference was not statistically significant. The relative liver weight of centrally shunted animals in group 3 was significantly decreased in comparison with that of the other three groups of animals.

Discussion

These studies demonstrate that the magnitude of metabolic changes resulting from portocaval venous drainage of small-bowel transplants parallels the degree of anatomic and hemodynamic alteration in the portal vascular system. As Fig. 1 illustrates, small-bowel transplantation with portal venous anastomosis is anatomically equivalent to the normal physiologic state. The data obtained confirm our expectations, i. e., that portal venous drainage is also physiologically equivalent to the normal state. The temporary reductions in weight gain and serum triglyceride levels in rats undergoing transplantation with portal venous drainage or with caval drainage probably result from disturbances in bowel function in the early post-transplantation period. These disturbances may be caused by transient and reversible ischemic injury, postoperative ileus, mesenteric lymphatic disruption, or intestinal denervation.

In contrast, central portocaval shunting totally diverts portal blood flow away from the liver and causes severe metabolic derangements. The abnormalities observed in group 3 rats with central portocaval shunts are consistent with the observations of other investigators (Herz et al. 1972; Lauterburg et al. 1976).

The abnormalities observed after intestinal transplantation with systemic venous outflow parallel the changes seen after central portocaval shunting, but are less severe. As shown in Fig. 1, systemic venous drainage of small-bowel grafts is anatomically equivalent to an incomplete mesocaval shunt, diverting small-bowel venous outflow into the systemic circulation but leaving gastric, duodenal, pancreatic, and proximal colonic venous outflow undisturbed. Our studies demonstrate that systemic venous drainage of small-bowel grafts results in a physiologic state which is between total portal diversion and the normal state or its equivalent, the small-bowel graft with portal venous drainage.

In the rat model of orthotopic intestinal transplantation, caval venous drainage causes an elevation of serum ammonia levels which is statistically significant, but is much less prominent than the elevation that occurs after total shunting. It can be assumed that the various metabolic changes induced by a portocaval shunt (for example, alteration of the enterohepatic cycle, impaired clearance of drugs and metabolites) also occur, but to a lesser degree with the partial shunt created by small-bowel transplantation and a portocaval anastomosis. Although we did not observe the marked liver atrophy that results from a total portocaval shunt, a minor reduction in the relative liver weight, although statistically not significant, appeared to accompany portocaval anastomosis in our series of experiments. Major liver atrophy is probably averted by preservation of pancreatic venous flow or by adequate portal hepatic blood flow in this partial shunt. These changes may not have clinical significance as long as the functional reserve of the liver is adequate, but may evolve into real clinical concerns should liver function deteriorate because of other diseases.

In summary, this study demonstrates that portal venous drainage is physiologically equivalent to the normal state, whereas systemic venous drainage causes metabolic disturbances consistent with a partial portosystemic shunt. These changes are less marked than those following complete portosystemic shunting and, in this model, do not provide a compelling reason to favor portal drainage to caval drainage. In clinical intestinal transplantation, however, the magnitude of these disturbances may be sufficient to warrant use of portoportal rather than portocaval venous anastomosis. In addition, pre-existing liver insufficiency of the small-bowel graft recipient, such as might result from chronic total parenteral nutrition or from the use of hepatotoxic pharmacologic agents, may magnify the significance of these disturbances and thereby lead one to favor the use of portal venous drainage.

References

Boeckx W, Sobis H, Lacquet A, et al (1975) Prolongation of allogeneic heart graft survival in the rat after implantation on portal vein. Transplantation 19:145–149

Herz R, Sautter V, Robert F, et al (1972) The Eck fistula rat: Definition of an experimental model. Eur J Clin Invest 2:390–397

Kort WJ, Westbroeck DL, MacDicken I, Lameijer LDF (1973) Orthotopic total small bowel transplantation in the rat. Eur Surg Res 5:81–89

Lauterburg BH, Sautter V, Preisig R, Bircher J (1976) Hepatic functional deterioration after portacaval shunt in the rat. Effects on sulfobromophthalein transport-maximum, indocyanine green clearance and galactose elimination capacity. Gastroenterology 71:221–227

Sakai A (1970) Role of the liver in kidney allograft rejection in the rat. Transplantation 9:333–334

Schraut WH, Abraham VS, Lee KKW (1985) Portal versus systemic venous drainage for small-bowel allografts. Surgery 98:579–585

Schraut WH, Rosemurgy AS, Riddell RM (1983) Prolongation of intestinal allograft survival without immunosuppressive drug therapy. J Surg Res 34:597–607

Session 1: Summary

E. DELTZ

It seems unequivocally clear that experiments concerning immunologic fundamentals of small-bowel transplantation should preferably be carried out in rat models by microsurgical operative methods. Since various inbred strains of rats with well-defined histocompatibility properties are available, transplantation experiments can be carried out in a specific immunogenetical situation.

In principle, small-bowel transplantation in the rat can be carried out both heterotopically in an accessory manner and orthotopically. Accessory models are most suited for pure immunologic investigations in basic research, because, even in the case of strong immunologic reactions, e. g., graft-versus-host (GvH) reaction and rejection reaction, the recipient does not succumb to GvH disease or rejection of the heterotopically transplanted graft immediately. This allows for long observation periods and the performance of different in vitro studies. However, accessory models do not represent the physiologic state of small-bowel function. For evaluation of small-bowel function in a preclinical model, orthotopic small-bowel replacement should be performed. Beyond that, these orthotopic models facilitate the corelation of immunologic and functional investigations.

The operative procedure for orthotopic small-bowel transplantation, with immediate interposition of the intestine has a relatively high operative mortality. In order to minimize these complications, the two-step procedure with secondary interposition of the small bowel 3 weeks after heterotopic transplantation seems to be appropriate.

The route of drainage of venous blood from the graft must be investigated further. Portal venous drainage seems to have a certain immunologic influence on graft survival. In contrast to systemic drainage, portal venous drainage after heterotopic small-bowel transplantation delays rejection and leads to chronic graft fibrosis rather than acute rejection with perforation of the graft.

The underlying mechanisms, i. e., the function of the liver in antigen elimination or antigen presentation, remains unclear at the present moment.

Metabolic disturbances, especially in respect of the increase of serum ammonia, are more profound with systemic blood drainage than with portal drainage, which represents the physiologic situation.

However, a decision as to which route of drainage for graft circulation should be preferred in clinical small-bowel transplantation cannot be founded on conclusions drawn from rat experiments.

Session 2
Experimental Models in Large Animals

*Small-Bowel Transplantation in the Pig**

T. J. PRITCHARD[1], W. A. KOLTUN, J. L. MADARA, and R. L. KIRKMAN

The availability of the new immunosuppressive agent cyclosporine (CsA) has produced a burst of enthusiasm for studies of experimental small-bowel transplantation. The unique ability of CyS to prevent both rejection and graft-vs-host disease suggests that this agent should be ideal for small-bowel transplantation, in which both phenomena have been shown to occur (MONCHIK and RUSSELL 1971; COHEN et al. 1976; DELTZ et al. 1981). Indeed, (CsA) has been remarkably effective in rat models of small-bowel transplantation (THIEDE et al. 1982; KIRKMAN et al. 1984). However, it has been much less satisfactory in large-animal models. Although a statistically significant prolongation of graft survival compared with untreated controls can usually be shown, only a few long-term survivors have been produced in either the dog or pig (CRADDOCK et al. 1983; DILIZ-PEREZ et al. 1984; RICOUR et al. 1983). In all large-animal series, the immunologic failures were caused by rejection, not graft-vs-host disease, and technical failure rates were high.

We have employed two models of small-bowel transplantation in the pig for a variety of technical and immunologic studies. The two models differ in the route of venous drainage; in the heterotopic model, drainage is into the systemic circulation, while in the orthotopic model, it is into the portal circulation. The utility of CsA in preventing rejection has been examined in both models, as have technical issues. This report will review our experience with these models; a portion of the data has been published elsewhere (PRITCHARD et al. 1985).

Materials and Methods

Animals

Outbred female pigs weighing 10–15 kg were obtained from Earle Parsons and Sons, Inc., Hadley, Massachusetts.

Histocompatibility typing was not performed. The animals were maintained in accordance with the United States Public Health Service policy on the humane care and use of animals and the *Guides for the Care and Use of Laboratory Animals* (DHEW 1978).

* Supported by NIH Grants AM 33040 and AM 35929 and by Sandoz, Inc.

[1] Dr. Pritchard is a Dudley P. Allen Research Fellow from the Department of Surgery, Case-Western Reserve University, Cleveland, Ohio.

Pre- and Postoperative Care

Food was withheld for 24 h prior to surgery; water was given ad lib. All animals were premedicated with ketamine (10 mg/kg IM) and atropine (0.4 mg IM) prior to induction of general anesthesia with a mixture of oxygen, nitrous oxide, and halothane. Intravenous fluids were given through a cannula placed in an ear vein. Cephalothin (500 mg IV) was injected prior to surgery.

Animals received water but no solid food for 2 days postoperatively. On the 1st postoperative day, 500 ml Ringer's lactate solution and cephalothin (1 g) were given intravenously. Feeding with standard pig chow was resumed on the 3rd postoperative day.

Operative Technique

In the heterotopic model, the graft consists of a 250 cm segment of proximal small intestine from midjejunum to midileum. The vasculature consists of the superior mesenteric artery and vein; their large size at this location facilitates subsequent anastamosis. Heparin (4000 I. U.) is given intravenously prior to vessel division. After harvest, the intestinal graft is placed into a sterile plastic bag and perfused by gravity through the artery with 500 ml ice-cold lactated Ringer's solution containing 2000 I. U. heparin. The graft is stored in an ice bucket during preparation of the recipient. Because the remaining small bowel is devascularized by this procedure, the donor must be sacrificed following harvest. In the recipient animal, the graft is anastamosed in an end-to-side fashion with the superior mesenteric artery attached to the aorta and the superior mesenteric vein connected to the vena cava just inferior to the native renal vessels. Each end of the bowel is externalized with the stomas located in each lower quadrant.

In the orthotopic model, each pig serves as both donor and recipient, with the animals being operated upon simultaneously. This reciprocal transplantation is made possible by removing the graft from a more distal segment of small bowel in a manner which preserves circulation to all remaining proximal bowel, thus avoiding the need to sacrifice the donor. The graft is perfused and stored as described for the heterotopic model. While the graft is being perfused, a single-layer bowel anastamosis is performed between the proximal and distal ends of the native bowel using interrupted sutures. The graft can then be positioned anterior to the native bowel. The allograft artery and vein are next anastamosed to the recipient mesenteric artery and vein in an end-to-end fashion using interrupted 6-0 Prolene sutures (Ethicon, Inc., Somerville, N.J.). The bowel ends are exteriorized as stomas as in the heterotopic technique.

Animal groups

Six groups of pigs were studied:

I.) Untreated heterotopic controls (n = 10) received no immunosuppression.

II.) Untreated orthotopic controls (n = 14) received no immunosuppression.

III.) Treated animals with a heterotopic transplant (n = 11) received daily oral CsA (25 mg/kg per day) beginning on preoperative day 1. The CsA was dissolved in olive oil and administered by pharyngeal lavage.

IV.) Treated animals with a heterotopic transplant (n = 10) received CsA as in group III and underwent donor graft irradiation (50 rad from a cesium source) and recipient splenectomy.

V.) Treated animals with an orthotopic transplant ($n = 12$) were given oral CsA (25 mg/kg per day) dissolved in olive oil by pharyngeal lavage commencing on preoperative day 1, as in group III.

VI.) Treated animals with an orthotopic transplant ($n = 8$) were injected with CsA 25 mg/kg per day IM on preoperative day 1, were given CsA (8 mg/kg per day IV) on the day of surgery, and were then administered CsA (25 mg/kg per day IM) beginning on postoperative day 1. When serum CsA levels were excessive (> 700 ng/ml), the daily drug dose was reduced to either 20 mg/kg per day or 15 mg/kg per day, depending on the values of subsequent determinations.

Postoperative Monitoring

Animals were evaluated daily in the postoperative period to assess their clinical characteristics and the appearance of the transplant stomas. They were sacrificed with an overdose of barbiturate if any three of the following criteria were observed: stomal discoloration, presence of a stomal exudate, lethargy, ear and/or nose discoloration, weight loss, anorexia, or vomiting. All recipients which succumbed or were sacrificed were autopsied to determine the cause of failure. Technical complications were defined as nonimmunologic events which led to host death.

Histology/Pathology

At 3-day intervals in the postoperative period, animals were sedated with ketamine (10 mg/kg IM) and mucosal biopsies of the transplant segments obtained using a suction biopsy instrument (Quinton Instruments, Seattle, Washington). Specimens were fixed in 10% phosphate-buffered formalin and embedded in paraffin. Subsequently, 6-μm sections were stained with hematoxylin and eosin and analyzed by light microscopy.

CsA Levels

At weekly intervals and just prior to administration of daily CsA, blood was obtained from an abdominal wall vein, allowed to stand for 1 h, and centrifuged for 5 min. The serum was stored at $-20°$ C until processing. Serum CsA levels were determined using the radioimmunoassay kit provided by Sandoz, Inc, Basel, Switzerland. These were considered trough levels of the drug.

Survival Data

Survival times were calculated using either the postoperative day of death (few instances) or time of sacrifice when clinical illness was apparent (most instances). In addition, several animals appeared clinically healthy, but their transplant mucosal biopsies consisted of necrotic fragments of tissue. In these cases, animals were sacrificed despite their apparent thriving condition.

Statistics

Survival times were compared using rank sum analysis.

Results

Survivals

The survival times of all 65 pigs undergoing small-bowel transplantation in this series are listed by group in Table 1. Technical failures, defined as all events other than rejection which led to death of the animal, are listed separately. All immunologic failures were caused by rejection; graft-vs-host disease was not identified in any animal.

Table 1. Survival time of pig small-bowel transplants by treatment group (n = 65)

Group		Cause of failure	Survival in days
I	Heterotopic, control	Technical	0, 3, 7, 10
		Immunologic	14, 15, 19, 20, 33, 35
II	Orthotopic, control	Technical	1, 1, 1, 6, 9, 10, 10
		Immunologic	6, 6, 6, 8, 9, 10, 11
III	Heterotopic, oral CsA	Technical	0, 4, 7, 9, 10
		Immunologic	7, 11, 14, 28, 36, 40, 104
IV	Heterotopic, oral CsA, X-rax, splenectomy	Technical	0, 6, 7, 18
		Immunologic	14, 16, 19, 23, 43, 60
V	Orthotopic, oral CsA	Technical	0, 0, 1, 3, 10, 46, 72, 113
		Immunologic	6, 9, 9, 15
VI	Orthotopic, IM CsA	Technical	0, 10, 15, 24, 38, 39, 50, 64
		Immunologic	none

Of the various therapeutic options evaluated, only treatment with intramuscular CsA (group VI) produced prolongation of survival. When compared with either the technical or immunologic failures of the appropriate control (group II), this prolongation was significant at the $P < 0.05$ level. No rejection was noted in any of the eight animals of this group. Of those animals surviving more than 2 weeks, three died from transplant intussusception, two from pneumonia, and one was sacrificed after repeated injections of CsA produced hind limb paralysis. As described below, these animals did not show histologic evidence of rejection.

Survival was not significantly prolonged in any of the other treatment groups. There were, however, occasional long-term survivors in each group. A single animal with a heterotopic transplant treated with oral CsA (group III) appeared well with pink stomas at 104 days, when it was sacrificed for histologic examination. The graft was thickened and fibrotic, but the mucosa was grossly intact. Likewise, one apparently healthy animal in group IV was sacrificed at 60 days with similar findings. One animal in group V survived 113 days before succumbing to pneumonia, without mucosal changes suggestive of acute or chronic rejection. Of interest, CsA administration to this animal was discontinued on postoperative day 36.

When only immunologic failures are considered, survival of untreated controls was greater in the heterotopic model than in the orthotopic model ($P < 0.01$). This result is probably artifactual, as recognition that rejection had occurred was delayed in group I while its clinical correlates were being learned. For example, the two animals sacrificed at days 33 and 35 were clinically healthy, but subsequent analysis of sequential biopsy specimens suggested that rejection had occurred much earlier.

Technical Failures

The technical failure rate in this series was 55%; causes of technical failure are listed in Table 2. The most common problem was intussusception of the transplanted loop, which accounted for 22% of all failures. Next in importance was arterial thrombosis; five of the seven failures in this group occurred in the orthotopic model, in which the arterial anastamosis is performed in a relatively small vessel. Most of the late technical failures were caused by sepsis. In three of these cases, the animals developed pneumonia, while one had peritonitis of uncertain origin. One animal was thought to have expired from sepsis originating from bacterial overgrowth in an occluded loop of transplanted intestine.

Table 2. Technical complications in 65 porcine small-bowel transplants

Complication	% of total	Survival in days
Anesthetic	14	0, 0, 0, 0, 0
Exsanguination	6	1, 1
Arterial thrombosis	19	0, 1, 1, 3, 3, 6, 7
Venous thrombosis	6	9, 10
Transplant intussusception	22	4, 10, 10, 10, 10, 15, 24, 50
Transplant volvulus	3	7
Sepsis	14	18, 39, 64, 72, 113
Host bowel obstruction infarction	14	6, 7, 9, 10, 46
Paralysis secondary to injections	3	38

CsA Levels

The mean trough CsA levels were 202 ± 37 ng/ml in group III, 125 ± 18 ng/ml in group IV, 63 ± 8 ng/ml in group V, and 543 ± 102 ng/ml in group VI. Intramuscular CsA doses were decreased from 25 mg/kg per day to 15–20 mg/kg per day in four group VI animals when their serum trough levels measured greater than 700 ng/ml.

Histology

The histologic structure of the transplanted small-bowel loops was assessed by serial mucosal suction biopsies, as illustrated in Fig. 1. The baseline pig mucosal architecture is more variable than that seen in more routinely used laboratory animals. The ratio of villus height to crypt depth varied from 1:1 to 3:1, although no cytologic evidence of epithelial cell damage was present. Additionally, mucosal lymphoid follicles, a normal component of small-intestinal mucosal anatomy, are more numerous in pigs than in many other species.

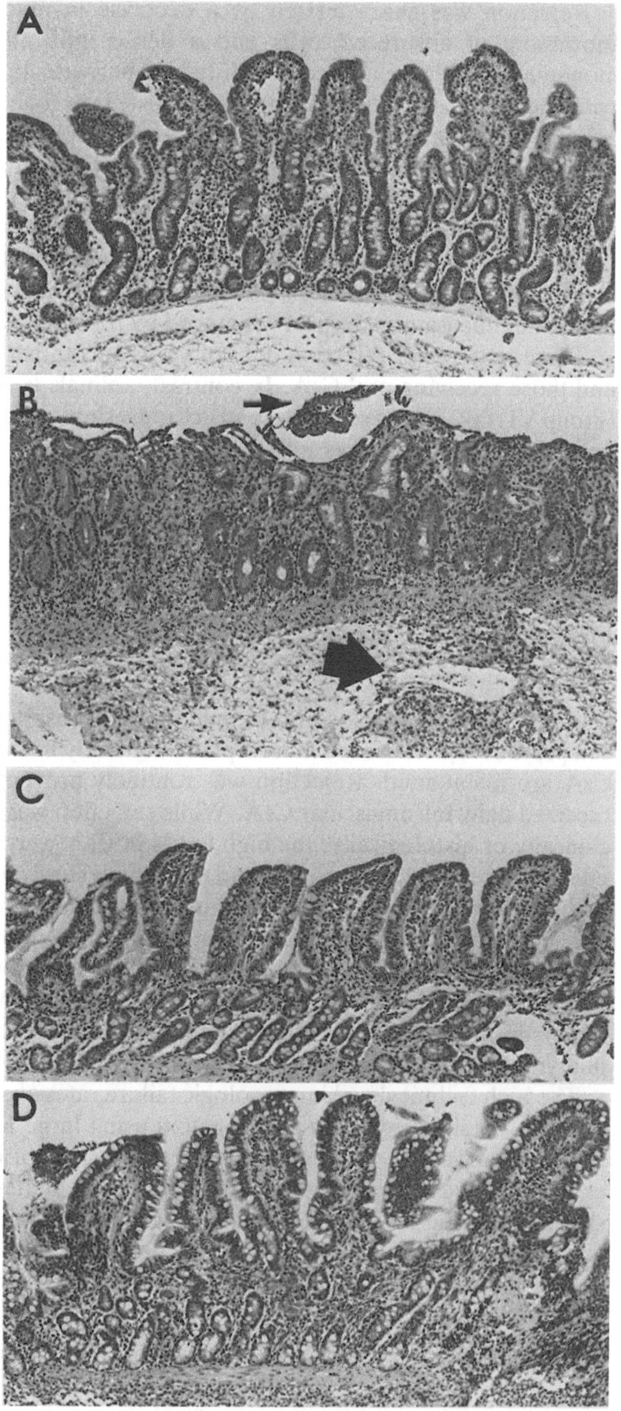

Fig. 1 A–D. Light photomicrographs of pig small intestinal mucosa. **A** Control mucosa taken from a pig before transplantation shows a normal villiform appearance. The villi are not quite as tall as in many other species, and some variation in villus height was noted in control tissues. **B** Mucosa from a transplanted loop in an untreated pig. The mucosa is flat and eroded as demonstrated by the presence of necrotic surface debris *(small arrow)*. Focally, submucosal vessels show associated mononuclear cell infiltrates *(large arrow)*. **C, D** Mucosa from a transplanted loop in a pig treated with CsA injections. Both 9 **(C)** and 34 **(D)** days after transplantation, a relatively normal villiform mucosal structure is retained. All magnifications approximately × 80

Rejection was characterized by a decrease in mucosal depth accompanied by shortening of absorptive cells and a dense infiltrate in the lamina propria of mononuclear inflammatory cells. Multifocal perivascular cuffing of mononuclear cells could be seen in vessels adjacent to the muscularis mucosa. As rejection progressed, erosion of the mucosal surface with loss of all epithelial cells occurred in a patchy fashion. These alterations were somewhat variable in a given loop. Moreover, the rejection process appeared to advance at differing rates in different animals. The earliest unequivocal structural features indicating rejection were seen at 6 days after transplantation, although this was occasionally delayed by as much as 12 days after transplantation. Focal mucosal necrosis could be found in most animals by 14 days; in many the mucosa was diffusely damaged by this time.

These features of rejection did not vary substantially between untreated animals and those receiving oral CsA. In contrast, animals treated with intramuscular CsA (group VI) failed to develop these structural lesions. These animals maintained nearly normal mucosal structures for periods of up to 33 days. The marked lamina propria and perivascular infiltrates by mononuclear cells seen in rejection were largely absent in this group.

Discussion

The data obtained in this series of small-bowel transplants in the pig suggest that CsA can prevent rejection of such transplants, but only if consistently high serum levels of CsA are maintained. Rejection was routinely prevented only in those pigs which received daily intramuscular CsA. While rejection was not seen in this group, either clinically or histologically, the high levels of CsA were associated with an increased number of septic complications, and no animals survived indefinitely. The CsA levels in this group were higher than those usually sought in human renal transplantation at this institution. None of the groups receiving oral CsA showed a significant prolongation of graft survival, although occasional longer-term survival occurred. CsA levels in the orally treated groups were significantly lower than the IM-treated group, despite monitored delivery of the drug to an intact host gastrointestinal tract by pharyngeal lavage.

The high technical and immunologic failure rates observed in this series are similar to those obtained by other investigators using large animal models of small-bowel transplantation with CsA immunosuppression (Craddock et al. 1983; Diliz-Perez et al. 1984; Ricour et al. 1983). Clinical trials of human small-bowel transplantation should await the development of improved immunosuppressive regimens.

References

Cohen Z, MacGregor AB, Moore KTH, Falk RE, Langer B, Cullen JB (1976) Canine small bowel transplantation: A study of the immunological responses. Arch Surg 111:248–253

Craddock GN, Nordgren SR, Reznick RK, Gilas T, Lossing AG, Cohen Z, Stiller CR, Cullen JB, Langer B (1983) Small bowel transplantation in the dog using cyclosporine. Transplantation 35:284–288

Deltz E, Muller-Hermelink HK, Ulrichs K, Thiede A, Muller-Ruchholtz W (1981) Development of graft-vs-host reaction in various target organs after small bowel transplantation. Transplant Proc 13:1215–15

Department of Health, Education, and Welfare (1978) Guides for the Case and Use of Laboratory Animals. DHEW publication no. NIH 78-23, Washington, D.C.

Diliz-Perez HS, McClure J, Bedetti C, Hong H, Santibanes E de, Shaw BW, Thiel D van, Iwatsuki S, Starzl TE (1984) Successful small bowel allotransplantation in dogs with cyclosporine and prednisone. Transplantation 37:126–129

Kirkman RL, Lear PA, Madara JL, Tilney NL (1984) Small intestine transplantation in the rat: Immunology and function. Surgery 96:280–286

Monchik GJ, Russell PS (1971) Transplantation of small bowel in the rat: Technical and immunological considerations. Surgery 70:693–702

Pritchard TJ, Madara JL, Tapper D, Wilmore DW, Kirkman RL (1985) Failure of cyclosporine to prevent small bowel allograft rejection in pigs. J Surg Res 38:553–558

Ricour C, Revillon Y, Arnaud-Battandier F, Ghnassia D, Weyne P, Lauffenburger, Jos J, Fontaine JL, Gallix P, Vaiman M (1983) Successful small bowel allografts in piglets using cyclosporine. Transplant Proc 15:3019–3026

Thiede A, Deltz E, Ulrichs K, Muller-Hermelink HK, Muller-Ruchholtz W (1982) Transplantation of small intestine in rats: Analysis and treatment of graft versus host reactions. J Microsurg 3:193

Lymphatic Regeneration Following Intestinal Transplantation in the Pig

N. Rotman, F. Michot, J.M. Hay, and P.L. Fagniez

Introduction

Lymphatic regeneration after small-intestinal autotransplantation has been shown to occur 2 weeks after transplantation and to be complete after 4 weeks (Goott et al. 1960; Ballinger et al. 1962; Kocandrle et al. 1966).

The Study of small-bowel allotransplantation has been impaired by the short survival of allotransplanted animals (Goott et al. 1960; Kocandrle et al. 1966).

The aim of this study was to evaluate the timing and pattern of lymphatic regeneration after orthotopic small – intestinal transplantation in the pig. The prolonged survival of SLA-compatible animals after allotransplantation allowed us to study lymphatic regeneration after small intestinal allotransplantation (Hay and Fagniez 1974).

Materials and Methods

Large White and Landrace pigs, 2–3 months old and weighing 25–35 kg, were used. The technique for orthotopic auto- and allotransplantation has been described previously (Kunlin et al. 1972). All animals were compatible in the SLA and AO systems.

Lymphatic regeneration was studied by lymphography performed under general anesthesia at 7, 15, 21, 30, 60, and 210 days after transplantation. Five autotransplanted and eight allotransplanted pigs were compared with three normal animals which served as controls. A fatty meal was given to the animals 6–10 h before lymphography. After performing a midline incision, a catheter was introduced into a lymphatic duct located just distal to the proximal mesenteric nodes. Three ml contrast medium and Evans blue were injected through the catheter during a 15-min period. The injection was done manually with a syringe, and injection pressure was not recorded. X-ray pictures were taken after 1 ml and 3 ml contrast medium were injected. In two allotransplanted pigs, a 16-mm film was taken 30 and 210 days after transplantation. At the end of the procedure, pigs were either killed or kept alive for further investigations. Some animals underwent an ileoportography just after lymphography in order to visualize the portal venous system.

Results

In the control animals, lymphography showed the normal route of lymphatic drainage with a brief visualization of the thoracic duct, but without visualization of the liver. In the transplanted pigs, there were no chylous ascites, no lymphangiectasia, and no fat malabsorption (HAY and FAGNIEZ 1974). Before the 30th day post-transplantation in the autotransplanted animals and before the 60th day in the allotransplanted animals, the thoracic duct was not able to be detected at lymphography. The contrast medium passed from the mesenteric lymphatic vessels to the venous portal system as confirmed by ileoportography. Lymphographies performed later on showed both the thoracic duct and the portal venous system. Films taken 210 days after transplantation showed that the visualization of the portal venous system was due to lymphovenous anastomosis.

Discussion

Lymphography did not show a specific lymphatic accessory route to the porta hepatis, but the topography of the hepatic vessels seen at lymphography was strictly comparable to the intrahepatic portovenous system distribution seen at ileoportography. Furthermore, lymphovenous anastomosis could be clearly defined on 16-mm films. The absence of fat malabsorption in the transplanted pigs can be partly explained by the opening of these lymphovenous anastomoses (HAY and FAGNIEZ 1974). Too small to be visualized in the normal animal, these anastomoses develop when there is obstruction in lymphatic circulation. In our study, the injection pressure of contrast medium was high, but cannot be responsible for the artificial opening of the lymphovenous anastomoses. In the control group, such anastomoses could not be visualized. The presence of lymphovenous anastomoses after small-bowel transplantation in the dog has not been reported consistently (BALLINGER et al. 1962; GOOTT et al. 1960; KOCANDRLE et al. 1966). Nonetheless, these anastomoses can explain why fat absorption is normal after small-bowel transplantation (KUNLIN et al. 1972; GRENIER et al. 1970).

Conclusion

After Orthotopic auto- or allotransplantation of the small intestine in the pig, lymphatic ciruclation to the thoracic duct is interrupted and develops through lymphovenous anastomoses in the porta hepatis. These anastomoses can be visualized 30 days after autotransplantation and 60 days after allotransplantation. Later on, the thoracic duct is seen at lymphography; however, up to 210 days post-transplantation, the lymphovenous anastomoses remain patent.

References

Ballinger WF, Christy MG, Ashby WB (1962) Autotransplantation of the small intestine: the effect of denervation. Surgery 52:151–163
Goott B, Lillehei RC, Miller FA (1960) Mesenteric lymphatic regeneration after autografts of small bowel in dogs. Surgery 48:571–575
Grenier JF, Doremieux J, Wong P, Botescu V (1970) Transplantation d'intestin grêle chez le chien: Enseignements tirés d'une statistique de 100 cas. Chirurgie 96:958–968
Hay JM, Fagniez PL (1974) Résultats de l'allotransplantation orthotopique de l'intestin grêle chez le porc. Ann Chir 28:1063–1070
Kocandrle V, Houttuin E, Prohaska JV (1966) Regeneration of the lymphatics after autotransplantation and homotransplantation of the entire small intestine. Surg Gynecol Obstet 122:587–592
Kunlin A, Hay JM, Fagniez PL (1972) Technique de la transplantation orthotopique de l'intestin grêle chez le porc. Ann Chir 26:505–510

Serum Lactic Dehydrogenase in Small-Bowel Transplantation in the Pig

N. ROTMAN, F. MICHOT, J.M. HAY, and P.L. FAGNIEZ

Introduction

An increase in serum lactic dehydrogenase (LDH) levels has been shown to be a good monitor of rejection in kidney and heart transplantation (ANDERSON et al. 1975; ROTTEMBOURG et al. 1977). The aim of this study was to evaluate the significance of the changes in serum LDH levels following small-bowel transplantation in the pig.

Material and Methods

A group of 61 Large White and Landrace pigs, 2–3 months old, weighing 25–35 kg, were used. In a control group of 12 laparotomized pigs, a Thomas cannula was inserted 20–30 cm distal to the duodenum. In a second group of 15 pigs, an orthotopic autotransplantation was performed and the same cannula inserted 20–30 cm distal to the duodenojejunostomy. A third group of 34 pigs with compatible AO and SLA systems underwent a cross-orthotopic allotransplantation and were cannulated according to the same procedure. Blood samples were harvested through an internal jugular catheter before surgery, before and after superior mesenteric occlusion, and for 1 month after operation. Histologic examinations were carried out on biopsies obtained through the Thomas cannula. Serum LDH levels were assessed according to the method described by KING (1965).

Results

Basal Values

In 59 pigs, serum LDH levels were below 500 U/ml with a mean value of 303 ± 138.4 U/ml. Only two pigs had values over 500 U/ml. The level of 500 U/ml was thus chosen as the upper limit for normal values.

Effect of Superior Mesenteric Occlusion

There were no statistically significant changes in serum LDH levels before and after superior mesenteric occlusion (259.75 ± 83.2 vs 246.61 ± 91.1 U/ml). All the values were below 400 U/ml whatever the duration of the occlusion was. Mesenteric occlusion varied from 22 to 100 min (mean, 53 ± 19 min).

Serum LDH in Transplanted Animals

A total of 14 allotransplanted pigs died within the first postoperative month from rejection or peritonitis related to a disinsertion of the Thomas cannula. Only two of these pigs showed a transient elevation of serum LDH levels above 500 U/ml during the immediate postoperative period.

In the transplanted animals that survied beyond the first postoperative month (14 autotransplanted and 20 allotransplanted), serum LDH levels were below 500 U/ml, except for two animals whose transient increase in serum LDH levels had returned to normal.

Four pigs died of necrosis of the graft (one autotransplanted and three allotransplanted). Two pigs died in the first few postoperative days of thrombosis of the vascular anastomosis; two animals died on the 10th and the 25th postoperative day respectively. In all these animals, serum LDH levels remained constantly above 500 U/ml until death.

Comments

The basal values of serum LDH observed in this study are comparable to the results obtained by Tegeris et al. (1965). The absence of changes in serum LDH levels before and after superior mesenteric occlusion suggests that a vascular occlusion of short duration does not influence the release of LDH by the small bowel.

Serum LDH levels are not good markers of rejection. The 12 allotransplanted pigs that died from rejection had serum LDH values below 500 U/ml, except for two animals in which a transient elevation was observed. The only significant change in serum LDH levels was observed in animals with necrosis of the graft. In these pigs, serum LDH levels remained elevated in successive measurements.

References

Anderson CB, Codd JE, Graff RJ, Gregory JG, Groce MA, Newton WT (1975) Serum lactic dehydrogenase and human allograft failure. Surgery 77:674–679

Rottembourg J, Gandjbakhch I, Guiraudon G, Mattei MF, Cabrol A, Cabrol C (1977) Aspects actuels de la transplantation cardiaque humaine: Surveillance postopératoire et résultats. Nouv Presse Med 6:819–823

King J (1965) Practical clinical enzymology. Van Nostrand, London, pp 85–88

Tegeris AS, Earl FL, Curtis JM (1965) Normal hematological and biochemical parameters of yong miniature swine: Swine in biomedical research. Busted, Washington, pp 575–595

In Vitro and In Vivo Studies of the Mucosal Immune Barrier After Long-Term Small-Bowel Allotransplantation in Pigs Using Cyclosporine

F. Arnaud-Battandier, H. Salmon, J.M. Aynaud, S. Bernard, Y. Révillon, and C. Ricour

Introduction

The intestinal mucosal barrier plays a major role in the body's local and general defense systems. Any alteration of the immune barrier can be responsible for severe diseases. This mucosal barrier consists of a large population of different cells, mainly lymphocytes, plasmocytes, macrophages, polynuclear cells, and mast cells (Arnaud-Battandier 1984), a fact which distinguishes small intestinal (SI) transplantation from that involving other organs. Surgical improvements and drug developments now enable long-term survival of animals that undergo SI transplantation, including large animals such as pigs (Ricour et al. 1983) or dogs (Cohen et al. 1983; Raju et al. 1984) and rodents (Thiede and Deltz 1978; Schraut et al. 1983; see review by Kirkman 1984). Before the use of immunosuppressive drugs, rejection of small-bowel allografts in experimental animals occurred within 10 days.

Considering the importance of the mucosal barrier in homeostasis, studies were undertaken in animals with total small-bowel allotransplantation under cyclosporine A (CsA) therapy following a two-step procedure: A first set of experiments was designed to evaluate in vitro the morphological characteristics and functions of the lymphoid cells isolated from the transplanted gut; a second set of experiments was performed in vivo after intestinal infection with two different viruses. Both in vitro and in vivo results demonstrated preservation of the mucosal immune barrier.

Materials and Methods

Animals and Transplantation

Eight Large White Pigs (weighing 20–60 kg) were used for transplantation as described by Revillon et al. (this volume). Briefly, SI segments (6 m long), histoincompatible for one haplotype, were immediately grafted in continuity with the small intestine of the recipient ($n = 4$). CsA (started 48 h before surgery) was given daily intravenously the first 15–20 days following surgery, after which it was administered orally. Animals were used for immunologic studies 10–18 months after transplantation.

We used 34 normal Large White Pigs for the in vivo experiments. They were divided into four groups, with two groups receiving CsA orally (20 mg/kg) and two groups undergoing no immunosuppressive therapy, as previously described (BERNARD et al. 1985).

Isolation of the Lymphoid Cells from the Transplanted Gut

Tissue samples were surgically obtained 10–12 months after grafting. Lymphocytes from blood and mesenteric lymph nodes (MLN) were isolated as described by SALMON (1982). Lymphocytes from the gut were isolated by mechanical procedures (SALMON and ARNAUD-BATTANDIER, submitted for publication). Rosette formations with different compounds were used for study of T and B cell surface markers according to SALMON (1982). Histocompatibility tests were performed using anti-swine leukocyte antigen (SLA) reagents as described by RICOUR et al. (1983).

Proliferation studies were performed after lectin stimulation (PHA, Con A, PWM). Interleukin 2 (IL-2) production was tested after a 48-h culture in the presence of PHA and was then tested on a mouse CTL line (ARNAUD-BATTANDIER et al. 1985).

In Vivo Infections with Enteropathogenic Viruses

Immunization with Sheep Red Blood Cells
Fourteen days after the beginning of CsA treatment each normal animal and each transplanted animal received an intraperitoneal injection of sheep red blood cells (SRBC).

Experimental Infection by a Swine Rotavirus
One group with and one group without CsA as well as the transplanted animals, were orally infected with 45 ml of a swine rotavirus suspension ($5 \cdot 10^4$ infectious units/ml) 14 days after beginning CsA therapy.

Experimental Infection by a Swine-Transmissible Gastroenteritis Coronavirus
Forty days after beginning CsA therapy, each of the 34 normal pigs and the transplanted animals received one oral dose of the swine-transmissible gastroenteritis coronavirus (TGE) (10^5 infectious units/ml) in suspension.

Blood and Fecal Sample Analysis
Serum levels of antibodies against SRBC and TGE coronaviruses, were monitored every week from day 0 to day 70 by hemagglutination and seroneutralization tests. Titration of TGE virus inducing interferon activity was carried out in vesicular stomatitis virus (VSV)-infected Madin-Darby bovine kidney (MDBK) cells (LA BONNARDIÈRE and LAUDE 1981).

From day 0 to day 70, stool samples were tested twice a week by ELISA for rotavirus antigen levels and for levels of antirotavirus antibodies with corresponding immunoglobul in classes.

Results and Discussion

Morphological Characteristics of Isolated Lymphoid Cells from Transplanted Gut

Lymphoid populations isolated from the transplanted gut mucosa contained a high proportion of T cells (87% ± 5%) with few B cells (2%), and some Fc-positive cells (12% ± 4%), similar to the proportions observed in normal animals. No difference was demonstrated between isolated cells from the donor or recipient MLNs. Granulated lymphoid cells (ARNAUD-BATTANDIER 1982) were equally present in the grafted and recipient gut (approximately 50%).

Study of the SLA phenotypes of the isolated cells from the different tissues showed that transplanted MLNs contained only cells with the phenotype of the recipient, as did the recipient MLN cells. Within the gut, 10%–30% of the isolated cells possessed the SLA phenotype of the donor; this proportion correlated roughly with the proportion of nonlymphocytic cells that contaminated the mucosal cell suspension.

Proliferative Responses to Polyclonal Mitogens

Long-term CsA treatment did not affect the mitogenic proliferation of cells isolated from the donor and recipient MLNs. Mucosal lymphocytes isolated from the transplanted gut were also able to proliferate and to marked quantities of produce IL-2 after PHA stimulation (four times more than the results observed in stimulated blood cells). Similar results were observed in normal pigs.

These results support the success of the earlier use of CsA in SI allografts in piglets (RICOUR et al. 1983). There grafts were well tolerated and CsA well absorbed, as was also demonstrated in dogs (COHEN et al. 1983). In addition, lymphocyte populations present within the gut mucosa did not seem affected, either by the graft or by CsA treatment, in their morphological characteristics or in their functions (i. e., proliferation and IL-2 production). Therefore, it seems that these cells are able to function in the mucosal immune barrier, as confirmed by a lack of infections even more than 18 months after transplantation.

In Vivo Responses to Viral Infections

Experiments were designed to compare the responses of three animals which had undergone transplantation more than 12 months previously with those of the four groups of eight normal animals, of which two received the same dasage of CsA as the transplanted pigs.

To check their capacity for antibody response an intraperitoneal injection of SRBC was given. All 37 animals had anti-SRBC antibodies 10 days after the injection, and the antibody titer reached a plateau value of 2.5 $\log_2$. Therefore, CsA did not alter the capacity for response to an antigen injection, and humoral immune response following viral infections was able to take place and be interpreted. Transplanted animals had a similar response.

Rotavirus antigen excretion in the stools was statistically higher in the two groups of animals that had received the virus, independently of CsA treatment. No significant difference was observed in the transplanted group. Antirotavirus IgG and IgM were practically absent in any group. Only antirotavirus IgA could be detected; controls with or without CsA therapy had the same antibody levels (on day 28 respectively, 16 ± 10 μg/ml and 19 ± 9 μg/ml) as the transplanted animals (Fig. 1) (with a maximum value of 30 μg/ml). CsA did not alter the excretion of antigens in the stools, nor was there any change in the kinetics of the antirotavirus coproantibody excretion.

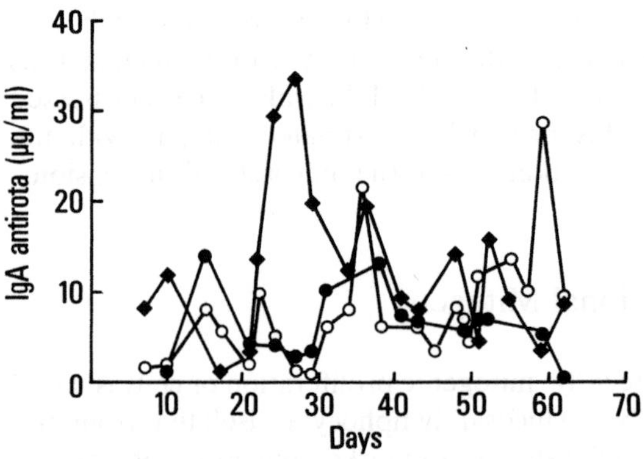

Fig. 1. IgA antirotavirus antibodies in the stools of the three transplanted pigs (○, pig no. 22; ◆, pig no. 60; ●, pig no. 06) following rotavirus oral infection on day 20. Pigs had previously been in contact with the virus, as shown by the presence of antibodies before day 20

After TGE coronavirus infection, only four controls had slight diarrhea. Interferon activity was observed between days 2 and 4, while neutralizing anti-TGE coronavirus antibodies appeared 9 days after oral virus administration and reached a plateau on day 20 (titer 1/128) in all groups. The transplanted animals presented no clinical manifestations, nor were their biological responses different from those of the controls (Fig. 2).

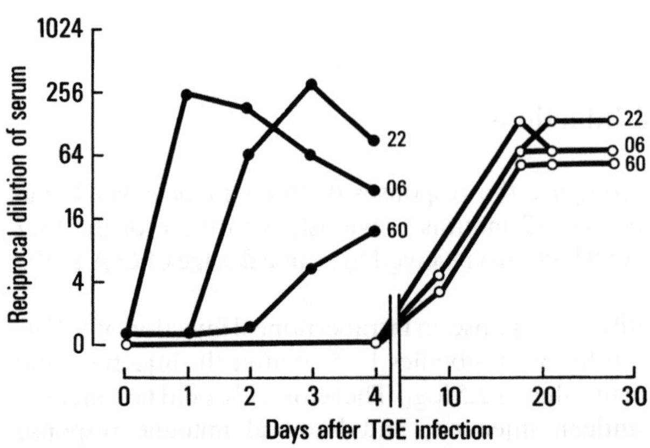

Fig. 2. Serum interferon activity *(left panel)* and anti-TGE coronavirus antibody titer *(right panel)* following TGE coronavirus oral infection (*22, 06* and *60* are the code numbers of the three transplanted animals)

Oral CsA did not alter the proliferation or IL-2 production of cells isolated from the gut mucosa of transplanted small intestines. There was also no difference observed in the humoral immune response against enteropathogenetic virus. Different responses were observed after infection with vaccinia virus or herpes simplex virus, depending in part on the activity of T cells; it has been demonstrated (Cole et al. 1983) that CsA is responsible for a decrease in the animal resistance to these viruses.

To our knowledge, no information was previously available on the role of CsA in viral enteric infection. Our results seem to indicate the absence of CsA influence on the antibody response of pigs to the two swine-specific enteropathogenetic viruses.

Intestinal allotransplantation also did not alter the ability of the mucosal immune barrier to react against viral infections. Therefore, in vitro and in vivo studies demonstrated that the mucosal immune barrier is preserved after intestinal transplantation, bringing in a new argument in favor of human intestinal transplantation.

References

Arnaud-Battandier F (1982) Immunologic characteristics of isolated gut mucosal lymphoid cells. In: Strober W, Hanson LA, Sell KW (eds) Recent advances in mucosal immunity. Raven, New York, pp 287–299

Arnaud-Battandier F (1984) Le système lymphoïde intestinal: conceptions actuelles. Gastroenterol Clin Biol 8:632–640

Arnaud-Battandier F, Salmon H, Vaiman M, Revillon Y, Gallix P, Olivier M, Ricour C (1985) Small intestinal allotransplantation in swine with cyclosporine treatment: Studies of the intestinal lymphoid populations. Transplant Proc 17:1440–1441

Bernard S, Lantier I, Bottreau E, Aynaud JM, La Bonnardière C, Ricour C, Arnaud-Battandier F (1985) Influence de la cyclosporine A sur la réponse du porc à l'infection expérimentale par le rotavirus et le coronavirus G.E.T. In: Journées de la recherche porcine en France. Institut Nationale de la Recherche Agronomique Symp Ser 17:173–202

Cohen Z, Nordgren SR, Mackenzie RD, Lossing AG, Stiller CR, Langer D (1983) Pharmacokinetics of cyclosporine in a canine intestinal transplantation model. Transplant Proc 15:3013–3018

Cole GA, Nickell SP, Mokhtarian F, Scheibel LW (1983) Effects of cyclosporine on experimental infections. Transplant Proc 15:2271–2277

Kirkman RL (1984) Small bowel transplantation. Transplantation 37: 429–433

La Bonnardière C, Laude H (1981) High interferon titer in newborn pig intestine during experimentally induced viral enteritis. Infect Immun 32:28–31

Raju S, Didlake RH, Cayirli M, Turner MD, Grogan JB, Achord J (1984) Experimental small bowel transplantation utilizing cyclosporine. Transplantation 38:561–566

Ricour C, Revillon Y, Arnaud-Battandier F, Ghnassia D, Weyne P, Lauffenburger A, Jos J, Fontaine JL, Gallix P, Vaiman M (1983) Successful small bowel allografts in piglets using cyclosporine. Transplant Proc 15:3019–3026

Salmon H (1982) Characterization of pig lymphocyte receptors for allogeneic and nonallogeneic erythrocytes. I. Apparent common identity of both receptors. Clin Exp Immunol 48:574–580

Thiede A, Deltz E (1978) Morphological reaction in transplanted small intestine using immunogenetically defined rat strain combinations. Langenbecks Arch Chir 346:119

Schraut WH, Rosemurgy AS, Riddell RM (1983) Prolongation of intestinal allograft survival without immunosuppressive drug therapy. Transplantation of small bowel allografts. J Surg Res 34:597–607

Orthotopic Segmental Small-Intestinal Transplantation in the Dog

J. Collin, A. R. Dennison, R. M. Watkins, and P. J. Morris

Introduction

Small intestine for total small-intestinal allografts can only be obtained from cadaveric donation, and graft-vs-host disease is liable to be a major problem in the recipient. Segmental small-intestinal allografts do not induce graft-vs-host disease and can be taken from living or dead donors.

The aim of this study was to discover if a 100-cm segment of terminal ileum functioned well enough to maintain the health of the recipient when transplanted orthotopically as an autograft or an allograft.

Materials and Methods

From the outset, a three-stage study was planned.

Stage 1

In outbred, unrelated dogs, a 100-cm segment of terminal ileum was orthotopically transplanted as a Thiry-Vella fistula by vascular anastomosis between the graft vessels and the superior mesenteric artery and vein of the recipient. The 14 dogs having intestinal allografts were operated on in pairs, each animal receiving its ileal graft from the other animal being operated on at the same time. The 24 ileal autografts were carried out in exactly the same way as allografts, except that the Thiry-Vella segment was reimplanted in the same dog from which it had been removed.

All dogs were given oral neomycin 500 mg b.i.d. for 2 days before the operation and 250 mg cefuroxime at operation and three times daily for 5 subsequent days. Dogs receiving allografts were given oral cyclosporine A (CsA) 20 mg/kg 24 h before operation and IM CsA 20 mg/kg daily for 2–3 days until they were eating again when daily oral administration was restarted.

Post-operatively, intestinal absorption from six auografts and six allografts was studied by luminal perfusion with an isotonic solution of sodium chloride, glucose, l-alanine, lauric acid and medium-chain triglycerides. Perfusion was at 2.9 ml/min, and after a 30-min stabilisation period, effluent volumes were recorded, and concentrations of nutrients in the effluent measured. Mucosal biopsies were taken from 6–7 cm inside the proximal and distal stomas of the transplanted Thiry-Vella segment to monitor post-operative histological changes.

Stage 2

In ten dogs with autografts and seven with allografts, the stomas were freed from the abdominal wall 5–6 weeks after intestinal transplantation of a Thiry-Vella segment. The anastomosis for the restoration of intestinal continuity of non-transplanted small intestine was resected and the original anatomy restored by end-to-end anastomosis of transplanted and non-transplanted intestine (Fig. 1).

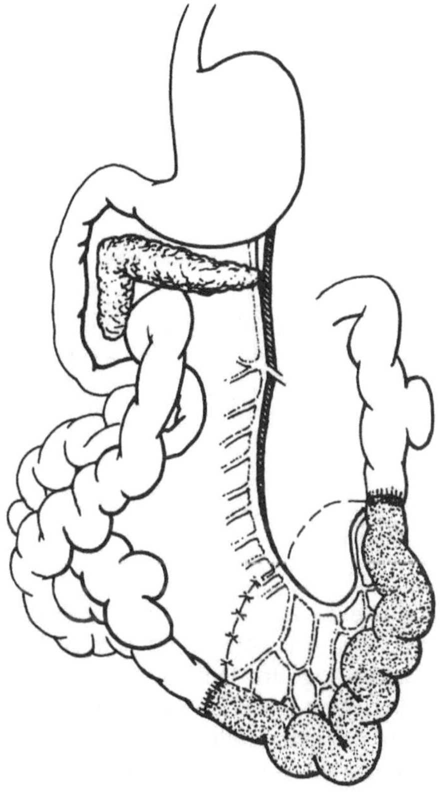

Fig. 1. Establishment of intestinal continuity through the transplanted ileal segment in its normal anatomical position

In all ten dogs with autografts subjected to the stage 2 operation, a third operation was performed 3–4 months after intestinal transplantation. At this operation, all the non-transplanted small intestine from the mid-duodenum to the autograft was excised and intestinal continuity restored by anastomosing duodenum to the ileal autograft (Fig. 2).

After this operation, maintenance of adequate nutrition in the animal was almost totally dependent on absorption from the intestinal autograft.

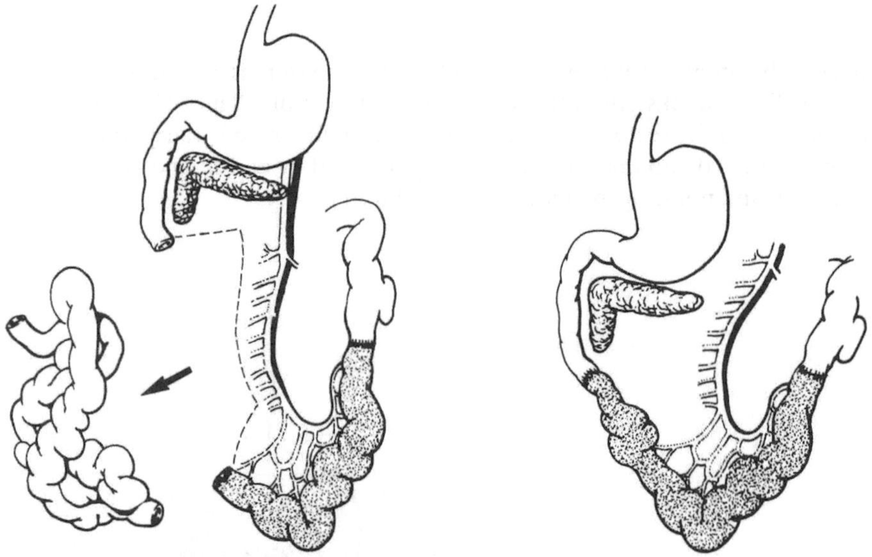

Fig. 2. Ablation of all non-transplanted small intestine distal to mid-duodenum and re-establishment of intestinal continuity by enteroanastomosis between the duodenum and the proximal end of the intestinal autograft

Results

The mean duration of intestinal ischaemia was similar for the autografts and allografts. Anastomosis times were 77 ± 4 min (mean ± SE) for autografts and 75 ± 6 min for allografts. Difficulty was encountered with several of the allografts because of a disparity between the sizes of the donor and recipient mesenteric vessels.

Six autografts failed, one graft was unsuccessful because of the small calibre of the mesenteric vessels, one dog bled to death from the arterial anastomosis, and four grafts infarcted within 5 days. Three animals with allografts died within the 1st week, two from intussusception and one from intestinal volvulus.

The intestinal stomas of the Thiry-Vella transplants were initially oedematous, but after the first 2 days, the stomas of autografts became increasingly healthy in appearance, bled freely and produced clear secretions. In contrast, allograft stomas were increasingly unhealthy from the 3rd–4th days after transplantation, becoming progressively paler and granular in appearance with granulomas forming around sutures. The stomas of all allografts became stenosed and in several animals became completely occluded.

Intestinal Absorption from Thiry-Vella Transplants

In perfusion studies of the Thiry-Vella segments during the first 28 days after transplantation, the pattern of volume absorption was similar in autografts and allografts. Absorption increased progressively for the first 8 days after transplantation but decreased again by the 28th day. Intestinal absorption from allografts was always less than from autografts but only significantly different on the 14th day post-transplantation.

When the Thiry-Vella segments were not being perfused, fluid exudation from their distal stomas occurred throughout the day. It was not possible to make a complete collection of this effluent to measure its volume over 24 h but it was noted that the abdominal wall of dogs with allografts was always wet with the exudate. The total protein concentration in the exudate was significantly greater in allografts (mean ± SE, 15.6 ± 1.7 g/l) than in autografts (mean ± SE, 2.1 ± 0.5 g/l; $t = 7.46$; $P < 0.0001$).

Histology of Mucosal Biopsies

In all autografts for the first 10 days after transplantation, there was sloughing of the tips of some villi, dilatation of lacteals, prominence of goblet cells and a cellular infiltrate of the lamina propria. All these changes have been described in the early stages of acute rejection but are likely to be a response to acute intestinal ischaemia.

In allografts, the same appearances noted in autografts were present for the first 10 days, but thereafter the histology varied, depending on whether the dog was a long- or short-term survivor. In grafts with short survival, marked necrosis of the lamina propria and shedding of the mucosa were present at 10–14 days. In dogs surviving longer, flattened mucosa and perivascular mononuclear cell infiltrates were seen on day 28.

Survival and Post-mortem Findings

All 18 technically successful autografts survived indefinitely and were eventually sacrificed. All 10 dogs survived the stage 3 operation for 4–6 months in good health, and at autopsy, the graft was completely normal, apart from some physiological dilatation consistent with adaptation to the short-bowel syndrome.

Mean survival of dogs with allografts was 63 ± 16 days (mean ± SE). In dogs surviving fewer than 60 days, death was from peritonitis following allograft rejection. The three animals which survived more than 15 weeks after intestinal allografting all died from starvation and pulmonary oedema. At autopsy, all intestinal allografts were shrunken and thickened with gross lymph node enlargement in the allograft mesentery. The seven dogs in which intestinal continuity through the allograft had been established at the stage 2 operation all had marked dilatation of the non-transplanted intestine proximal to the allografted segment.

Conclusions

A 100-cm ileal autograft provides sufficient intestinal function to allow indefinite survival of a dog with no other small intestine.

Segmental ileal allografts in dogs receiving oral CsA immunosuppression initially retain intestinal absorptive function but soon become shrunken and stenosed and cause intestinal obstruction. In addition, the allografted intestine develops a severe protein-losing enteropathy.

Duodenal Histology During Rejection of Whole-Organ Pancreaticoduodenal Allografts in the Pig

W.H. Marks, A. Borgstrom, D.C. Dafoe, D. Campbell Jr., and J.G. Turcotte

Introduction

The behavior of small-bowel allografts in the porcine model has not been well investigated to date. The pig is an excellent model for this type of research for several reasons: Compared with dogs, pigs are relatively inexpensive to purchase and board; they require no preconditioning for handling; a diverse genetic pool is available; their size and anatomy approach those of man. Therefore, we have chosen to study the gross and microscopic appearances of the duodenum in our porcine whole-organ pancreaticoduodenal allograft model during rejection.

Materials and Methods

Animals

Farm-bred pigs were used. Genetic diversity in the population was assured by using donor-recipient pairs from separate litters.

Surgical Method

A total of 20 pairs of animals were successfully transplanted. The donor organs were harvested intact with complete duodenal loops. The graft was immediately flushed with iced Ringer's lactate solution through the graft aorta. The vascular pedicle consisted of a section of aorta (with the celiac and mesenteric branches intact) and the portal vein. Storage prior to revascularization was from 1 to 4 h. The graft was placed in the recipient's abdomen with the aorta and portal vein anastomosed to the recipient's aorta and vena cava respectively. The proximal duodenum was closed, and the distal duodenum was anastomosed to a loop of ileum in an end-to-side fashion (Fig. 1).

Immunosuppression

Recipients were treated with cyclosporine (Sandoz Pharmaceuticals, East Hanover, N.J.), 6 mg/kg intravenously, and prednisolone, 1.5 mg/kg intravenously, before transplantation. Prednisolone was then tapered off over 7 days to the maintenance dose of 0.5 mg/kg per day for an additional 21 days.

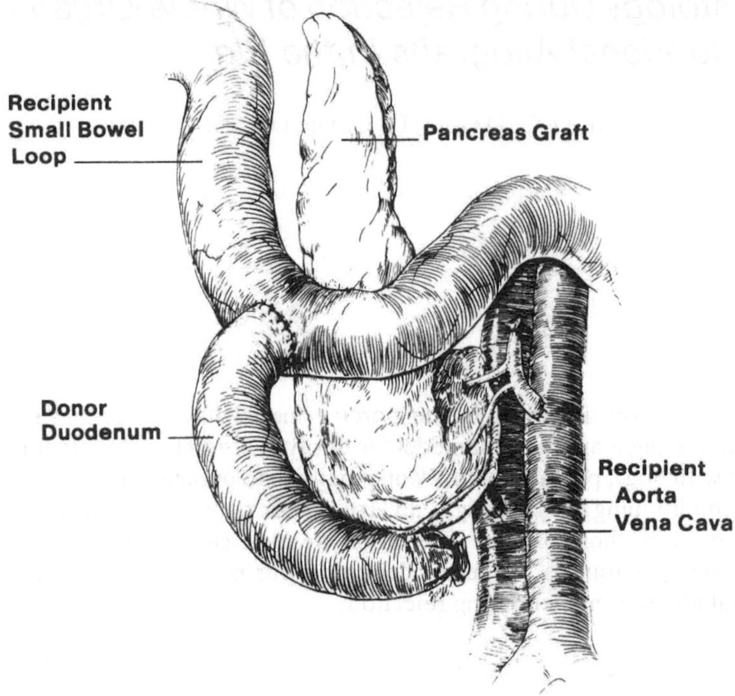

Fig. 1. Artist's rendering of the whole-organ pancreaticoduodenal allograft in the pig

Sampling
Daily serum samples were obtained and analyzed for glucose and amylase. Eighteen of the 20 animals were sacrificed either when they became glucose intolerant ($n = 16$) or when their circulating amylase levels fell significantly below baseline, although they remained glucose tolerant ($n = 2$). The remaining two animals were sacrificed on postoperative days 59 and 80 respectively, having no evidence of rejection. Specimens were harvested from anesthetized animals prior to sacrifice. Biopsies of the pancreatic gland and duodenum were immediately performed and the gross appearance of the graft noted. Specimens were fixed in buffered formalin.

Results

Of these 20 animals, 19 maintained normal glucose levels through out the period of immunosuppressive treatment. One animal became glucose intolerant while receiving immunosuppressive treatment.

Fig. 2A-D. Duodenal histology in the pig. **A** Normal (x 10); **B** Nonrejecting animal (x 10); **C** Early rejection (x 10); **D** Late rejection (x 10) ▷

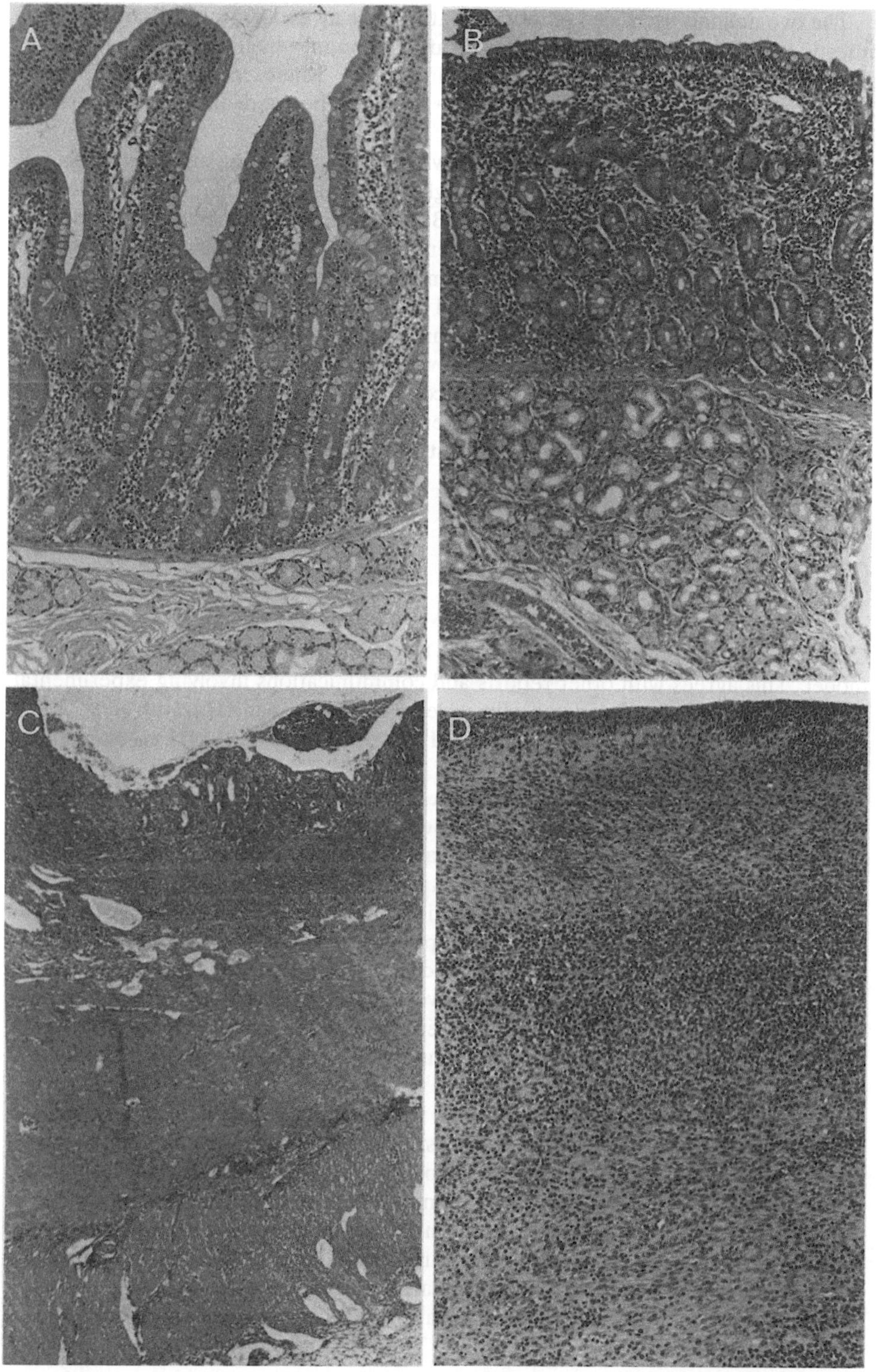
A
B
C
D

The two animals sacrificed on postoperative days 59 and 80 were without signs of rejection. Each had a normal appearing graft duodenum which was indistinguishable from that of the native bowel upon gross inspection. Microscopic examination was also unremarkable, except that a loss in the height of the duodenal villi was apparent (Fig. 2b).

The two animals that were sacrificed when their circulating amylase levels fell significantly below baseline values, although the animals remained glucose tolerant, had grossly thickened and adhesed bowel. Both the pancreas and bowel were encased in an inflammatory process. Microscopy demonstrated that the mucosa was denuded and that there was remarkable intramural mononuclear cell infiltration (Fig. 2c).

The 16 remaining animals were sacrificed when they became glucose intolerant. All had remarkable inflammatory reactions surrounding their grafts. At necropsy, the grafts were difficult to identify, as they were involved in a dense inflammatory response and appeared infarcted. Microscopy demonstrated extensive cellular necrosis in the pancreas with large numbers of mononuclear cell infiltrates. The duodenum showed transmural involvement with a similar process (Fig. 2d).

Discussion

Cyclosporine and prednisolone proved to be adequate immunosuppressives in this model. This agrees with other reports and communications involving experimental studies in rat, dog, and pig and clinical experience in man (Reznik et al. 1982; Kirkman et al. 1984; Sutherland 1984; Timmermann et al. 1984; Dafoe et al., to be published).

In our model, the rejection process in the pancreas parallels that in the duodenum. Early in the rejection process, the duodenal mucosa is heavily involved in a mononuclear attack. This takes place at a time when the recipient is still glucose tolerant but reveals a dramatic fall in circulating amylase levels. Later in the rejection process, the entire duodenum and pancreatic graft are involved in an intense reaction. Both organs have extensive cellular disruption, and at the same time the recipient becomes glucose intolerant. Currently, except for serial biopsy, there is no reliable means of monitoring rejection in small-bowel allografts. Since the severity of changes in the pancreas and duodenum are apparently parallel in this model, alterations in serum amylase may be used to signal simultaneous rejection in the duodenal and pancreatic portions of the graft.

A similar tactic has been used by some for monitoring rejection of the pancreas during clinical trials. These investigators simultaneously transplant the kidney and pancreas from donor to recipient. Elevations in creatinine signaling rejection in the kidney allograft are assumed to reflect a similar process in the pancreas. Although in these studies no biopsy proof of rejection is available, graft survival is reportedly improved. This improvement has been attributed to early detection of the rejection process using the kidney graft as an early warning device. We have recently demonstrated the efficacy of monitoring amylase to signal rejection in our porcine whole-organ pancreaticoduodenal model. Therefore, this model may offer a means by which to study the response of the duodenal allograft to antirejection therapy, as well as its post-treatment healing.

A further advantage of this model is that it minimizes experimental variables by leaving a nutritionally intact animal which is not in jeopardy of graft-vs-host disease.

References

Dafoe DC, Campbell D, Marks W, Wilson G, Turcotte JG Karyotypic chimerism and rejection in a pancreaticoduodenosplenic transplant. Transplantation (to be published)

Kirkman RL, Madara J, Lepir P, Yrhier A (1984) The utility of cyclosporine in small bowel transplantation. 10th international congress of the Transplantation Society, August, 1984, Minneapolis, MN

Reznik R, Craddock G, Langer B, Gilas T, Cullen J (1982) Structure and function of small-bowel allografts in the dog: Immunosuppression with cyclosporine A. Can J Surg 25:51

Sutherland DER (1984) Selected issues of importance in clinical pancreas transplantation. Transplant Proc 16:95–104

Timmermann W, Schang T, Thiede A (1984) The course of pancreatic allografts with physiologic secretion drainage in rats temporarily treated with cyclosporine A. Transplant Proc 16: 228–230

Segmental Small-Bowel Replacement by Gastric Tube in the Pig

M. Walter, U. Brenner, W. Holzmüller, H. W. Keller, and J. M. Müller

The short-bowel syndrome which has an incidence of one to two cases per million of the general population, has been established as a specific symptom complex. Its treatment and prognosis have been favorably improved with the introduction of long-term parenteral nutrition (Broviac et al. 1973). This is, however, an elaborate and complicated procedure with a high complication rate. Although the majority of affected patients can adapt fully with a suitable diet and resume oral nutrition, a small group of patients remain permanently dependent on parenteral nutrition. During their hospital stay, patients are taught to make their own nutritional solutions, which they can infuse themselves at home. Needless to say, certain psychological and social preconditions have to be met for patients to have this degree of independence. In cases where this is not possible, the patients are given prepackaged nutrients ready for infusion. Parenteral nutrition requires that the central venous catheter system be kept clean and free of bacteria to avoid catheter infections, the most common complication in this form of nutrition. While this can quite often be treated conservatively, it is often necessary to remove the entire catheter system (Jeejeebhoy et al. 1976; Müller et al. 1984).

For these patients, small-intestine transplantation would be the ideal method of treatment, although immunologic problems have prevented its use so far. Other procedures, such as the construction of a jejunal-colonic valve require a minimal length of remaining small intestine and have so far only been tested in animals. When this procedure fails, small intestinal segments that could be used for absorption are lost, explaining why this method is seldom used clinically.

In 1955, Heimlich described a procedure where a tube-like structure was formed from the greater curvature of the stomach as an esophagus replacement (Heimlich and Winfidd 1955). Based on this technique, we have attempted to develop a method of extending the functional length of small intestine using an autogenous material.

In 1965, Thall demonstrated that after covering defects in the esophagus with the serasal layer of the stomach, metaplasia of the mucous membrane occurred. Within several weeks, however, this initial irregularity was completely replaced by esophagal epithelium. We considered this technique, which is described below, quite promising, as the ability of the mucous membrane in the gastrointestinal tract to regenerate is well known. We then projected that metaplasia of the mucous membrane in the small intestine would also occur.

Materials and Methods

Experimental animals were ten domestic pigs of both sexes with body weights of between 25 and 30 kg. Access to the small intestine was gained via median incision, and the greater curvature of the stomach with its blood supply intact was dissected away. The gastrotomy was closed in two layers. The dissected area usually measured approximately 10 × 25 cm. After careful dissection of the stomach mucous membrane, a cylinder was formed with the serosa facing outward. This segment was anastomosed to a loop of small intestine in the direction of peristalsis. Both ends of the small-intestinal loop were brought to the skin surface as a double stoma. A perforated silicone tube 2.5 cm in external diameter was used as a splint and to continually perfuse the anastomosed segment during the first 10–14 days. A central venous catheter was introduced into the internal jugular vein and then tunnelled under the skin to exit at the back of the neck. Using this catheter intravenous nutrition was administered until the 3rd postoperative day, and during the next 2 days oral nutrition was gradually introduced. Biopsies were taken after 8 and 10 weeks. Histologic studies were carried out after fixation in 10% formaldehyde in the usual manner. The specimens were stained according to the hematoxylin-eosin and Elastica van Gieson methods.

After 8 weeks, the borders of the anastomoses were covered with conformed mucous membrane structures, which in some cases were confluent and continued the

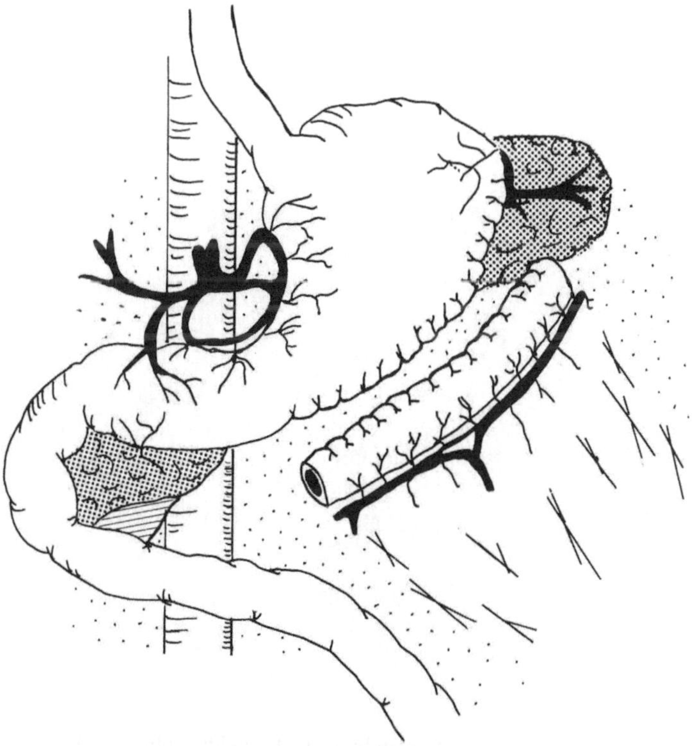

Fig. 1. Surgical technique for segmental small-bowel replacement in the pig

length of the transplant as an avenue of mucous membrane. Between these structures, islands of well-vascularized granulation tissue could be recognized. Early formations of submucosal structures were also evident. After 10 weeks, the mucous membrane covering of the transplants was complete, and macroscopically, there was almost no difference between the new mucous membrane surface, and the normal mucous membrane of the small intestine. Only in the area of the anastomoses was the tissue somewhat firmer than normal, and some isolated remnants of the polydioxanoneacid (PDA) suture material were also recognizable. In three cases, after 8 and 10 weeks, there was a decrease in the area near the anastomoses. The lumina were reduced to only a few millimeters at this point, but could still be dilated without any marked resistance.

The method which we have described permits the construction of an autogenous cylinder for the purpose of increasing the usable length of small intestine, in this case 15–20 cm. It is important to note that in the pig, the blood supply to and from the stomach is principally via epiploic vessels. To guarantee the blood supply to the remaining stomach, the left gastroepiploic vessels have to be left intact. This permits the surgeon much less dissection than in man.

The removal of the stomach mucous membrane proved to be easier than expected, owing to rapid mucosae edema. The mucosa was freed mainly by blunt dissection, and bleeding from small vessels was quickly controlled. Of particular importance for the success of the operation in our opinion is the careful and complete removal of the

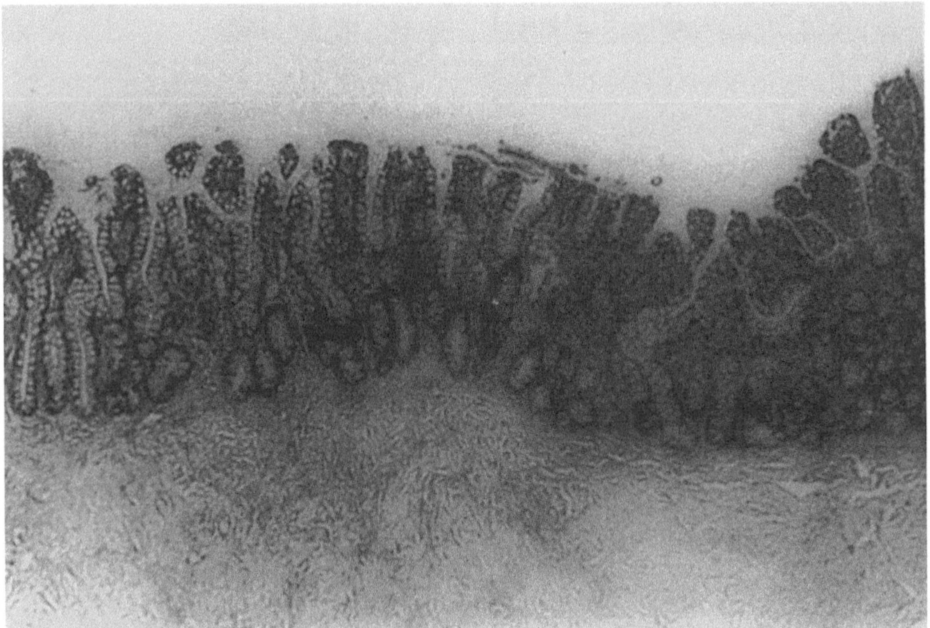

Fig. 2. Formation of mucous membrane in the middle of the gastric tube at 10 weeks postoperatively (hematoxylin and eosin staining method)

stomach mucous membrane in order to prevent later ulceration or the proliferation of any remaining stomach mucosa.

The insertion of a perforated silicone tube after anastomosis and the creation of a double stoma from a small-intestinal loop was very useful for several reasons. Firstly, using the tube to perfuse the anastomoses with normal saline once a day during the first 10–14 days prevented the accumulation of blood clots and cell debris. The silicone cuff also prevented accumulations on the wound surface, which would have quickly led to adhesions and then to complete obstruction of the lumen. By using a temporary splint, the danger of circular shrinkage in the area of anastomoses is also reduced. This circular shrinkage can be a voided to a large extent by careful surgical technique and by using only the minimal amount of absorbable suture material required for surgery. If an oblique anastomosis is made instead of an end-to-end anastomosis, the lumen is even larger. After 8 weeks, the mucous membrane cylinder that we had inserted was two-thirds covered with small-intestinal mucous membrane; after 10 weeks, the cylinder was completely covered. Thus, the main precondition for absorption in the transplant was achieved. However, until further studies are carried out, no definitive statement can be made on the absorptive capabilities of this newly formed small-intestinal mucous membrane.

References

Broviac JW, Cole JJ, Scribner BH (1973) Silicon rubber art. catheter for prolonged parenteral alimentation. Surg Gynecol Obstet 136:602

Heimlich HJ, Winfidd JM (1955) The use of a gastric tube to replace or bypass the esophagus. Surgery 37:549

Jeejeebhoy KN, Langer B, Tsallas G, Chu RC, Kuksis A (1976) Total parenteral nutrition at home: Studies in patients surviving 4 months to 5 years. Gastroenterology 71:943

Müller JM, Keller HW, Brenner U, Walter M (1984) Die ambulante parenterale Dauerernährung bei Kranken mit Kurzdarm-Syndrom. Internist (Berlin) 25:292

Session 2: Summary

C. Ricour

The aim of this session was to determine the possibilities for using small-bowel transplantation in large animals such as pigs and dogs and to present these experimental models. The technical procedures for total or segmental, allo- or autotransplantation have been described by the different groups from Europe and North America. The functions of absorption and adaptation of the remaining small bowel after large resection have been presented and compared with the results observed after allo- or autograft; the importance of anatomical and functional lymphovenous anastomosis in pigs is described. In these animal models, the immunologic problems – rejection/tolerance or graft-versus-host (GVH) reaction – have been studied by the most of participants. GVH reaction was not described in those models. Conflicting results concerning graft rejection with cyclosporin A (CsA) therapy have been observed; the modalities of CsA administration probably explain these discrepancies, and the essential role of intravenous CsA infusion, correlated with plasma CsA levels, is clearly shown. Finally, in vitro and in vivo studies have demonstrated that the mucosal immune barrier is preserved after intestinal allotransplantation.

Session 3
Intestinal Absorption and Adaptation

*Absorption and Graft Function After Small-Intestinal Transplantation**

Z. Cohen, R. Wassef, S. Nordgren, and R. Silverman

Introduction

As a result of recent literature resports, there has been renewed interest in small-intestinal transplantation. Studies from both our own laboratory and others have shown that there has been increased survival following small-intestinal transplantation, particularly with the use of cyclosporine as an immunosuppressant. However, in reviewing the literature of long-term animal survivors, little work has been done in large animals to answer questions regarding absorptive function following small-intestinal transplantation.

Therefore, this manuscript will address the problems of absorptive function in long-term survivors following total small-intestinal transplantation as well as absorption of cyclosporine in a model in which isolated allograft pouches have been constructed to represent events that occur in an in-continuity intestinal transplant.

Small-Intestinal Transplantation in a Canine Model

The techniques for canine auto- and allotransplantation of the small intestine have remained similar throughout the years in various laboratories (Craddock et al. 1983; Lillehei et al. 1959). The entire small bowel on its vascular pedicle of superior mesenteric artery and vein is transplanted in a heterotopic position owing to the nature of the vascular anastomoses. The superior mesenteric artery is anastomosed end to side to the aorta, while the superior mesenteric vein is anastomosed end to side to the recipient inferior vena cava.

In our early experiments, where survival was the main consideration, the animals were divided into three groups. Group A represented control animals, who lived for an average of approximately 12 days (Craddock et al. 1983). No immunosuppression was given in this group, which numbered 11 dogs. In group C (13 dogs), animals received cyclosporine (25 mg/kg per day orally) through the graft itself and lived for a mean of 30 days. Group B animals were those 11 dogs which received parenterally administered cyclosporine initially and then oral cyclosporine after 4 weeks of intramuscular administration. The graft survival was significantly prolonged to a

* This work was supported by grants from the Medical Research Council of Canada and the Lawrence and Elsie Pifko Foundation, Toronto, Canada.

mean of over 100 days in those animals which received parenteral and oral cyclosporine. There was a statistically significant improvement in survival if one compares this group of animals with those which received no immunosuppression and with those historical controls on which more conventional immunosuppressant techniques were used. However, if one scrutinizes our results closely, there were only three long-term survivors: Two lived for more than 200 days, and one lived for more than 400 days.

Overall in the world literature, there are very few long-term (more than 200 days) canine intestinal transplant survivors. It is therefore extremely difficult to assess the absorptive capacity of the graft when only a few long-term survivors have been reported. This fact has obvious important clinical applications because to this date, we have not been able to arrive at an adequate long-term physiologic assessment of a canine model following small-intestinal allotransplantation.

The three long-term survivors discussed above initially lost weight, but subsequently regained a significant proportion of it. However, even after 180 days, their weight had not reached their preoperative state. Although their weight did return to approximately 90% of the preoperative weight, there still appears to be some defect in the absorptive capacity of the long-term survivors which limited their ability to regain all of their lost weight. In other reports, there is also a slight diminution in the overall weight of the animal, again leading to the suspicion that the graft does not function normally even though the animals survive for a long period of time. This also has important clinical implications in that, when one considers intestinal transplantation in a human case, one may have to utilize more small intestine because of the fact that, thus far, no one has been able to demonstrate normal graft function in long-term survivors following experimental intestinal transplantation. Recipients of autografts will far exceed their own original body weight in the long-term; the diminution in weight gain is thus limited strictly to the allograft situation.

The studies reported thus far for D-xylose have also given similar results in that the absorption of D-xylose never returns to normal in long-term allograft survivors (Ruiz et al. 1972; Holmes et al. 1971).

More recently, we have been encouraged by the confirmatory report of Starzl's group on the increased survival in a canine small-intestinal transplantation model using both cyclosporine and prednisone (Diliz-Perez et al. 1984). In their report, two dogs lived for over 500 days. They reported on the percentage of fat excreted in the stools in normal controls, allotransplanted dogs, and short-bowel controls. However, only two long-term survivors were studied, and the percentage of fat excreted in the stool was significantly elevated compared with normal controls, as one might expect following transplantation. Similarly, when this group studied the long-term survivors over 500 days, one dog survived 525 days and another 530 days. The weights of these animals never returned to a perfectly normal level. There was always a slight decrease of approximately 10% of the total body weight, which would be in keeping with the results reported above.

Absorption of Cyclosporine in Canine Small-Intestinal Transplantation

Both autotransplanted and allotransplanted animals can absorb an oral dose of cyclosporine (COHEN et al. 1983). In five normal animals, cyclosporine was given as an oral dose of 25 mg/kg. The peak absorption occurred 6 h after oral administration. Similarly, in five dogs who had had a massive small-bowel resection, there was virtually no cyclosporine absorption following an oral dose. This shows that the site of cyclosporine absorption is a functioning small bowel. In the autotransplants that were tested with oral cyclosporine, there was a significant decrease in the ability of autotransplants to absorb the drug initially. Even though there are long-term surviving autotransplanted animals that have the ability to thrive and gain weight, their absorptive capacity within the first 4–6 weeks is diminished to approximately 40%–50% of the degree of cyclosporine absorption occuring in normal animals.

We also noted that, after small-intestinal autotransplanted, there was persistent malabsorption of oral cyclosporine and persistent diarrhea, which continued for up to 10 weeks following transplantation. We have therefore hypothesized that, because cyclosporine is a lipophilic agent carried in a lipid vehicle, we were causing a significant amount of diarrhea and, possibly, cyclosporine malabsorption. We felt that the cause of the diarrhea might be the oily vehicle itself. In order to answer this question, the three autotransplanted dogs were treated with repeated administrations of olive oil alone, and cyclosporine levels were measured again on a weekly basis after orally administered doses of cyclosporine.

In this experiment, in the dogs that were pretreated with olive oil, there was a significant increase after weeks 1, 2, and 4 in their ability to absorb cyclosporine following an oral test dose. We therefore concluded that, following the administration of the oily compound alone, there was indeed some mechanism leading to adaptation, which would allow for an increase in the absorption of cyclosporine and possibly have some importance as far as experimental intestinal transplantation using cyclosporine is concerned. This does not seem to have significant clinical applicability, as cyclosporine is given in a low volume in most transplant situations and there have been no reports of its causing significant diarrhea which might lead to impaired cyclosporine absorption.

The cause of this cyclosporine malabsorption is multifactoral. With transplantation, there is complete denervation at the level of the vascular pedicle, hypermotility produced in the bowel, and disruption of the lymphatics. All of these factors might contribute to decreased absorption of the orally administered agent.

In order to try to find the underlying causes of the cyclosporine malabsorption, we attempted to cannulate the thoracic duct and create cutaneous fistulae in this structure. This was done in five animals and followed by the administration of cyclosporine in olive oil (COHEN et al. 1983). The result of this experiment demonstrated that there were very large levels of cyclosporine seen in the lymph of these anesthetized animals following administration of cyclosporine directly into the duodenum. We could also still demonstrate measurable amounts of cyclosporine in the plasma, although they were greatly diminished in comparison with the values found in the lymph. This demonstrates that the lymphatic system is probably the major, though certainly not the only, source of cyclosporine absorption, and we hypothesize that some cyclosporine is free in the peritoneal cavity and absorbed directly through the peritoneal membrane.

The lätter experiment was performed in anesthetized animals, in which it was certainly difficult to maintain patency of the thoracic duct cutaneous fistulae for a prolonged period of time. However, we were able to do that in one animal, to which cyclosporine was given orally the following day. The cyclosporine level in the lymph reached levels greater than 1800 mg/L. In the plasma, it also reached a level of 700 mg/L. Therefore, the major portion was again absorbed through the lymphatic system.

Absorption of Cyclosporine and ^{14}C-Labelled Glucose in Out-of-Continuity Allografts

In the experiments summarized here, we used an experimental model which has previously been described. In this model of total small-intestinal allotransplantation, the proximal jejunal end and the distal ileal end are brought to the skin surface as isolated intestinal allografted stomas (Lossing et al. 1982). The remainder of the bowel is placed back into continuity. The purpose of this model is to allow one access each to the proximal and distal ends of the allograft, while still maintaining continuity. It has been shown that the histologic course of rejection of the proximal and distal ends are similar and that biopsies from these isolated stomas represent the histologic sequence of rejection that is expected in in-continuity bowel (Lossing et al. 1982). In addition to daily biopsies, which are possible form these isolated stomas, one could also infuse these isolated pouches with compounds to test the absorptive capacity of the allograft itself and to compare this with the histologic course of rejection.

In the experimental design, four autotransplants and 15 allotransplants were performed (Nordgren et al. 1984). The allotransplants were treated with cyclosporine (7.5 mg/kg per day parenterally) in divided doses. On day 14, all immunosuppression was stopped, and the animals were allowed to proceed to rejection. During this period following cessation of the cyclosporine, an oral dose of cyclosporine (25 mg/kg) was given. These oral test doses of cyclosporine were given twice weekly. In addition, the isolated pouches were infused with ^{14}C-labelled glucose, and blood samples were taken at 0, 1, 2, 4, 6, and 12 h. The absorption of ^{14}C-labelled glucose would then be compared with the absorption of cyclosporine and the histologic results of the daily isolated pouch biopsies.

The ^{14}C-labelled glucose was instilled into the isolated pouches in 3 ml of an isotonic saline solution containing 2 μCi [^{14}C]glucose. The blood samples were taken according to the time schedule noted above, and the measurements were made using a liquid scintillation counter. Counts per minute (cpm) were used for the final analysis.

The absorption of an oral dose of cyclosporine was compared in animals with autotransplants, in animals which received allotransplants and demonstrated normal histologic results of daily pouch biopsies, and in allotransplanted animals which demonstrated evidence of rejection. When ohne compared the absorption of cyclosporine in autotransplants and in those allotransplants with normal graft histology, the patterns of absorption were similar. However, when the animals started to reject the graft, one could see a definite decrease in the absorption of cyclosporine itself. This was statistically significant at the $P < 0.05$ level.

This same pattern occurred when the results of the uptake of ^{14}C-labelled glucose from the allotransplanted jejunum were examined. We demonstrated that, when the pouch biopsies were normal histologically, the curve showing ^{14}C-labelled absorption was almost normal, although the peak of this curve occurred 4–5 min later than one would expect in normal animals. When there was evidence of rejection, the peak absorption of ^{14}C-labelled glucose was greatly diminished, and the time course was also prolonged.

This last experiment demonstrates that there is a correlation between absorptive function and histology, as one would expect, and that most likely histology is still the best parameter of function when considering small-intestinal transplantation from the clinical point of view. Furthermore, one can conclude that, when small-intestinal transplantation is performed clinically, there must be some form of stoma on the skin for biopsy purposes. Absorptive studies, whatever the ones chosen, will still not be as sensitive as the structural changes seen histologically.

Summary

As yet, there is little data on long-term surviving experimental animals to support the position that a small-intestinal allograft can function normally. Further experiments in both the canine and other large-animal models are necessary to ensure long-term survival so that proper physiologic studies can be carried out.

References

Cohen Z, Nordgren SR, Mackenzie RD, Lossing AG, Stiller CR, Langer B (1983) Pharmakokinetics of cyclosporine in a canine intestinal transplantation model. Transplant Proc [Suppl] 15 (4):3013–3018

Craddock GN, Nordgren SR, Reznick RK, Gilas I, Lossing AG, Cohen Z, Stiller CR, Cullen JB, Langer B (1983) Small bowel transplantation in the dog using cyclosporine. Transplantation 35:248

Diliz-Perez HS, McClure J, Bedetti C et al (1984) Successful small bowel transplantation in dogs with cyclosporine and prednisone. Transplantation 37(2):127–132

Holmes JT, Yeh SDJ, Winawer SJ, Kawana N, Fortner JG (1971) Absorption studies in canine jejunal allografts. Ann Surg 174:101–108

Lillehei RC, Goott B, Miller FA (1959) The physiological response prolonged in vitro preservation of the bowel with successful replacement and survival. Ann Surg 50:543–560

Lossing A, Nordgren S, Cohen Z, Cullen J, Craddock G, Langer B (1982) Histologic monitoring of rejection in small intestinal transplantation. Transplant Proc 14:643–645

Nordgren S, Cohen Z, Mackenzie R, Finkelstein D, Greenberg GR, Langer B (1984) Functional monitors of rejection in small intestinal transplants. Am J Surg 147:152–158

Ruiz JO, Uchida H, Schultz LS, Lillehei RC (1972) Problems in absorption and immunosuppression after entire intestinal allotransplantation. Am J Surg 123:297–302

Intestinal Preservation of Small-Bowel Grafts by Vascular Washout and Cold Storage

W. H. Schraut, K. K. W. Lee, and Y. Tsujinaka

Introduction

The development of an effective method for preserving the small intestine during the interval between harvesting and implantation is a key factor to the success of future clinical small-bowel transplantation. In particular, a method of small-bowel preservation which allows for functional graft survival after ischemic intervals of up to 24 h should be devised. Such an interval is desirable to permit unhurried graft procurement from cadaveric donors and recipient preparation until the actual implantation is completed.

At present, a tested and proven technique for small-bowel preservation which is suitable for clinical application is lacking. There is an abundance of conflicting literature on experimental approaches and models. Of the many techniques for preserving the small bowel, ranging from simple hypothermic storage in a hyperbaric oxygen chamber (Manax et al. 1965) to pulsatile normothermic perfusion (Hohenleitner and Senior 1969), intravascular flushing with a cold (4°C) crystalloid solution followed by cold storage appears to be technically easy and economical and promises effective short-term (6–18 h) preservation (Manax et al. 1965; Ricour et al. 1981). Procedures that are technically more difficult and involve continued intravascular perfusion may be required for extended periods of preservation (Toledo-Pereya and Najarian 1973). The small bowel may also be preserved by perfusion of the intestinal lumen; this can be used in conjunction with or even replace intravascular methods.

It was our objective to develop a simple but effective method for short-term preservation of the small intestine. The efficacy of intravascular flushing with cold Collins' solution followed by cold storage was evaluated, an approach which has been found to be highly effective for kidney preservation for periods of up to 24 h (Mozes et al. 1985).

Materials and Methods

The rat model of heterotopic (accessory) and of orthotopic small-bowel transplantation was used. The experiments were conducted in the Lewis (LEW) → LEW rat strain combination, i. e., isografts were transplanted. The harvesting and transplantation procedures have been described previously (Schraut et al. 1983). Harvesting involves dissection of the superior mesenteric artery and the portal vein, leaving the entire small intestine attached to the donor only at these two vessels and at the duodenum and ileum. After rinsing of the gut lumen with 20 cc normal saline containing 0.05% neomycin sulfate at 4°C, the portal vein is divided at its bifurcation at the porta hepatis. The vascular bed is then flushed with 5–10 cc cold (4°C) saline containing 10000 units of heparin per liter. During flushing, intravascular pressure is kept below 100 mmHg. The superior mesenteric artery is then divided, and the graft is immediately wrapped in cold, saline-soaked sponges and kept at 4°C until transplantation. Transplantation involves anastomoses between the mesenteric artery and abdominal aorta and between the portal vein and inferior vena cava. The total time of ischemia with this method ranges from 40 to 60 min. The small-bowel isograft is then either exteriorized via enterostomies (accessory graft) or placed into intestinal continuity following resection of the recipient's own small bowel (orthotopic graft). The success rate with this approach reaches 80% for accessory transplants and 70% for orthotopic grafts (one-stage procedure). Using this technique, eight experiments were conducted, each with accessory and orthotopic graft placement (control group).

The experimental protocol of small-bowel preservation involved harvesting of the entire small bowel according to the described surgical techniques and is listed as follows:

1) Harvesting
   a) Intravascular flushing with Collins' solution at 4°C
   b) Intraluminal flushing with normal saline and 0.05% neomycin at 4°C
2) Cold storage for 6, 12, or 18 h at 4°C
3) Implantation as heterotopic isograft; biopsy 30 min after revascularization
4) Orthotopic placement after 5–6 days; biopsy

For intravascular flushing Collins' solution containing 10000 units of heparin per liter at 4°C was used. Cold normal saline was used for intraluminal flushing. The intestine was then stored at 4°C for 6 h (group 1; $n = 8$), 12 h (group 2; $n = 14$), or 18 h (group 3; $n = 15$). After the preservation period, the graft was implanted as an accessory organ. Approximately 30 min after revascularization, a segment of small bowel was taken for histologic study prior to the formation of the enterostomies. After 5–8 days, surviving animals underwent relaparotomy, biopsy of the accessory graft, and orthotopic placement into gastrointestinal continuity. The nutritional status of the animals (weight gain, serum protein, serum triglycerides, maltose absorption) was followed for 4 months. The animals were then killed.

Preservation of the small-bowel graft was considered to be successful if the recipient survived with a functioning graft in orthotopic position or a histologically intact graft in accessory position. Preservation was also assumed to be adequate if the animal succumbed to other causes (pneumonia, hemorrhage) within days after transplantation, as long as the graft was histologically intact.

The determination of the precise cause of graft loss within 5 days of transplantation poses a dilemma. The macroscopic and microscopic appearance of an intestinal graft lost as a result of either insufficient preservation or technical failure of the anastomosis are similar and include mucosal sloughing, graft necrosis, and/or vascular thrombosis. In these situations, if the vascular anastomoses were smooth, intact, and widely patent on inspection (i. e., anastomotic failure was unlikely), we concluded that preservation was insufficient and the cause of graft loss.

Results

Control Experiments

Isografts of the entire small intestine transplanted immediately after harvesting (accessory or orthotopic position) sustained temporary histologic alterations limited to sporadic sloughing of the superficial villi tips and edema (Fig. 1). These alterations

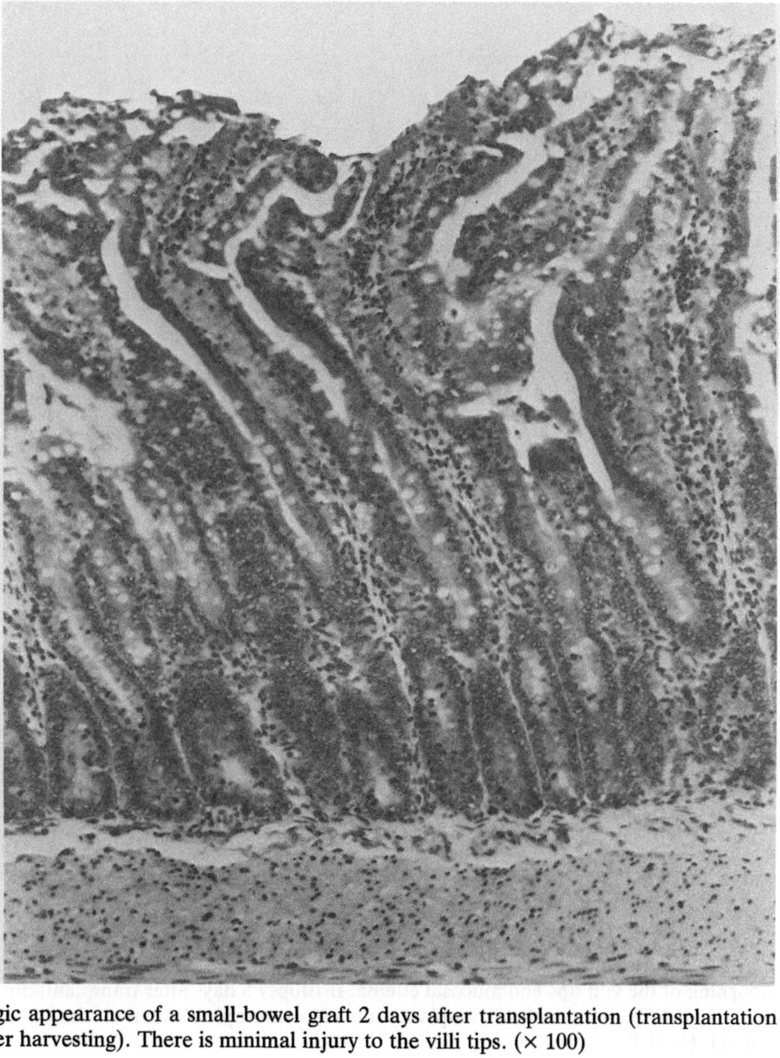

Fig. 1. Histologic appearance of a small-bowel graft 2 days after transplantation (transplantation immediately after harvesting). There is minimal injury to the villi tips. (× 100)

reversed within 3 days. Accessory grafts developed disuse atrophy, which became evident by shrinkage of the graft 3–6 weeks after transplantation. Orthotopic grafts behaved as normal in situ small intestine of the recipient. Light-microscopic findings in both of these grafts were unremarkable; alterations due to lymphatic interruption or denervation were not detected. Animals with orthotopic isografts exhibited normal weight gain and demonstrated normal nutritional parameters in comparison to age-matched controls (LEE and SCHRAUT 1986).

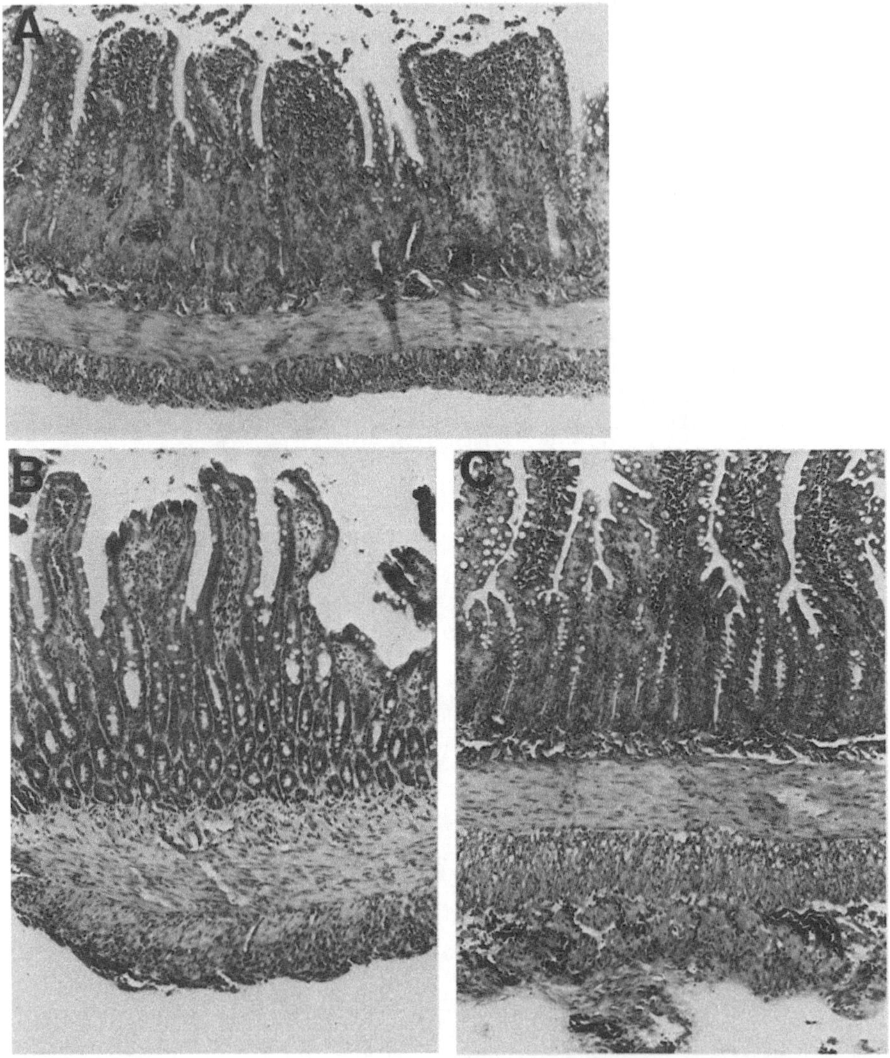

Fig. 2A–C. Isograft preserved for 6 h. **A** Biopsy obtained 30 min after revascularization shows sloughing of the villi tips and mucosal edema. **B** Biopsy 5 days after transplantation shows an intact mucosa. **C** Four months after transplantation and orthotopic placement, the bowel is histologically normal. (× 100)

Small-Bowel Preservation for 6 H (Group 1)

Six of the eight animals in this group survived with functioning isografts. Two grafts were lost as a result of vascular complications after the implantation procedure. One animal succumbed during relaparotomy and placement of the isograft in gastrointestinal continuity. This graft was histologically intact. Surviving animals (n = 5) had normal weight gain and showed normal nutritional parameters at 120 days post-transplantation.

The histologic alterations within days after revascularization paralleled those seen in grafts with immediate transplantation (control group), although sloughing of the villi tips and mucosal edema seemed to be more pronounced (Fig. 2). Five to 8 days

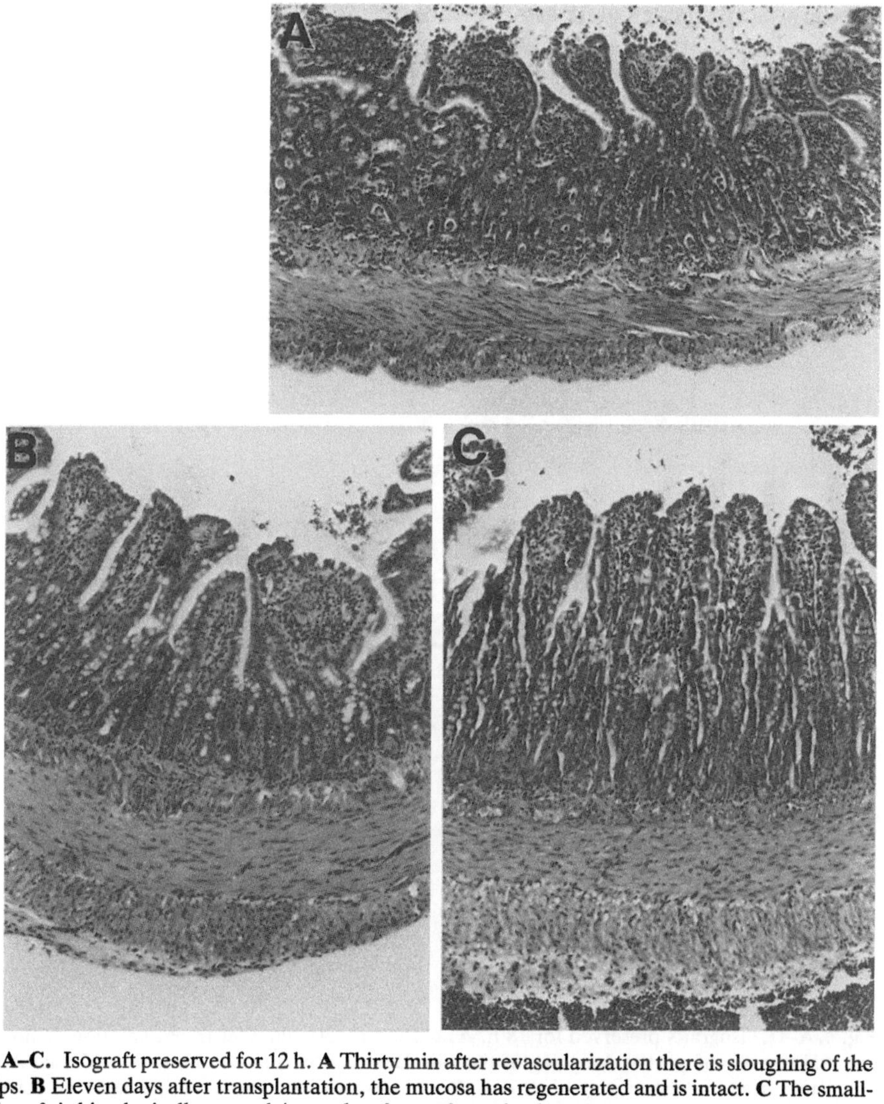

Fig. 3 A–C. Isograft preserved for 12 h. **A** Thirty min after revascularization there is sloughing of the villi tips. **B** Eleven days after transplantation, the mucosa has regenerated and is intact. **C** The small-bowel graft is histologically normal 4 months after orthotopic placement

post-transplantation and several months later at sacrifice, the grafts demonstrated normal histology.

Small-Bowel Preservation for 12 H (Group 2)

The results in this group of animals were variable. Seven out of 14 grafts could be transplanted successfully and survived beyond 6 days. Two of the seven animals died during relaparotomy and placement of the graft into gastrointestinal continuity and two died several months after the transplantation procedure as a result of a small-bowel obstruction. In these four animals, there was no evidence of graft necrosis or fibrosis due to ischemia (Fig. 3). The remaining seven animals succumbed 1–8 days after the transplantation procedure and presented a necrotic graft. The biopsies from these grafts, after revascularization, demonstrated more pronounced sloughing of the villi tips than that seen with grafts preserved for 6 h (Fig. 3A). In none of these

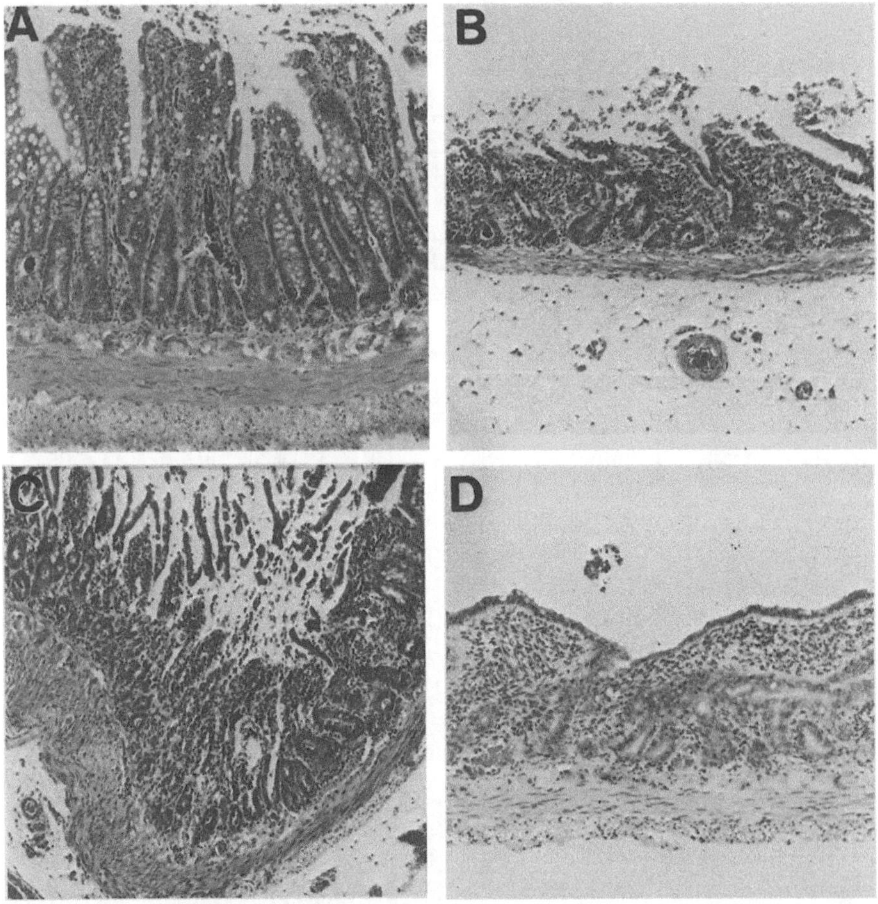

Fig. 4.A–D. Isografts preserved for 18 h. **A, C** Biopsies 30 min after transplantation demonstrate mucosal edema and partial sloughing of the villi. Destruction is more extensive in **C** than **A. B, D** Specimens from the respective grafts 1 day after transplantation. There is thinning of the bowel wall and extensive mucosal destruction. Remnant crypts are seen in **C.** (× 100)

specimens was complete mucosal loss seen. Extensive mucosal destruction was present in those grafts which led to the recipients' death within 8 days. In five of these seven animals, the vascular anastomoses were patent; we therefore attributed graft loss to insufficient preservation.

Small-Bowel Preservation for 18 H (Group 3)
All grafts in this group were implanted successfully, and the recipients survived 1–4 days. Evaluation of the biopsies obtained 30 min after revascularization demonstrated various degrees of mucosal destruction. However, in none of these grafts was complete mucosal sloughing and necrosis observed. Impairment was always limited to the villi tips. All grafts obtained 1–4 days after revascularization demonstrated severe necrosis with complete loss of the intestinal mucosa (Fig. 4). Vascular anastomoses of the transplants were patent in 12 of the 15 transplants.

Discussion

The small bowel and, particularly, its mucosa are as susceptible to the effects of ischemia as other organ grafts. Therefore, any method of small-bowel preservation must maintain the integrity of the intestinal mucosa or, at least, minimize ischemic damage so that regeneration may occur within a few days of the ischemic period. Structural damage of the small-bowel mucosa is observed as early as 30 min after the onset of ischemia; the upper two-thirds of the villi are denuded of epithelial cells, whereas the lower regions of the villi and crypts remain relatively intact (Robinson et al. 1966; Robinson and Mirkovitch 1972). If circulatory arrest persists for 1–2 h, then the crypt epithelium sustains ischemic damage as well (Gabbert et al. 1978).

Recovery of the intestinal mucosa from an ischemic event can occur, but depends on the duration of ischemia. In the rat, after ligation of the arterial inflow for 1 h, epithelial injury reverses within 48–72 h (Pitha 1971). When the period of normothermic ischemia is prolonged to 2 h, the structure of both villi and epithelial crypts require 7 days to return to normal (Wagner et al. 1979). We concluded from the reports of these investigators that histologic evaluation of the preserved bowel made 2–5 days after transplantation should indicate whether a particular method of preservation is effective or not. We have shown that biopsies obtained 5–7 days after transplantation demonstrate normal histology if preservation was adequate. Furthermore, these grafts performed satisfactorily when placed into gastrointestinal continuity.

In anticipation of small-bowel transplantation in the clinical setting, short-term (6–18 h preservation of the bowel graft is required. Hypothermia combined with various methods of perfusion has been shown to extend viability of the small intestine by several hours. We found that core cooling of the small bowel with Collins' solution, which is similar in composition to the intracellular milieu, followed by storage at 4°C allows safe preservation for 6 h. Preservation beyond 6 h can not be safely and consistently achieved with this technique. In contrast, Ricour et al. (1981) suggested that successful preservation for 20 h could be achieved with this technique in piglets.

These investigators based their conclusions on histologic findings and tissue culturing of mucosal biopsies obtained at the end of the preservation period (i. e., biopsies prior to revascularization) and on the successful transplantation which resulted in seven of 13 cases. However, we caution that biopsies prior to revascularization may not be predictive of the ultimate outcome. Our study indicates that biopsies, even after reperfusion for 30 min, fail to indicate whether or not the bowel graft will survive; the histologic alterations seen at that time are limited to the villi tips and do not reflect the total extent of ischemic mucosal damage. It takes several hours or even 1–2 days of reperfusion until the extent of ischemic injury becomes histologically evident. From our experience, we suggest that an observation period of several days is necessary before one can decide whether a preservation method is effective or not.

A common dilemma which arises in all organ preservation models requiring transplantation of the preserved graft with vascular anastomoses, lies in the fact that insufficient preservation leads to the same histologic changes in the organ graft (edema, cellular disruption, global necrosis, vascular thrombosis) as are seen after anastomotic failure. In our study, we attributed the failure of seven of the 37 preservation experiments to complications of the vascular anastomoses. It is conceivable that some of these experiments failed because of inadequate preservation, in combination with anastomotic vascular insufficiency. Approaches to circumvent this difficulty (i. e., methods which obviate vascular anastomoses), involve detailed histologic study of the graft without implantation, cell cultures, and study of biochemical and histochemical markers of cell injury. All of these approaches are valuable and provide information as to the effectiveness of a particular preservation method. However, conclusive evidence for successful preservation is obtained by graft transplantation, with the recipient's survival depending on unimpaired graft function. The second step of our experimental protocol (orthotopic placement of the viable isograft) fulfills this requirement. All recipients which underwent this second procedure successfully grew normally and remained healthy until they were killed. There was no evidence of nutritional impairment, nor were there any histologic findings of graft injury (fibrosis, strictures) at autopsy.

We conclude that preservation for 6 h utilizing core cooling and hypothermic storage is effective. Preservation for 12 h is sometimes effective and may be effective up to 20 h in the piglet. Ricour et al. (1981), after 20 h of preservation, transplanted the small-bowel graft into heterotopic and orthotopic position with a successful outcome in seven of 13 instances. Projecting these data into the clinical setting, one must realize that a partial success rate with this method of preservation is insufficient and continue to search for different methods of small-bowel preservation that can be used once ischemic intervals beyond 6–8 h are anticipated. There are possibilities which may safety prolong the period of preservation: Different solutions containing pharmacologic agents could be used, continuous or intermittent intravascular and/or intraluminal perfusion could be employed, and the solutions could be oxygenated with or without the use of oxygen carriers such as fluorocarbons. Further investigations into these possibilities will be a future task.

References

Gabbert H, Wagner R, Aust P, Höhn P (1978) Ischemia and post-ischemic regeneration of the small intestinal mucosa. An enzyme-histochemical investigation. Acta Histochem 63:197–213
Hohenleitner FJ, Senior JR (1969) Metabolism of canine small intestine vascularly perfused in vitro. J App Physiol 26:119–128
Lee KKW, Schraut WH (1986) Structure and function of orthotopic small-bowel allografts in rats treated with cyclosporin A. Am J Surg (in press)
Manax WG, Bloch JH, Eyal Z, Lillehei RC (1965) Experimental preservation of the small bowel. Am J Surg 109:26–30
Mozes MF, Finch WT, Reckard CR, Merkel FK, Cohen C (1985) Comparison of cold storage and machine perfusion of cadaver kidneys: A prospective, randomized study. Transplant Proc 17:1474–1477
Pitha J (1971) The fine structure of regenerating epithelium in the small intestine. Virchows Arch [Cell Pathol] 7:314–341
Ricour C, Revillon Y, Pletyncx M, Laufenburger A, Jehannin B, Ghnassia D, Duval C , Ghnassia J-C, Jos J, Fontaine J-L, Navarro J, Schmitz J, Gallix P (1981) Conservation hypothermique et autotransplantation du grêle chez le porcelet. Gastroenterol Clin Biol 5:977–986
Robinson JWL, Mirkovitch V (1972) The recovery of function and microcirculation in small intestinal loops following ischaemia. Gut 13:784–789
Robinson JWL, Antonioli JA, Mirkovitch V (1966) The intestinal response to ischemia. Naunyn-Schmiedebergs Arch Pharmacol 255:178–191
Schraut WH, Rosemurgy AS, Riddell RM (1983) Prolongation of intestinal allograft survival without immunosuppressive drug therapy. Transplantation of small bowel allografts. J Surg Res 34:597–607
Toledo-Pereyra LH, Najarian JS (1973) Small bowel preservation: Comparison of perfusion and nonperfusion systems. Arch Surg 107:875–877
Wagner R, Gabbert H, Höhn P (1979) Ischemia and post-ischemic regeneration of the small intestinal mucosa. A light microscopic and autoradiographic study. Virchows Arch [Cell Pathol] 31:259–276

Glucose Absorption After Heterotopic Small-Bowel Transplantation

P. Schroeder, F. Sandforth, and E. Deltz

In heterotopic transplantation, the grafted intestine is temporarily excluded from normal passage of the ingesta. Therefore, it seemed logical to examine the response of the organ during the period of functional inactivation, before the graft is brought into orthotopic position. The aim of this study was to show changes in graft function by measuring glucose and water absorption and by correlating these results to morphometric findings.

Methods

The technique of heterotopic small-bowel transplantation in syngeneic rates has been described previously by Deltz (1984). Male Lewis rats with a body weight of 250 g were used. Glucose and water absorption was measured in nonanesthetized rats using an in vivo recirculation system designed by Sheff and Smyth (1955), which was modified by Menge et al. (1970). Figure 1a shows the system, which allowed for the simultaneous perfusion of two intestinal loops in the same animal. The glucose was dissolved in Krebs-Henseleit buffer (Krebs and Henseleit 1932) with a concentration of 360 mg%. Absorption was expressed in terms of intestinal length. At the end of the perfusion period (45 min), the animals were killed, the intestine was quickly removed, and the length measured under constant tension of the small bowel.

Jejunal and ileal tissue samples were taken from identical locations in both the grafted and the recipient's own intestine. For morphometric investigations, microdissection was performed as described by Clarke (1970) and Lorenz-Meyer et al. (1976).

Experiments were performed on the 35th day after transplantation. There was a 24-h starvation period before transplantation and the perfusion experiment. For statistics, the Wilcoxon rank-sum test was used.

Results

The body weight of the animals rose from 250 g to an average of 331.3 g during the 35 days after transplantation. Upon macroscopic examination in situ, the grafts showed a reduction in diameter. Results of the morphometric studies are given in Table 1 and

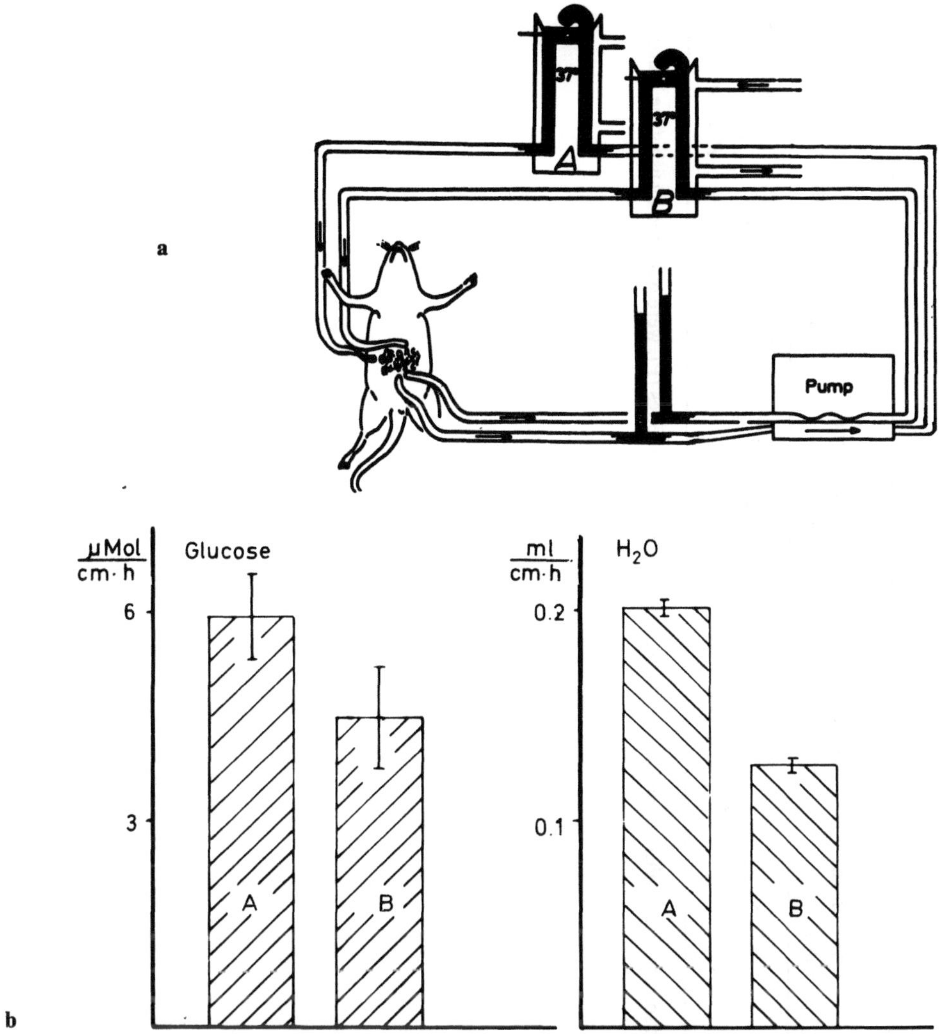

Fig. 1a, b. **a** Recirculation system for in vivo measurement of glucose and water absorption. **b** Glucose *(left)* and H_2O *(right)* absorption after heterotopic small-bowel transplantation ($n = 6$, 35 days after surgery). *A*, recipient small intestine; *B*, graft small intestine

Fig. 2b. The proximal-distal gradient of villus height was calculated for both the graft intestine and the recipient's own small bowel. When comparing graft and recipient intestinal villi, the difference in villus height was significant at the 5% level. Correspondingly, there was a decrease in crypt length at the jejunal and ileal loci, but this decrease was insignificant.

Figure 2a shows data on the calculated villus surface. In the graft, the surface area of jejunal villi is about 30% and the surface area of ileal villi is about 48% less than the respective areas in the recipient's own intestine. The difference is significant at the 1% level for ileal and at the 5% level for jejunal villi.

Table 1. Results of microdissection

	Parameter jejunum			Parameter ileum		
	villus height (µm)	crypt length (µm)	villus surface (mm^2)	villus height (µm)	crypt lenght (µm)	villus surface (mm^2)
Recipient small bowel	448.2 ± 91.48	218.9 ± 31.89	0.2518 ± 0.0311	264.3 ± 75.60	166.5 ± 21.49	0.148 ± 0.0205
Small-bowel graft	352.0 ± 80.54	176.8 ± 17.79	0.134 ± 0.035	230.4 ± 29.84	146.7 ± 37.32	0.065 ± 0.0148
Probability	$P < 0.05$	NS	$P < 0.05$	$P < 0.05$	NS	$P < 0.01$

The results are means ± SD of measurements in six rats. Probability values for the differences between the two series *(P)*, were obtained by using the Wilcoxon rank-sum test.

NS, not significant

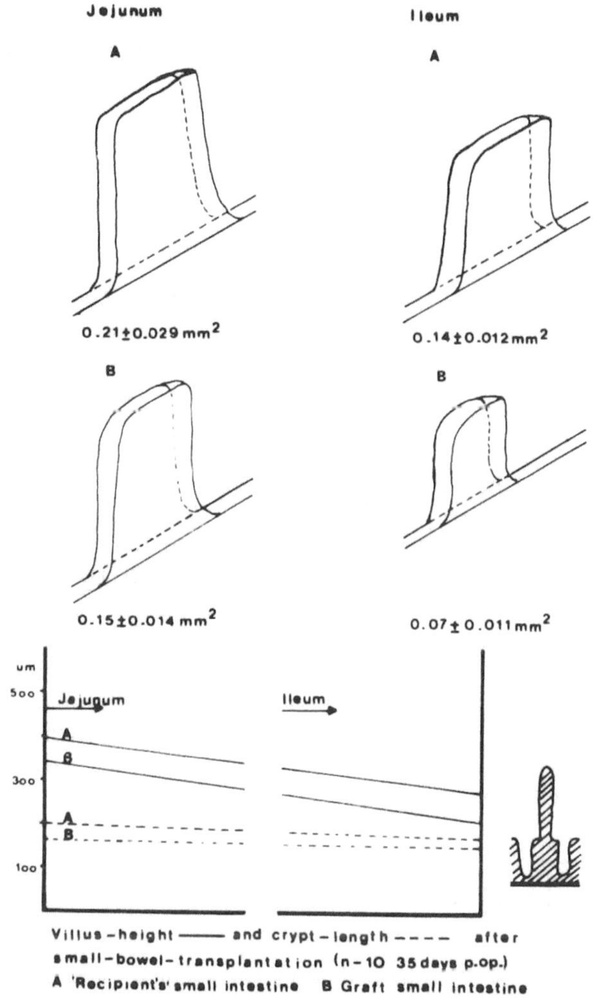

Fig. 2a, b. a Villus surface area (mean ± SEM) after heterotopic small-bowel transplantation (n = 10, 35 days after surgery). **b** Villus height (——) and crypt length (– – – –) after small-bowel transplantation (n = 10, 35 days after surgery). *A*, recipient small intestine; *B*, graft small intestine

Table 2. Measurements of glucose and water absorption

	Glucose (μmol/cm per h)	H_2O (ml/cm per h)
Recipient small bowel	6.1 ± 0.67	0.22 ± 0.088
Small-bowel graft	4.6 ± 0.77	0.126 ± 0.017
Probability	$P < 0.05$	$P < 0.01$

The results are means ± SD of absorption measurements in six rats. The probabilities for the difference between the two series *(P)* were obtained by using the Wilcoxon rank-sum test.

Table 2 shows the absorption data. Corresponding to morphometric changes, we found a significant reduction in water absorption at the 1% level, which is shown on the right side of Fig. 1b. Glucose absorption was only slightly reduced in the small-bowel graft yet even this amount was significant. Expressed in terms of villus surface, the capacity for glucose absorption in the grafted intestine was 1.9-fold better than in the small bowel of the recipient, in the graft was 1.4-fold better than in the recipient's small bowel.

Discussion

The morphometric results showed typical atrophy of the mucosa, which was not unlike the severe atrophy found in experimental, self-emptying blind loops that are deprived of all nutritive material (Menge et al. 1975). Reduced glucose and water absorption in heterotopically transplanted small bowel corresponds to mucosal atrophy (Menge et al. 1970). Earlier studies on self-emptying blind loops have shown that the proportion of functionally mature absorptive cells is greater in blind loop mucosa than in normal mucosa, so that the absorptive capacity is higher than expected in mucosal atrophy (Menge et al. 1978; Robinson et al. 1980). These findings may explain the increased glucose and water absorption in the grafted small bowel.

In animals in which the heterotopic small bowel is brought into orthotopic position, body weight drops for a few days, owing to impaired graft function. This corresponds to our observations of reduced absorption in connection with the morphometric data. However, this functional and morphometric irregularity is only briefly of concern, as the body weight of the animals with an orthotopic graft rises again after 7 days.

Heterotopically transplanted small bowel which is brought into orthotopic position takes on capacity for absorption which is sufficient for complete nutrition and the survival of the animal.

References

Clarke RM (1970) Mucosal architecture and epithelial cell production rate in the small intestine of the albino rat. J Anat 107:519–529

Deltz E (1984) Immunreaktionen nach allogener Dünndarmtransplantation. Fortschr Med 102:29–30

Krebs HA, Henseleit K (1932) Untersuchungen über die Harnstoffbildung im Tierkörper. Hoppe-Seyler's Z Physiol Chem 210:33–66

Lorenz-Meyer H, Köhn R, Riecken EO (1976) Vergleich verschiedener morphometrischer Methoden zur Erfassung der Schleimhautoberfläche des Rattendünndarms und deren Beziehung zur Funktion. Histochemistry 49:123–129

Menge H, Bloch R, Schaumlöffel E, Riecken EO (1970) Transportstudien, morphologische Untersuchungen zum Verhalten der Dünndarmschleimhaut im operativ ausgeschalteten Jejunalabschnitt der Ratte. Z Gesamte Exp Med 153:74–90

Menge H, Werner H, Lorenz-Meyer H, Riecken EO (1975) The nutritive effect of glucose on the structure and function of jejunal self-emptying blind loops in the rat. Gut 16:462–467

Menge H, Robinson JWL, Schroeder P (1978) Functional and structural correlations in the atrophic mucosa of self-emptying blind loops of rat small intestine. J Physiol 280:33–34P

Robinson JWL, Menge H, Schroeder P, Riecken EO, van Melle G (1980) Structural and functional correlations in the atrophic mucosa of self-emptying blind loops of rat jejunum. J Clin Invest 10:393–399

Sheff MF, Smyth DH (1955) An apparatus for the study of in vivo intestinal absorption in the rat. J Physiol 128:67

Absorption Studies After Orthotopic Small-Bowel Transplantation

J. SEIFERT and E. DELTZ

Recent research has shown that immunologic problems in small-bowel transplantation can be controlled by the use of certain immunosuppressive drugs, which thus makes it possible to investigate in more depth problems in intestinal function after small-bowel transplantation. The finding of WASSEF et al. (1985) that cyclosporine A absorption is impaired in the bowel of both autotransplanted and allotransplanted dogs allows us to speculate that the absorption of protein and carbohydrates in transplanted intestine is also reduced.

To investigate the absorption of both proteins and carbohydrates, orthotopically transplanted rats (see PREISSNER et al., "Microsurgical Techniques of Heterotopic and Orthotopic Small-Bowel Transplantation in the Rat," this volume), were tested in a syngeneic donor-recipient combination (Lewis on Lewis). For this purpose, 3- to 9-month-old rats with a small-bowel graft were fed a mixture of 100 mg radioactively labeled gamma globulin, together with 1 g maltose dissolved in 3 ml water by means of an intragastral tube. Rats remained conscious over the 6-h absorption period. Blood samples were taken from the tail veins before and after feeding at 10, 30, and 60 min and at 3 and 6 h. To determine protein absorption, radioactivity was measured in blood samples and expressed as the percentage of the applied dosage per ml blood. To determine the digestion and absorption of maltose, the glucose concentrations in the rats' serum were investigated. Glucose concentrations were measured in 10 μl serum for the time intervals described above. The results of absorption studies in animals with syngeneic orthotopic small-bowel transplants were compared with results of quite similar experiments with control animals of the same strain and age, but with a normal, intact intestine.

Table 1. Absorption of radioactively labeled proteins (mean ± SD) after small-bowel transplantation in rats

	Transplanted rats (% administered dosage in 1 ml)	Controls (% administered dosage in 1 ml)
Before transplantation	0 0	0 0
After transplantation		
10 min	0.01 ± 0.005	0.01 ± 0.009
30 min	0.02 ± 0.009	0.01 ± 0.008
60 min	0.03 ± 0.01	0.03 ± 0.02
3 h	0.08 ± 0.01	0.07 ± 0.003
6 h	0.1 ± 0.02	0.09 ± 0.02

Table 1 shows the result of protein absorption. There was no difference in radioactivity between transplanted and control animals, indicating that protein absorption is not impaired in transplanted animals. It can, however, be argued that radioactivity is an unreliable indicator for protein absorption, as the label can be separated from the original protein by enzymatic digestion. Since the absorption of the label alone is much faster than the absorption of protein by products, it seems likely that the digestion and absorption of proteins was similar in both groups because the statistical values do not differ radically. A simple calculation with these values shows the amount of dose that can be found in the blood 6 h after administration. If this amount is multiplied by the blood volume, approximately 2.5% of the administered dose can be detected in the blood of both the transplanted and the control animals. Since the animals survived we chose not to study any other organs.

Similar results were obtained in our observations of carbohydrate digestion and glucose absorption (Table 2).

Table 2. Maltose absorption after small-bowel transplantation in rats (mean ± SD)

	Transplanted rats (Glucose concentration in mg/dl)	Controls (Glucose concentration in mg/dl)
Before transplantation	66 ± 16	133 ± 33
10 min	200 ± 57	300 ± 56
30 min	300 ± 57	766 ± 133
60 min	1000 ± 127	1000 ± 157
3 h	266 ± 33	500 ± 151
6 h	260 ± 30	200 ± 58

Differences in the glucose concentration before maltose application are rapidly equalized during absorption. In both groups, maximum concentration was reached after 60 min and during the next 5 h, this concentration decreased at the same rate for both groups. Since at no time was the difference statistically significant, it can be postulated that the digestion and absorption of maltose also remains unimpaired in syngeneic bowel-transplanted animals.

Thus long-term survivors of orthotopic small-bowel transplantation in a syngeneic strain combination show normal protein and carbohydrate digestion and absorption.

Reference

Wassef R, Cohen Z, Nordgren S, Langer B (1985) Cyclosporin absorption in intestinal transplantation. Transplantation 39:496–499

Functional Adaptation of the Small-Intestinal Mucosa After Experimental Small-Bowel Transplantation: A Quantitative Histochemical Study

F. SANDFORTH, P. SCHROEDER, E. DELTZ, S. GUTSCHMIDT, and E. O. RIECKEN

In studies conducted in recent years, DELTZ and his coworkers have shown (THIEDE and DELTZ 1978; DELTZ et al. 1981; DELTZ 1984) that, after allogeneic small-intestinal transplantation, both graft rejection and graft-vs-host reaction are dependent on the histoincompatibility grade, graft length, and the amount of lymphatic tissue grafted. In syngeneic transplantation, however, it was not possible to detect histologic alterations of the mucosal architecture in the small bowel of either the graft or the recipient. Since these studies did not show major alterations in villus size, and since it is well known that villus height is a representative parameter of nonelectrolyte transport, it is conceivable that syngeneic transplantation does not alter either the structure or function of the small intestine.

In order to validate this hypothesis, more sophisticated methods for the analysis of mucosal architecture and function were applied. The results of three-dimensional morphometric evaluation of the mucosal architecture using microdissection, and measurement of glucose absorption by in vivo perfusion of the small bowel have been presented in another paper (see SCHRÖDER et al., "Glucose Absorption after Heterotopic Small-Bowel Transplantation," this volume). The following presentation will deal with the histochemical part of the study.

Methods

Thirteen male Lewis rats were investigated after syngeneic heterotopic accessory small-bowel transplantation. Details concerning the experimental design and operative technique have been presented in another contribution (see PREISSNER et al., "Microsurgical Techniques of Heterotopic and Orthotopic Small-Bowel Transplantation in the Rat," this volume). The quantitative histochemical methods applied imply a biochemical technique which allows measurements of enzyme activities in the V_{max} range of substrate hydrolysis in situ, i.e., to be taken directly in the histochemical section. Enzyme activities were measured at apical and basal villus positions in both the jejunum and ileum of the grafts and were compared with the corresponding values or the recipients' small intestines. The activity of the following enzymes was measured: neutral α-glucosidase in jejunum and ileum and lactase/β-glucosidase and alkaline phosphatase in the jejunum (GUTSCHMIDT 1981; GUTSCHMIDT et al. 1979; 1981). Calculations were performed using a factorial analysis of variance (repeated-measures design).

Results and Comments

The neutral α-glucosidase (Fig. 1) shows a marked proximodistal and apicobasal activity gradient in both controls (hosts) and grafts. There is no difference due to transplantation.

Lactase/β-glucosidase and alkaline phosphatase (Fig. 2) were measured only in the jejunum, as there was no acitivity in the distal ileum. As shown for neutral α-glucosidase, the normal apicobasal gradient can be demonstrated in both hosts and grafts without any significant differences between the two groups.

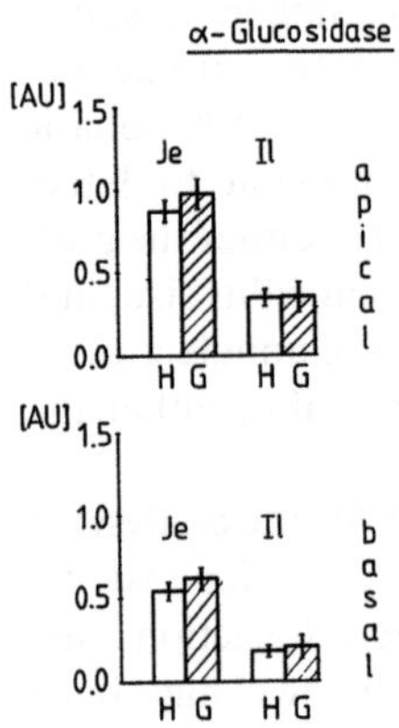

Fig. 1. In situ activities (mean ± SEM) of neutral α-glucosidase of grafts *(G)* and hosts *(H)*, measured at apical and basal villus positions in the jejunum *(Je)* and ileum *(Il)*. Activities are expressed as absorbance units *(AU)* at a wave length of 480 nm

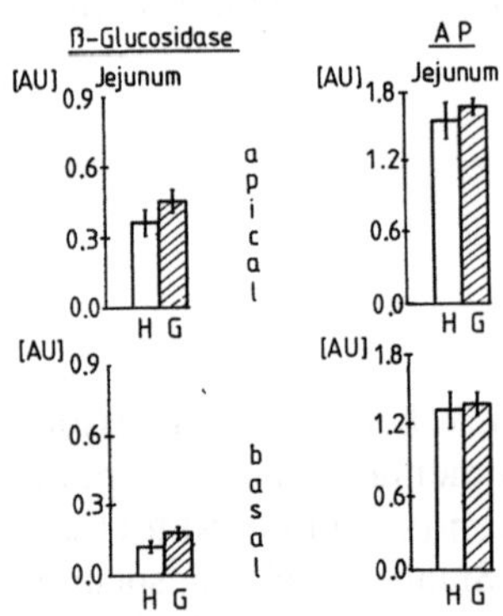

Fig. 2. In situ activities (mean ± SEM) of lactase/β-glucosidase (*left,* wave length = 640 nm) and unspecific alkaline phosphatase (*AP, right:* wave length = 550 nm), measured at apical and basal villus positions in the jejunum. *H,* hosts; *G,* grafts; *AU,* absorbance units

In summary, there are normal proximal-to-distal and apical-to-basal gradients of enzyme activities in the controls (hosts). There is no decrease in activity in the grafts due to the transplantation procedure when a comparison is made with the corresponding values in the hosts' small intestines. These findings support our initial hypothesis that syngeneic heterotopic small-bowel transplantation does not alter small-intestinal structure or function.

Nevertheless, one should keep in mind that slight mucosal atrophy can be detected in the grafts when using three-dimensional analysis of mucosal architecture after microdissection (see SCHRÖDER et al., this volume, "Glucose Absorption after Heterotopic Small-Bowel Transplantation"), a more sensitive parameter than the ratio villus to crypt of determined in histologic sections. As is known from previous studies of self-emptying small-intestinal blind loops (MENGE et al. 1970; GUTSCHMIDT et al. 1982) – an experimental design which in some repects is similar to the grafted intestine – when this type of atrophy is pronounced, it is accompanied by a decrease in brush border enzyme activity. The preservation of enzyme activity revealed in this study may be due to the fact that there is only small amount of mucosal atrophy, or it may be the result of mechanisms involved in the transplantation procedure that are still undefined.

References

Deltz E (1984) Immunreaktionen nach allogener Dünndarmtransplantation. Fortschr Med 102:760–762

Deltz E, Müller-Hermelink K, et al (1981) Development of graft-versus-host reaction in various target organs after small intestinal transplantation. Transplant Proc 13:1215–1216

Gutschmidt S (1981) "In situ" determination of apparent Km and V_{max} of brush border disaccharidases along the villi of normal jejunal biopsy specimens. A quantitative histochemical study. Histochemistry 71:451–462

Gutschmidt S, Kaul W, Riecken EO (1979) A quantitative histochemical technique for the characterisation of α-glucosidases in the brush-border membrane of rat jejunum. Histochemistry 63:81–101

Gutschmidt S, Lange U, Riecken EO (1981) Kinetic characterization of unspecific alkaline phosphatase at different villus sites of rat jejunum. A quantitative histochemical study. Histochemistry 69:189–202

Gutschmidt S, Menge H, Riecken EO (1982) The kinetic properties of neutral α-glucosidase (EC 3.2.1.20) in the atrophic mucosa of self-emptying blind loops of rat jejunum: A microdensitometric study at two different villus sites. Lab Invest 46:476–480

Menge H, Bloch K, Schaumlöffel E, Riecken EO (1970) Transportstudien, morphologische, morphometrische und histochemische Untersuchungen zum Verhalten der Dünndarmschleimhaut im operativ ausgeschalteten Jejunalabschnitt der Ratte. Z Ges Exp Med 153:74–90

Thiede A, Deltz E (1978) Morphological reaction in transplanted small intestines using immunogenetically defined rat strain combinations. Langenbeck's Arch Klin Chir 346:119–127

Patterns of Gastrointestinal Hormone Distribution After Small-Bowel Transplantation

J. H. Gebhardt, W. Ch. Preissner, E. Deltz, E. Kaiserling, and H. K. Müller-Hermelink

Small-bowel transplantation causes a severe disturbance of the integrity and physiologic function of the gut. It is therefore of great interest to investigate how orthotopic and heterotopic transplantation of the small bowel changes the distribution patterns of gastrointestinal (GI) hormone-producing cells, particularly if one considers that the gut has been called the largest endocrine organ of the body (Thompson and Marx 1984). The aim of our studies is to find out how the donor and recipient small bowel react to altered neural and luminal stimuli after heterotopic transplantation. Because the heterotopically transplanted small bowel is shunted off from intestinal passage and is completely deprived of neural and luminal stimuli, GI hormone distribution in the graft's mucosa and circular muscle layer might be altered. Furthermore, we shall attempt to investigate whether the heterotopic graft acts as a hormonal organ after having been brought into the orthotopic position and linked up with normal physiologic intestinal passage. In so doing, we shall attempt to observe how heterotopic small-bowel transplantation changes the distribution of GI hormone-producing cells and whether or not orthotopic small-bowel transplantation leads to normal function and distribution of GI hormone-producing cells.

Syngeneic heterotopic and orthotopic transplantation were performed as previously described by Preissner et al. (see "Microsurgical Techniques of Heterotopic and Orthotopic Small-Bowel Transplantation in the Rat," this volume). The heterotopically transplanted rats ($n = 5$) were killed on the 21st day postoperatively and samples of the donor and recipient small bowel preserved. Also on the 21st day postoperatively, another group of heterotopically transplanted rats ($n = 5$) underwent a second operation and the donor small bowel was brought into the orthotopic position. These rats were killed on the 40th day postoperatively. The gastrointestinal tracts of sham-operated rats were taken as a control ($n = 5$) for the other groups. Small samples bowel were collected, and the tissue was fixed in Bouin's solution and embedded in wax. Micron sections were immunostained using rabbit anti-rat antibodies. The hormone-producing cells of cholecystokinin (CCK), neurotensin (NT), glucagon-like immunoreactivity (GLI), and vasoactive intestinal peptide (VIP) were stained, and the bound antibodies were localized using the peroxidase-antiperoxidase method (Sternberger 1974) and counterstained with hematoxylin. The number of immunoreactive cells were measured by counting 20 high-power fields.

Results

The normal distribution of these cells is demonstrated in Table 1. CCK is normally present throughout jejunum and ileum, but the largest amount of CCK is in the jejunum. VIP fibers are found throughout the entire length of the gut, most prominently in the lamina propria in close contact with the circular muscle layer and around blood vessels. In contrast, the vast majority of NT cells are found in the ileum and to a lesser degree in the jejunum. GLI-containing cells are most numerous in the mucosa of the ileum and proximal colon (Bloom and Pollak 1981).

Table 1. Normal distribution of GI hormone-producing cells in the rat

Hormone	Location	
Cholecystokinin (CCK)	Jejunum	Ileum
Vasoactive intestinal peptide (VIP)	Jejunum	Ileum
Neurotensin (NT)	Ileum	Jejunum
Glucagon-like immunoreactivity (GLI)	Ileum	Colon

Heterotopic Transplantation

The initial results after evaluation of heterotopically transplanted small bowels indicate that there is no change in distribution, but that there is a quantitative change. After heterotopic transplantation (Fig. 1), recipient and donor organs differ most in CCK- and VIP-producing cells and fibers. The recipient organ shows normal amounts of these hormone-producing cells, but the missing neural and luminal stimuli seem to lead to a decrease in CCK and VIP throughout the donor organ. GLI seems to differ between recipient and donor ileum, but not jejunum. On the other hand, NT shows no change in distribution or quantity, and it looks as if it does not react to these manipulations of the small bowel. In accordance with these findings the donor organ shows atrophy of the villi and crypts which is similar to that described by Sandforth et al. (this volume).

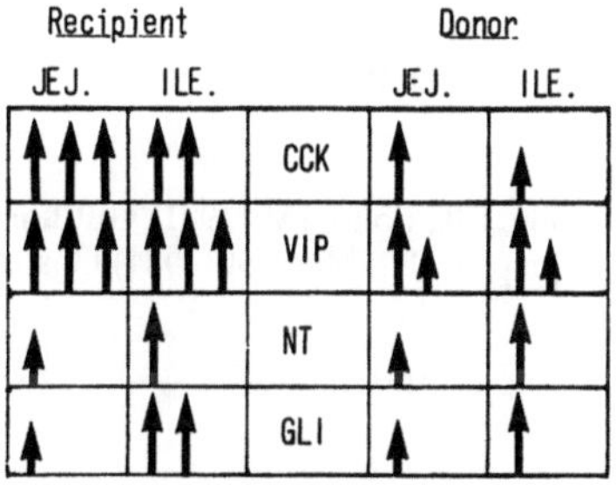

Fig. 1. Distribution of GI hormone-producing cells after heterotopic small-bowel transplantation. (21 days after transplantation) *JEJ*, jejunum; *ILE*, ileum

Orthotopic Transplantation

When the heterotopically transplanted small bowel is brought into normal position, thus establishing an orthotopic small-bowel replacement, the decrease in CCK- and VIP-containing cells can no longer be seen (Fig. 2). The hormone-producing cells are found in almost normal amounts and can be counted about twice as often as in the donor organ still in heterotopic position. NT, on the other hand, again shows normal distribution and quantity. GLI-producing cells do not differ in the jejunum, but are more frequently observed in the orthotopically transplanted ileum than in the ileum of the heterotopic graft. In accordance with these findings, no atrophy of the villi and crypts can be demonstrated after orthotopic transplantation.

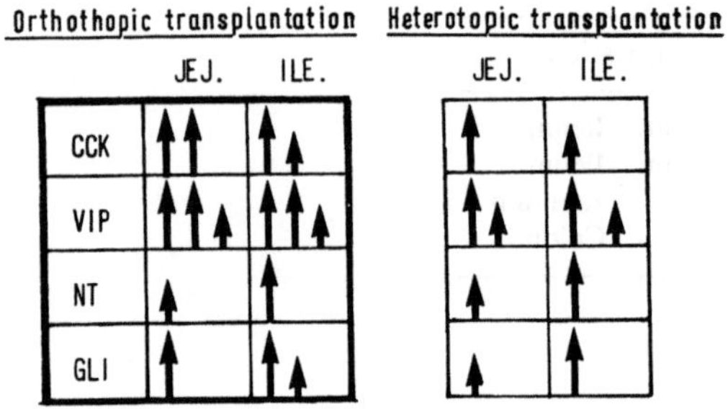

Fig. 2. Distribution of GI hormone-producing cells after orthotopic small-bowel transplantation and in heterotopically transplanted small bowel (donor, 40 days after transplantation). *JEJ,* jejenum; *ILE,* ileum

Discussion

Since these are still preliminary results, conclusions have to be carefully drawn. However, our findings support the view that the absence of challenge by chymus and other gastrointestinal stimuli (e.g., neural stimulation) may be responsible for the decrease in CCK and VIP in the donor organ still in heterotopic position. The increase in these hormone-producing cells after orthotopic small-bowel transplantation indicates that the transplanted gut is working again as a hormonal organ and might be linked to the neurohormonal axis. Intestinal adaptation after small-bowel transplantation therefore seems to be interdependent on the activity and distribution of gastrointestinal hormones.

References

Bloom SR, Polak JM (1981) Gut hormones, 2nd edn. Churchill Livingstone, Edinburgh
Thompson JC, Marx M (1984) Gastrointestinal hormones. Curr Probl Surg 21(6):

Session 3: Summary

H. MENGE

Session 3 was mainly devoted to the function of the transplanted small intestine and to correlations between functional and morphological findings in this situation. Four presentations dealt with these subjects. Two further communications were concerned with the distribution of gastrointestinal hormones in the grafts and with a method for short-term preservation of the explanted small intestine.

In the first presentation, COHEN et al. pointed out that, until now, only a very small number of dogs surviving over the long term after small-intestinal allotransplantation have been reported in the literature. As far as can be concluded from this small number of animals, preoperative body weight is not regained, and malabsorption of D-xylose and fat is observed. To explain these findings, the authors performed small-intestinal allotransplantations and brought the proximal jejunal ends and the distal ileal ends as stomas to the skin surface, while the remainder of the bowel was replaced in continuity. These isolated pouches – which with regard to rejection behave like small bowel in continuity – were subjected to combined morphological and functional studies (absorption of D-xylose and cyclosporine). A good correlation was observed between morphological alterations (arising from the rejection of the grafts) and functional impairments. These results help to explain the above-mentioned malabsorption after allotransplantation of the small bowel. Another interesting finding of the authors' investigation is the fact that cyclosporine was mainly absorbed by the lymphatic system.

Three presentations dealt with morphometric and/or functional findings after small-bowel transplantation in syngeneic rats. SCHROEDER et al. demonstrated that heterotopically transplanted small bowel exhibits a significant reduction in villus height (both in jejunum and ileum) and a less pronounced decrease in crypt length compared with the recipients' own intestines. These findings were paralleled by a decrease in D-glucose and water absorption (measured by using a perfusion system in vivo). SANDFORTH et al. observed that, in this situation, several enzyme activities (neutral alpha-glucosidase, lactase/beta-glucosidase, alkaline phosphatase) remained unchanged, as measured by quantitative histochemical techniques. Thus, heterotopic grafts in syngeneic rats display mucosal atrophy with a concomitant decrease in D-glucose and water absorption. Though these findings are statistically significant, the mucosal atrophy observed is only of moderate extent when compared with intestinal atrophy observed in other conditions. SEIFERT and DELTZ reported that orthotopically transplanted small intestines in syngeneic long-term surviving rats display no alterations in protein and maltose absorption (measured by indirect techniques) when compared with control animals with intact small bowels.

In the following communication, GEBHARDT et al. presented their preliminary results concerning the distribution of gastrointestinal hormone-producing cells in heterotopically and orthotopically transplanted small intestines (syngeneic rats). While orthotopically transplanted grafts do not show any differences when compared with the recipient's organs, heterotopically transplanted small bowels exhibit a decrease in CCK- and VIP (jejunum and ileum)-producing cells and in cells containing glucagon-like immunoreactivity (ileum) (neurotensin-producing cells were unchanged). Thus, it seems that the absence of luminal stimuli leads to a nonuniform reduction of hormone-producing cells in heterotopically transplanted small intestines. SCHRAUT et al. studied the method of intravascular flushing with cold Collins' solution followed by cold storage (4°C) for the short-term preservation of explanted small intestine (heterotopic and orthotopic isografts in rats). The authors were able to demonstrate that by using this technique, preservation for up to 6 h is possible, but that preservation for up to 12 h is not dependable.

Reference

Menge H, Bloch R, Schaumlöffel E, Riecken EO (1970) Transportstudien, morphologische, morphometrische und histochemische Untersuchungen zum Verhalten der Dünndarmschleimhaut im operativ ausgeschalteten Jejunalsegment der Ratte. Z Ges Exp Med 153:74–90

Session 4
Immunology

Early Intestinal Lesions of Graft-vs-Host Reaction and Allograft Rejection in Rodents, Identified by Quantitative Histological Techniques

A. FERGUSON and A. G. CUMMINS

Introduction

In our investigations of intestinal mucosal lymphocytes, we have used models of T-cell–mediated, delayed-type hypersensitivity (DTH) reactions in the small intestinal mucosa of rodents. Secondary effects in addition to DTH have been reduced by transplanting sterile foetal tissue and by avoiding irradiation in animals with graft-vs-host reaction (GvHR). The evolution of the pathology of the reactions has been examined in various ways, using quantitative techniques whenever possible. The epithelium has been studied by measuring villi, crypts, crypt cell production rate (CCPR) by a stathmokinetic technique, cell migration rate and the number of crypts associated with each villus. Enterocytes have been examined by electron microscopy, assays of brush border enzymes and measurements of labelled amino acid uptake. In the case of lymphoid cells, intra-epithelial lymphocytes (IEL) have been counted in all experiments, work on mast cells is described in a separate paper (see A. FERGUSON, et al., this volume), and we are currently investigating plasma cells and IgA in these models.

Rejection of Small-Intestinal Allografts

The work referred to here was done some years ago, using foetal rodent intestine transplanted heterotopically under the kidney capsule (FERGUSON and PARROTT 1973; MACDONALD and FERGUSON 1976, 1977). Such grafts are sterile and have not been exposed to dietary or other antigens. Because the donor tissue is collected before seeding of the Peyer's patches and mucosa with lymphoid cells, the lymphoid cells of established grafts are of host and the stroma and epithelium of donor origin. Isografts of mouse small intestine have short villi and crypts, and the CCPR is on the order of two cells per crypt per hour. Mucosal lymphocytes and plasma cells appear in the 3rd week after implantation.

The earliest sign of rejection noted in allografts of mouse small intestine was a lymphocyte infiltrate in the graft lamina propria, followed a day or two later by the appearance of IEL. In the rejecting allografts, the crypts were not only longer, but by the 3rd day after transplantation, the CCPR was fourfold greater than in isografts and the difference between isografts and allografts was statistically significant on days 7 and 9. Lengthening of crypts preceded villus flattening by several days.

Graft-vs-Host Reaction

In most strain combinations of mice and rats, GvHR can be measured as the ratio of spleen weight per unit body weight in experimental and control animals (SIMONSEN 1962). We use semiallogeneic chimaeras in which parental strain lymphocytes are infused into an F_1 hybrid host. A preliminary study of neonates showed a reduction in villus height from day 7 of the GvHR, with the CCPR increased to above that of controls from the 5th day. GvHR had no effect on the ratio of the numbers of crypts to villi, and epithelial cell height in histological sections was normal in rejecting allografts (MACDONALD and FERGUSON 1976, 1977).

When GvHR is induced in young (aged 5 days) mice of the CBAxBALB/c strain combination, the clinical effects are mild, with normal weight gain and no diarrhoea. By using the spleen index as a measure of GvHR, highly significant correlations were obtained between crypt length, CCPR, and the magnitude of the GvHR as measured by spleen index, even though there was no villus atrophy. The striking rise in CCPR is shown in Fig. 1. IEL counts rose significantly above those of controls within 24 h of induction of the GvHR and significantly correlated with the spleen index during the proliferative phase of the reaction (MOWAT and FERGUSON 1982) (Fig. 2). Counts of lamina propria cells have not been performed. However, a late increase in mucosal mast cell numbers was noted, and the absence of both plasma cells and polymorphonuclear leucocytes was a feature of all of the experiments described above.

Since villus atrophy often occurs in allograft rejection or GvHR, it would be anticipated that deficiencies of enterocyte enzymes and malabsorption would parallel the histological changes described above. We have found that uptake of isotope-labelled phenylalanine by jejunum is reduced in neonatal mice with GvHR and villus

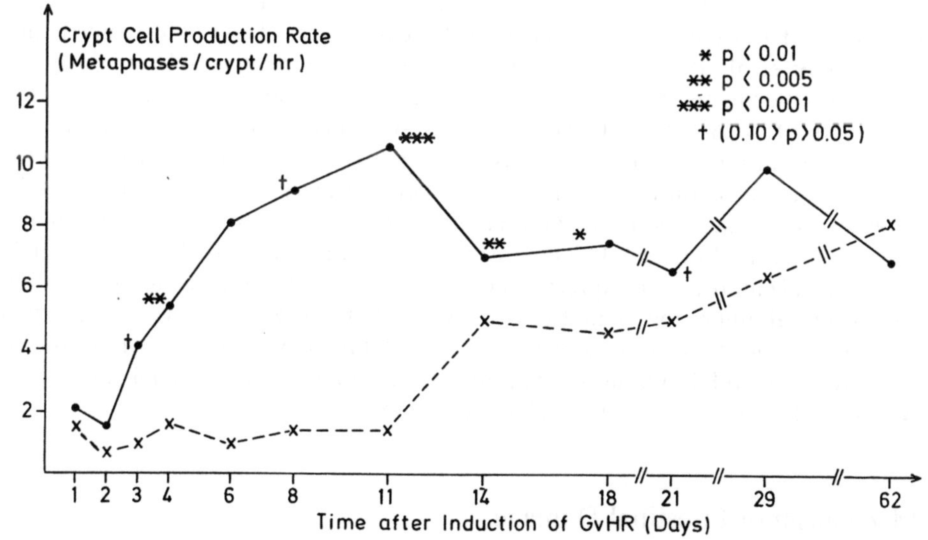

Fig. 1. CCPR in neonatal mice with GvHR. ●-●- GvHR; x-- controls. For each experimental group, the result is expressed as a single point, the value for the slope of the regression line of metaphases per crypt against time after colchicine injection

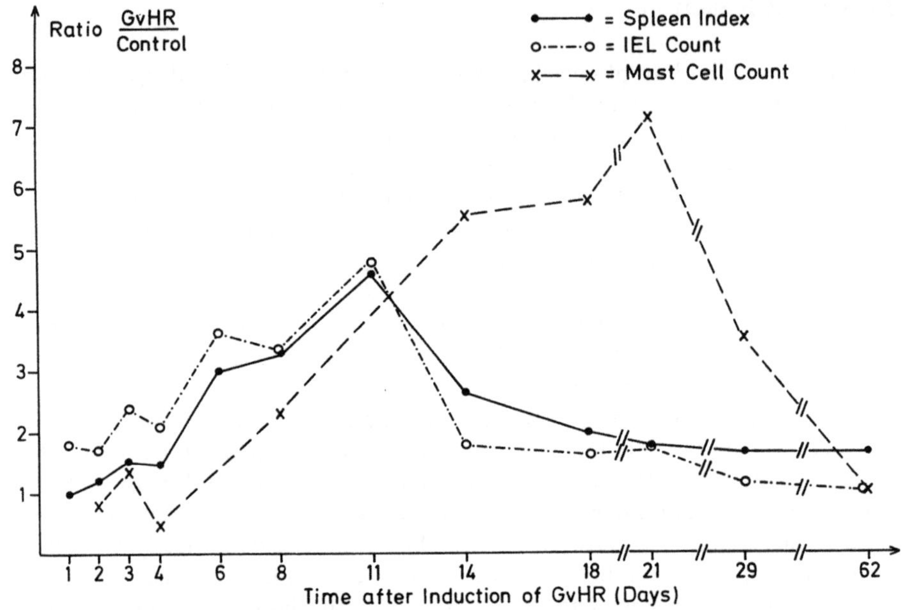

Fig. 2. Correlation of IEL and mast cell counts with the spleen index throughout the course of the GvHR in neonatal mice. The IEL count closely follows the spleen index, whereas the rise in mast cell count is delayed and prolonged

flattening, but not in those animals with crypt hyperplasia and normal villi (ZIEGLER and FERGUSON, unpublished).

We have also examined in some detail the developmental profiles for enterocyte expression of disaccharidase activity during the early stages of GvHR in neonatal mice (FERGUSON et al. 1985). In these animals, significant relative splenomegaly was present on the 5th day after injection of parental strain spleen cells. From this time, the crypts of GvHR animals were significantly longer than those of litter mate controls. From the 6th day, there was significantly lower lactase activity in GvHR animals, but reduction in villus length was delayed until day 8. The rate at which enterocytes migrated along the villi, as measured by the incorporation of tritiated thymidine, showed a threefold increase in GvHR mice (days 7–8). The time taken by an individual enterocyte to express lactase activity at maximal rate decreased by about 10 h when cell migration along the villi was rapid, but these adaptive changes were nevertheless insufficient to prevent an overall fall in net lactase synthesis. We conclude that GvHR initiates a pattern of development in neonatal enterocytes similar to that which occurs normally at weaning.

Mechanism of Intestinal Damage

Rejection of mouse intestine is unrelated to the presence of antigraft cytotoxic antibodies (ELVES and FERGUSON 1975), and antihost cytotoxic T cells were not detected among IEL populations during the GvHR in mice (BORLAND et al. 1983). On the other hand, evidence favouring damage via lymphokines is provided by sophisticated experiments in which GvHR was induced in mice bearing heterotopically transplanted isografts of small bowel (ELSON et al. 1977; MOWAT and FERGUSON 1981). Histopathological features of GvHR were found in parental strain grafts of foetal gut in F_1-hybrid animals. The host mice had GvHR induced by injection of the same parental strain spleen cells. Thus, changes in the crypts and IEL infiltration of the parental strain grafts were considered to be the effects of mediators released by activated donor T cells as they recirculated in the gut graft lamina propria, where they would have encountered host-derived lymphocytes and macrophages. MOWAT et al. further clarified the nature of the T cell effect in intestinal GvHR in unirradiated mice by examining the phenotype of the T cells responsible (A. Mc. I. MOWAT, A. BORLAND, D. M. V. PARROTT, The delayed type hypersensitivity reaction in the intestinal mucosa of mice undergoing a graft-versus-host reaction is due to I. A. restricted Lyt1+ cells, to be published). These experiments showed that the mucosal pathology characteristic of GvHR is due to Lyt1+ T cells restricted by antigens coded by the IA region of the major histocompatibility complex (MHC). Thus, the intestinal pathology of GvHR is produced by class 2 MHC-restricted DTH effector T cells.

GvHR in Irradiated Mice

We have recently completed an experiment which illustrates the greatly accentuated effects on the intestinal mucosa when mice are irradiated prior to induction of GvHR. Adult BDF_1 mice were used half of which were irradiated with 450 rad; groups of mice had GvHR induced either by IP injection of 10^7 parental spleen cells or, as controls, by BDF_1 spleen cells. Results for the spleen index and villus and crypt measurements are summarised in Table 1. Unirradiated mice had significant splenomegaly, but at

Table 1. Features of GvHR in adult mice

Group	Spleen index	Villus length (μm)	Crypt length (μm)	CCPR (cells/h)
Untreated		769	106	10.8
GvHR	2.34	720	112	12.2
Irradiated		712	107	9.9
Irradiated/GvHR	0.61[a]	478	282	34.0

[a] Host response, impaired after irradiation, is an important component of the splenomegaly.

the time studied, mucosal architecture was normal; on the other hand, the irradiated mice with GvHR had villus atrophy and striking crypt hyperplasia. Several factors are likely to have contributed to the enhanced mucosal damage associated with irradiation, including bacterial colonisation of the irradiated intestine, irradiation effects on the enterocytes and stem cells, as well as the absence of an effective host lymphocyte response.

Conclusions

The early manifestations of allograft rejection and GvHR in mouse small intestine include the appearance of lamina propria lymphocytes and, within a day, IEL. Crypt hyperplasia also appears followed by changes in the expression of brush border enzymes. In our GvHR experiments, villus atrophy has been a late and inconsistent feature. Crypt hyperplasia *is not* merely a repair response to villus or enterocyte damage, and the mechanism of crypt hyperplasia is likely to be via soluble factors secreted by activated T_{DTH} lymphocytes.

References

Borland A, Mowat AMcI, Parrott DMV (1983) Augmentation of intestinal and peripheral natural killer cell activity during the graft-versus-host reaction in mice. Transplantation 36:513–519

Elson CO, Reilly RW, Rosenberg IH (1977) Small intestinal injury in the graft versus host reaction: an innocent bystander phenomenon. Gastroenterology 72:886–889

Elves MW, Ferguson A (1975) The humoral immune response to allografts of foetal small intestine in mice. Br J Exp Pathol 56:454–458

Ferguson A, Parrott DMV (1973) Histopathology and time-course of rejection of allografts of mouse small intestine. Transplantation 15:546–554

Ferguson A, Lund EK, Pickering MG, Smith MW (1985) Lymphocyte-induced changes in disaccharidase expression by neonatal mouse enterocytes. J Physiol 364:84P

MacDonald TT, Ferguson A (1976) Hypersensitivity reactions in the small intestine. 2. Effects of allograft rejection on mucosal architecture and lymphoid cell infiltrate. Gut 17:81–91

MacDonald TT, Ferguson A (1977) Hypersensitivity reactions in the small intestine. 3. The effects of allograft rejection and of graft-versus-host disease on epithelial cell kinetics. Cell Tissue Kinet 10:301–312

Mowat AMcI, Ferguson A (1981) Hypersensitivity reactions in the small intestine. 6. Pathogenesis of the graft-versus-host reaction in the smal intestinal mucosa. Transplantation 32:238–243

Mowat AMcI, Ferguson A (1982) Intraepithelial lymphocyte count and crypt hyperplasia measure the mucosal component of the graft-versus-host reaction in mouse small intestine. Gastroenterology 83:417–423

Simonsen M (1962) Graft versus host reactions: Their natural history, and applicability as tools of research. Prog Allergy 6:349–367

*Mucosal Mast Cells in Experimental Graft-vs-Host Reaction**

A. FERGUSON, A. G. CUMMINS, G. H. MUNRO, and S. GIBSON

Heterogeneity of Mast Cells

All mast cells have large, electron-dense cytoplasmic granules made up of heparin (or related glycosaminoglycans) and protein. Mast cells vary in their morphology, histochemistry, sensitivity to fixatives and pharmacological properties. This heterogeneity has been studied in detail in the rat, and two major sub-populations have been defined in this species. Connective tissue mast cells (CTMC) are found in skin, muscle and the peritoneal cavity, and mucosal mast cells (MMC) predominate in the mucosa of the gut (ENERBAK 1981). The discovery of distinct proteases in rat mast cells has allowed clear differentiation between the two major subsets. Rat mast cell protease 1 (RMCPI) is present in CTMC; rat mast cell protease 2 (RMCPII) is found in MMC (WOODBURY et al. 1978).

MMC in Mice with Graft-vs-Host Reaction

In our detailed study of the evolution of graft-vs-host reaction (GvHR) in neonatal mice (MOWAT and FERGUSON 1982; see also FERGUSON and CUMMINS, this volume), we found an increase in MMC counts, but this occurred late in the evolution of GvHR. MMC counts remained high after other features such as crypt hyperplasia and intra-epithelial lymphocyte (IEL) count had dropped towards normal (see FERGUSON and CUMMINS, this volume, Fig. 2). In order to examine in more detail the relevance of MMC in GvHR, it has been necessary to set up similar experiments in the rat.

GvHR in Adult Rats

GvHR was induced in adult F_1 PVGRTI$^{u/c}$ rats by IP injection of 10^8 parental strain spleen cells. There were no clinical signs of graft-vs-host disease, but the GvHR was confirmed by measurements of relative spleen weight. Details of the spleen index (GvHR vs controls) and tissue RMCPII content are given in Table 1. It is evident that

* This work has been supported by grants from the Wellcome Trust and Fisons Pharmaceuticals.

the tissue content of RMCPII rose as GvHR evolved, with the values on days 10, 14 and 21 all being significantly higher than in controls.

Table 1. Tissue levels of RMCPII in rats with GvHR

Group	Spleen index	Tissue RMCPII (μg/g tissue)
Control	—	516 ± 56
Day 10	1.99	735 ± 152
Day 14	1.64	1035 ± 240
Day 21	1.84	1230 ± 345

A further experiment was conducted using recipients of the DAxPVG^c F_1 strain given DA strain spleen cells. Some of the rats were treated with cyclosporine A (25 mg/kg daily) subcutaneously on day −1, day 0 and day 1 and on alternate days until day 13 of GvHR. Results of spleen index, MMC counts in villi and crypts and RMCPII assays are given in Table 2. GvHR, as measured by the spleen index, was prevented in cyclosporine A-treated rats. Counts of MMC were high in the GvHR animals and lower in the cyclosporine A-treated GvHR group. RMCPII content of the tissues parallelled MMC counts as shown.

Table 2. MMC counts and tissue RMCPII in rats with GvHR

Group	Spleen index	MMC per mm²		Tissue RMCPII
		villi	pericrypt	(μg/g tissue)
Control	—	91.5	142.5	470
GvHR	1.56	185.2	218.6	620
CsA	—	93.6	142.7	430
GvHR/CsA	1.09	125.5	184.5	520

Day 14 of GvHR; counts on four rats per group
CsA, cyclosporine A

Conclusions

These experiments in the rat confirm our observations in the mouse that the number of mast cells in the intestinal mucosa increases during GvHR. Furthermore, the increased tissue content of RMCPII provides evidence that this expansion involves MMC. Assaying tissue RMCPII provides an easy method for quantitation of MMC in the rat. We have preliminary data on serum levels of RMCPII which suggest that the amount of protease in the serum reflects the number and state of activation of MMC.

References

Enerback L (1981) The gut mucosal mast cell. Monogr Allergy 17:222–232

Mowat AMcI, Ferguson A (1982) Intraepithelial lymphocyte count and crypt hyperplasia measure the mucosal component of the graft-versus-host reaction in mouse small intestine. Gastroenterology 83:417–423

Woodbury RG, Gruzenski GM, Lagunoff D (1978) Immunofluorescent localization of a serine protease in rat small intestine. Proc Natl Acad Sci USA 77:2785–2789

*Clinicopathologic Differentiation of Rejection and Graft-vs-Host Disease Following Small-Bowel Transplantation**

W. H. SCHRAUT and K. K. W. LEE

Introduction

Graft-v-host (GvH) reactions or GvH disease may be a complicating event after clinical small-bowel transplantation for two main reasions. Firstly, possibly as a result of malnutrition, the immune system of the recipient of a small-bowel allograft may be primarily compromised. Secondly, as a result of immunosuppressive therapy, the immunocompetence of the recipient might bei impaired more severely than that of the lymphoid tissues which are transferred with the allogeneic graft. Experimental evidence for the latter possibility is available in a report by KIRKMAN et al. (1984), who found that, in rats, cyclosporine A treatment limited to 1 week suppressed the rejection of small-bowel allografts, but did not prevent the occurrence of GvH disease in the parent → F_1-hybrid combination. Thus, it is conceivable that the immunocompetent allogeneic lymphocytes within the graft could overcome the immune resistance of the host and induce GvH disease.

Other studies in the rat model of small-bowel transplantation indicated that GvH disease is not a complicating factor of cyclosporine therapy (LEE and SCHRAUT 1986), and strong evidence has been obtained from clinical bone marrow transplantation that GvH disease can be controlled by cyclosporine A therapy (POWELS et al. 1980). However, the possibility that GvH disease will become a complicating factor of small-bowel transplantation cannot be discounted completely. Therefore, methods have to be devised that will allow a differentiation between a rejection reaction and GvH disease in small-bowel transplantation, as both situations may arise at the same time. In preparation for developing such a differential-diagnostic strategy, we undertook a comparison of the clinical and histopathologic course of these two immunologic reactions. Small-bowel transplantation in the rat, with a parental-strain allograft transferred into an F_1-hybrid recipient or vice versa, provides an ideal model for the study of the changes that occur in GvH disease and during the rejection of small-bowel allografts.

* Supported by The National Institutes of Arthritis, Metabolism, and Digestive Diseases (Grant No. AM27332).

Materials and Methods

The rat models of heterotopic (accessory) and of orthotopic small-bowel transplantation were used. The transplantation techniques were described previously (SCHRAUT et al. 1983; LEE and SCHRAUT, "Small-Bowel Transplantation in the Rat: Graft Survival with Heterotopic vs Orthotopic Position," this volume). The rats were adult males, weighing from 200 to 300 g, of the inbred Lewis (LEW) and Lewis x Brown-Norway hybrid (LBN-F_1) strains (Table 1). Details on the course of investigation are listed as follows:

	n
1) LEW → LBN-F_1 (GvH disease)	
a) Accessory grafts	
Followed to death	13
Sacrificed for study	30
b) Orthotopic grafts	
Followed to death	6
2) LBN-F_1 → LEW (rejection reaction)	
a) Accessory grafts	
Followed to death	25
Sacrificed for study	12
b) Orthotopic grafts	
Followed to death	14
Sacrificed	12

For the study of GvH disease, LEW rats were the donors of the small-intestinal grafts, and LBN-F_1 rats were the recipients ($N = 49$; heterotopic position, $n = 43$; orthotopic position, $n = 6$). With this combination, since the recipient is genetically incapable of rejecting the parental-strain graft, an uninhibited GvH reaction is assured. In this group, 19 rats (13 with accessory and 6 with orthotopic grafts) were followed until they died of GvH disease. The remaining 30 rats with accessory grafts were killed on various days after transplantation.

For the study of the rejection reaction, LBN-F_1 rats were the donors of the small-intestinal graft and LEW rats the recipients ($N = 63$; heterotopic position, $n = 37$; orthotopic position, $n = 26$). With this combination, an uninhibited rejection is guaranteed. In this group, 39 rats were followed until they died from rejection, and the other 24 rats were killed on various days after transplantation.

Pathologic Evaluation

At time of killing or at autopsy after death from GvH disease or rejection, the animals' spleen weights (relative to body weight) were determined, and organ specimens (intestinal allograft, recipient's own small bowel, liver, spleen, lymph nodes, and skin) were obtained and processed for light-microscopic examination.

Results

GvH Disease

Clinical Course

The first signs of GvH disease appeared between the 8th and 11th days and consisted of redness and swelling of the ears, snout, paws, and periocular region. These skin changes progressed over the following days, with scaling and hair loss and were paralleled by diarrhea and weight loss, both of which became precipitous in the days before death (Fig. 1). In the terminal stage, the rats were emaciated and listless and sat hunched on their hind legs. This course was the same in animals with orthotopic allografts and in those with accessory allografts. Death of the recipient as a result of GvH disease occurred after 14.4 ± 2.9 days for heterotopic grafts and after 14.0 ± 0.7 days for orthotopic grafts.

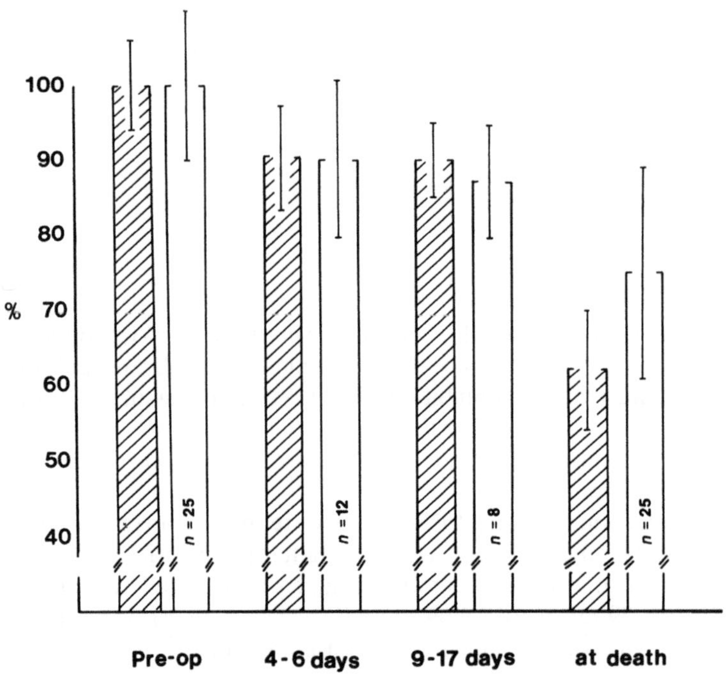

Fig. 1. Body weight in the course of fatal GvH disease and allograft rejection after small-bowel transplantation. In both situations, there is a progressive weight loss, which becomes precipitous just before death. □, GvH disease; □, rejection

Autopsy Findings

In rats that died of GvH disease, marked enlargement of all lymphoid tissues was a consistent finding. The host's ileum and colon always had a thinned wall and were filled with yellow, frothy material. All animals showed evidence of peritonitis. Rats

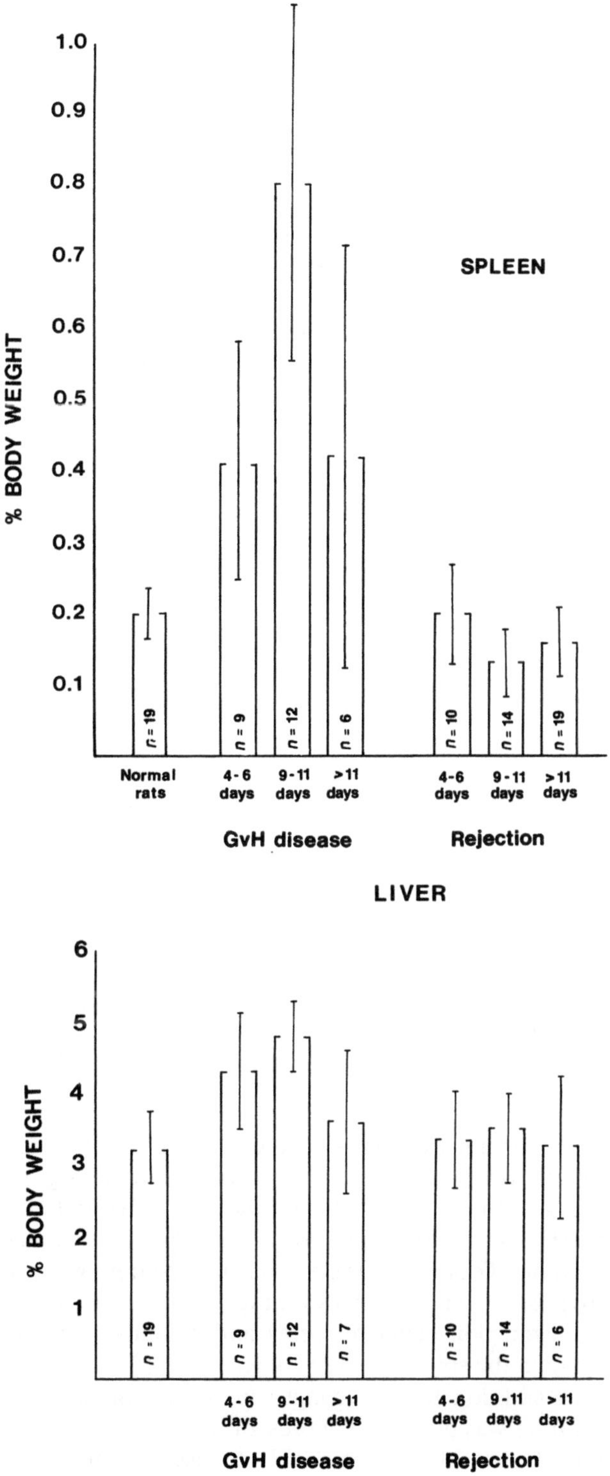

Fig. 2. During GvH disease, the spleen weight increases considerably over preoperative normal levels until the 11th day. Splenomegaly is not a feature of allograft rejection. At death, the spleen weight is low in both groups compared with prior days, probably an agonal change. The relative liver weight increases temporarily with the development of GvH disease, probably because of involvement of the reticuloendothelial system. Rejection is not accompanied by hepatomegaly

that were killed on the 3rd–9th postoperative day did not disclose any organ abnormalities except for splenomegaly (Fig. 2) and lymph node enlargement in both the graft and the host, which became evident by the 5th postoperative day. Macroscopic evidence of enteritis (serosal hyperemia and dilatation of the distal ileum) was found in the animals killed on the 11th postoperative day.

Histopathologic Findings

Rats that died of GvH disease had enteritis (reduced villous height, sloughing of the villi tips, polymorphonuclear cell infiltration of mucosa and submucosa) which involved their own small bowel and colon. Histologic evidence of this enteritis arose between the 10th and 14th postoperative days (Fig. 3A). The LEW allograft, in both the orthotopic and the heterotopic position, appeared normal on microscopic inspection (Fig. 3B).

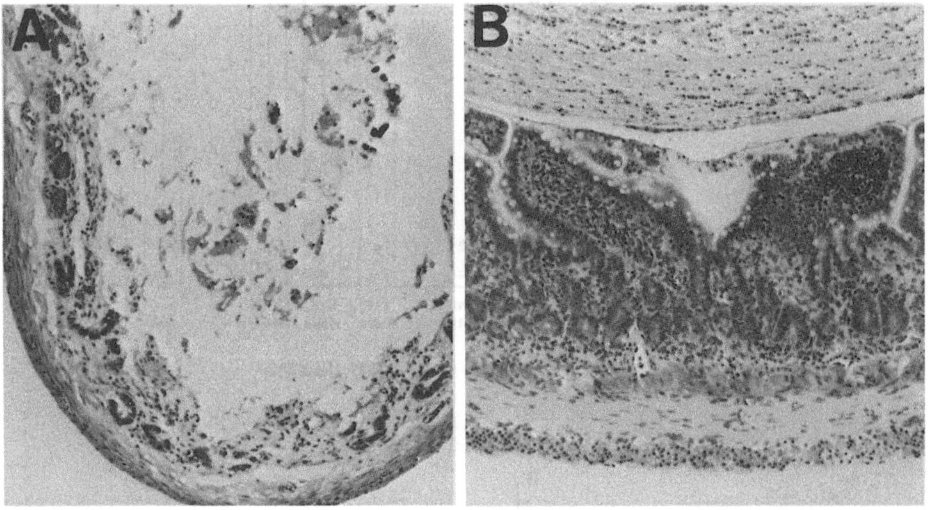

Fig. 3A, B. **A** Severe enteritis (thinned bowel wall, sloughing of villi tips, and cellular infiltration) is seen in the LBN-F_1 host's own small intestine. **B** In the LEW allograft, the histologic appearance is unchanged. (Sections for **A** and **B** were taken on the 14th postoperative day; × 100)

The lymphatic tissues of the LEW grafts (Peyer's patches, mesenteric lymph nodes), as well as those of the host, underwent progressive lymphoid depletion which began on the 5th postoperative day (Fig. 4B). Initially, this depletion was accompanied by scattered proliferation of histiocytoid cells and immunoblasts in the paracortical areas. These cellular elements disappeared over the following days, giving way to progressive lymphopenia with the disappearance of the germinal centers and loss of the distinction between cortex and medulla (Fig. 4C). These same changes were found in the spleen of the recipient (Fig. 5).

In addition to the changes in the lymphoid tissues, a periportal lymphocytic infiltrate was occasionally present in the livers of the rats dying of GvH disease. In animals with fulminant GvH disease, histologic examination showed that the

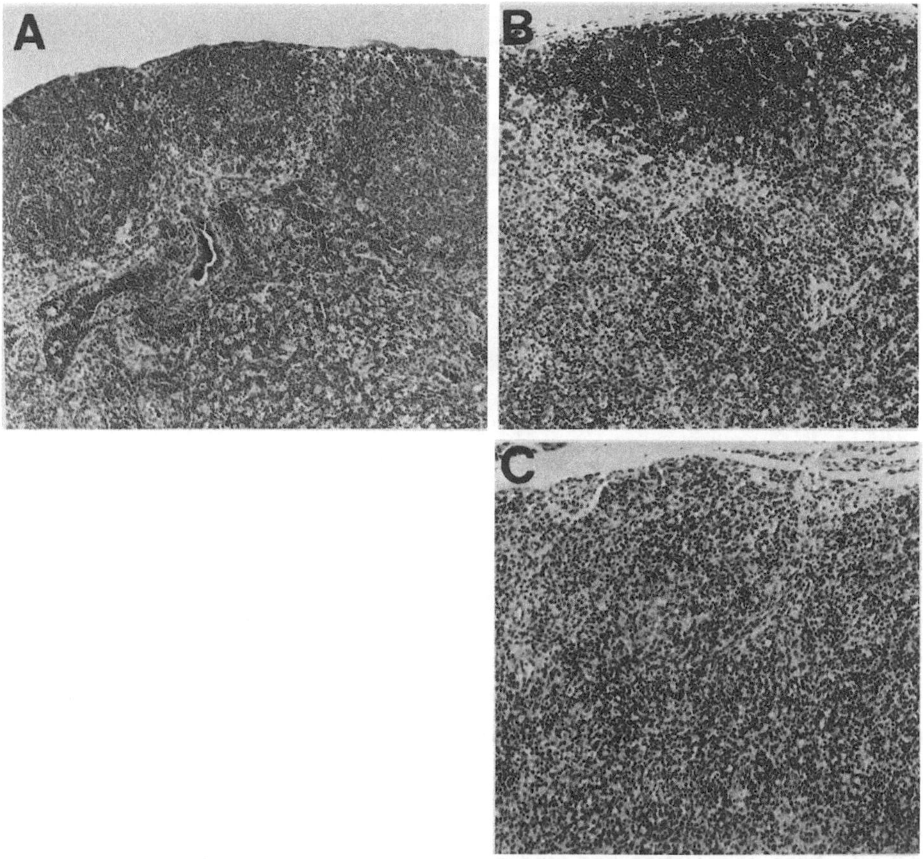

Fig. 4A–C. A Normal rat lymph node. **B** Mesenteric lymph node obtained from the LEW graft 5 days after transplantation shows mild lymphopenia and preserved nodal architecture. **C** Extensive lymphopenia with loss of germinal centers and nodal architecture ("empty" lymph node) characterizes this mesenteric node from a LEW graft (14th postoperative day; × 100)

epidermis was thickened, and in some cases the subcutaneous tissues were infiltrated by mononuclear cells.

Rejection of Small-Bowel Allografts

Clinical Course

The initial signs of allograft rejection evolved on the 7th–8th postoperative day and consisted of diarrhea, progressive inanition, and a hunched posture of the recipient. This course, similar to that of GvH disease, continued and was accompanied by progressive weight loss, culminating in the recipient's death (Fig. 1). The mean survival time of the rats with accessory allografts ($n = 25$) was 11.4 ± 0.4 days and that of the rats with orthotopic allografts ($n = 14$) was 12.4 ± 1.7 days.

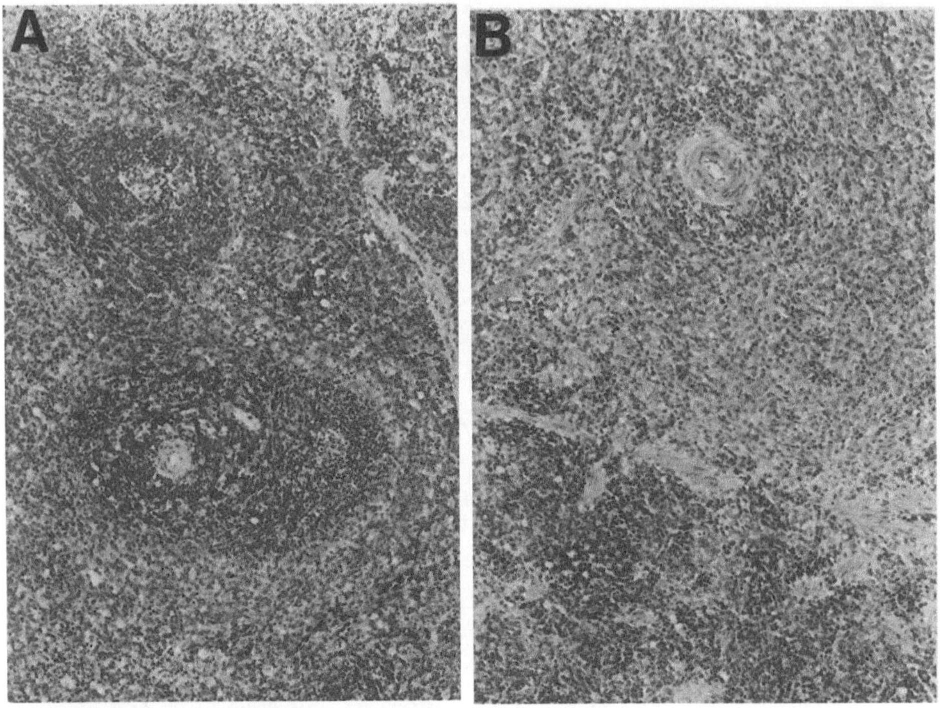

Fig. 5A, B. **A** Normal spleen. **B** Lymphogenic spleen from an LBN-F_1 host dying of GvH disease

Autopsy Findings

All rats dying of rejection had evidence of peritonitis. The allograft was severely thinned, and areas of necrosis and perforation were noted. Rats with orthotopic allografts had intact, patent intestinal anastomoses. The relative spleen weights were normal, except for an agonal reduction in the rats dying of rejection. The mesenteric lymph nodes of the allografts were always enlarged and discolored, whereas the lymphatic tissues of the recipients were unremarkable. Rats that were killed at various intervals after transplantation showed evidence of allograft rejection (patchy, serosal erythema; intestinal distention) and enlargement of the graft's mesenteric lymph nodes. The host's tissues were always unremarkable. Instead of splenomegaly, there was a slight decrease in the relative spleen weight. The liver weight remained stable (Fig. 2).

Histopathologic Findings

Allografts which were followed to complete rejection, a course associated with the host's death, showed mucosal sloughing, polymorphonuclear infiltration, and thinning of the bowel wall as described previously (see LEE and SCHRAUT, "Small-Bowel Transplantation in the Rat: Graft Survival with Heterotopic vs Orthotopic Position," this volume). The lymphatic tissues of the allograft underwent a progressive course of lymphopenia and loss of normal architecture. These changes began on the 7th–9th postoperative day and followed a progressive course terminating in complete

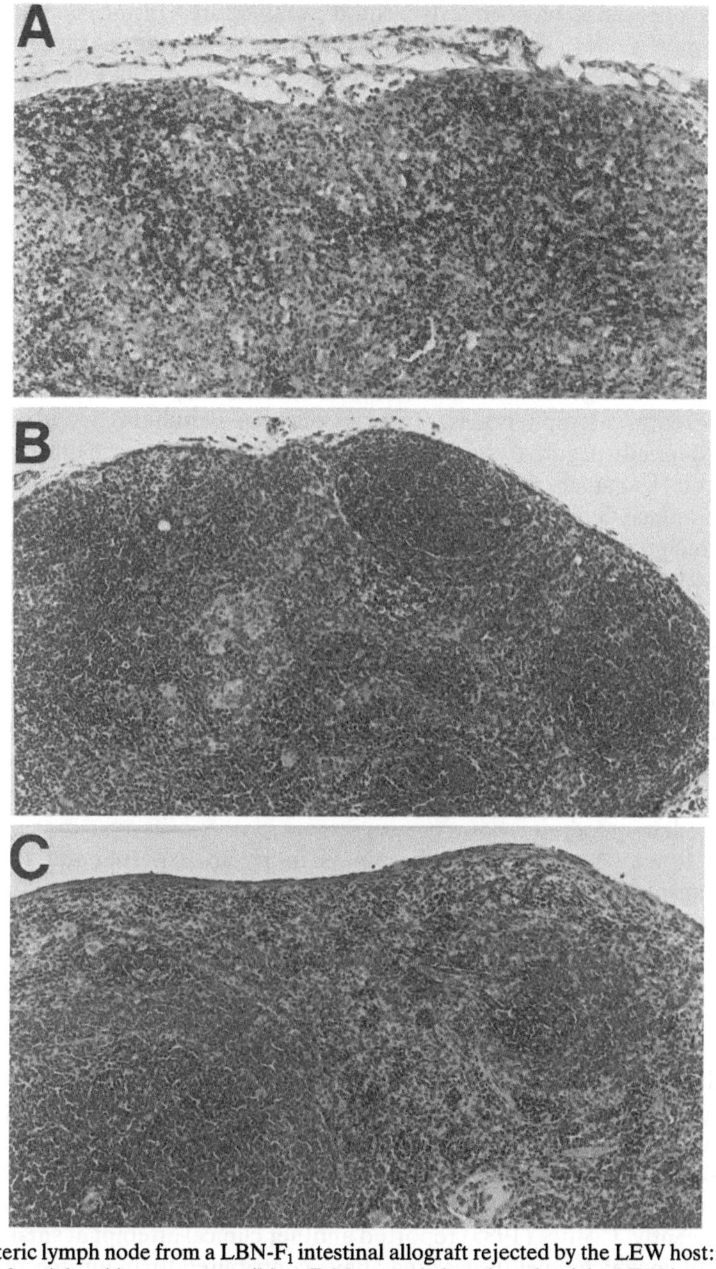

Fig. 6 A–C. A Mesenteric lymph node from a LBN-F_1 intestinal allograft rejected by the LEW host: lymphopenia and loss of nodal architecture are striking. **B** Mesenteric lymph node of the LEW host: normal cellularity and enlarged lymph follicles are evident. **C** Spleen of the LEW recipient of a LBN-F_1 intestinal allograft: normal architecture with prominent lymph follicles is apparent. (× 100)

disappearance of normal lymphoid architecture (Fig. 6A). The lymphatic tissues (lymph nodes, spleen) of the LEW host appeared normal or showed areas of stimulation, as indicated by enlarged lymph follicles that were replete with lymphocytes and immunoblasts (Fig. 6B, C).

The liver, pancreas, kidneys, native bowel, and skin of the rats succumbing to the rejection process were histologically normal.

Discussion

The small-bowel allograft is unique among vascularized organ allografts in that it includes large amounts of lymphoid tissue in the form of Peyer's patches and mesenteric lymph nodes. The presence of lymphoid tissue in the graft has two potentially negative consequences. Firstly, it may increase the immunogenicity of the graft (LAFFERTY 1980), and secondly, alloreactive cells in the graft have the potential to induce GvH disease. This potential has been clearly documented in inbred rats in which parental grafts were transplanted into the F_1-hybrid recipient (MONCHIK and RUSSELL 1971; DELTZ et al. 1981; LEE and SCHRAUT 1985). However, these allografts have the capability of inducing GvH disease because they reside in recipients unable to reject the graft; consequently, these studies tend to overemphasize the potential role of GvH disease in clinical practice. The studies on GvH disease in the dog model of small-bowel transplantation came to varied results for unexplained reasons; LILLEHEI et al (1959) and COHEN et al. (1976) found that GvH disease was an inevitable consequence of transplantation of the entire small bowel, whereas RESNICK et al. (1982) reported that rejection of the bowel allograft predominated.

It may be that GvH disease is more an experimental facet of small-bowel transplantation than a clinical reality. When fully allogeneic donor-recipient combinations were studied in the rat model (KORT et al. 1973; SCHRAUT et al. 1985), rejection rather than GvH disease was prevalent. In the clinical situation with fully allogeneic donor-recipient pairs, one would also anticipate that the host would be capable of reacting against the graft; in addition, of course, the host would receive immunosuppressive therapy, which would also interfere with the expression of GvH disease. To what degree, if at all, GvH disease would be a complication of human small-bowel transplantation remains unknown. One of the two long-term human survivors of small-intestinal grafts (FORTNER et al. 1972) was thought, on the basis of clinical signs, to have had an episode and possibly to have died of GvH disease while being treated with antilymphocyte serum, prednisone, and azathioprine. More recently, COHEN (1985) reported another clinical attempt at small-bowel transplantation in which GvH disease may have contributed to an unsuccessful outcome. These cases, although not providing conclusive evidence for the occurrence of GvH disease in clinical small-bowel transplantation, provide a true impetus for the study of this potential obstacle to the success of such a procedure in man.

With the assumption that GvH disease may develop after small-bowel transplantation, strategies and methods have to be developed which make it possible to distinguish between GvH disease and exacerbation of the rejection process, with the

Table 1. Rejection vs GvH disease in small-bowel transplantation

	Rejection	GvH disease
Dermatitis	(?, drug-induced?)	++++
Diarrhea	++++	++++
Lymphadenopathy	+/−	++++
Splenomegaly	+/−	++++
Fever	++++	++++
Skin biopsy	Negative	Positive (late)
Lymph node biopsy	Normal	"Empty" node

++++, frequent and marked; +, slight; −, absent

knowledge that the two may occur separately or simultaneously. Most of the clinical signs and symptoms of the two processes are similar (Table 1). Splenomegaly, which is seen only in GvH disease, may not be easily ascertained by physical examination until late in the course of GvH disease, when marked splenic enlargement has occurred. In the rat, the earliest clinical signs of GvH disease are diarrhea and dermal erythema with scaling. It may not be possible to distinguish GvH disease from a rejection episode on the basis of these signs. Diarrhea is an imminent sign and symptom of small-bowel graft rejection (SCHRAUT et al. 1983), and dermatitis may be drug-induced or may arise from other causes. A skin biopsy which demonstrates lymphocytic infiltration at the dermal-epidermal junction together with basal cell degeneration might make the distinction possible. This approach has been useful in clinical bone marrow transplantation in confirming the suspicion of GvH disease (SLAVIN and SANTOS 1973). However, it has been our experience in the laboratory that the early dermal changes observed clinically are difficult to substantiate by a skin biopsy. Only in the presence of fulminant GvH disease is the dermatitis (and also enteritis of the host's native bowel) histologically prominent. In small-bowel transplantation, one would certainly biopsy the allograft and perform a function test of the graft in order to verify the development or delineate the progression of a rejection episode. Then, by exclusion, in the absence of any evidence of graft rejection, one might make the diagnosis of GvH disease. However, if a graft biopsy is equivoval and a biopsy of the host's remnant small bowel is inconclusive or unavailable, biopsy of a recipient lymph node will allow a definitive differentiation between a GvH reaction and a rejection episode. The histopathologic changes seen in the host's lymphatic tissues are characteristic of GvH disease and do not occur with rejection, as is borne out in our experimental study.

The question arises of what course of therapy would be advisable in the event that GvH disease should arise, either alone or in conjunction with exacerbation of small-bowel graft rejection. The experimental studies by SILVERS and BILLINGHAM (1969) indicate that established GvH disease can be alleviated by administration of antilymphocyte serum. One must also keep in mind that, in clinical bone marrow transplantation, GvH disease has been prevented by prolonged cyclosporine A therapy (POWELS et al. 1980). For lack of different, newer immunosuppressive drugs, it thus appears that aggressive immunosuppressive therapy with increased doses of cyclosporine A, most likely given parenterally, together with prednisone and possibly antilymphocyte serum, would prevent the progression of a GvH reaction. The best possible approach to this problem, however, would be to preempt the development of GvH disease in small-bowel transplantation from the outset by irradiating the allograft in vitro before transplantation (Lee and Schraut 1985).

In summary, if the clinical triad of diarrhea, diffuse dermatitis, and lymphoid hypertrophy arises in clinical small-bowel transplantation, the physician should be alerted to the possible development of GvH disease. The suspicion of GvH disease can be confirmed by a lymph node biopsy which, together with a biopsy of the intestinal allograft, should allow a clear differentiation between GvH disease and rejection of the intestinal graft.

References

Cohen Z (1985) Immunosuppression in experimental and clinical small-bowel transplantation. Paper presented at experimental and clinical fundamentals of small-bowel transplantation symposium, 11–12 Oct 1985, Kiel, Federal Republic of Germany

Cohen Z, MacGregor AS, Moore KTH, Falk RE, Langer B, Cullen JB (1976) Canine small bowel transplantation. A study of the immunological responses. Arch Surg 111:248–253

Deltz E, Müller-Hermelink HK, Ulrichs K, Thiede A, Müller-Ruchholtz W (1981) Development of graft-versus-host reaction in various target organs after small intestine transplantation. Transplant Proc 13:1215–1216

Fortner JG, Sichuk G, Litwin SD, Beattie EJ Jr (1972) Immunological responses to an intestinal allograft with HL-A-identical donor-recipient. Transplantation 14:531–535

Kirkman RL, Lear PA, Madara JL, Tilney NL (1984) Small intestine transplantation in the rat: Immunology and function. Surgery 96:280–287

Kort WJ, Westbroek DL, MacDicken I, Lameijer LDF (1973) Orthotopic total small bowel transplantation in the rat. Eur Surg Res 5:81–89

Lafferty KJ (1980) Immunogenicity of foreign tissues. Transplantation 29:179–182

Lee KKW, Schraut WH (1985) In vitro allograft irradiation prevents graft-versus-host disease in small-bowel transplantation. J Surg Res 38:364–372

Lee KKW, Schraut WH (1986) Structure and function of orthotopic small-bowel allografts in rats treated with cyclosporin A. Am J Surg (to be published)

Lillehei RC, Goott B, Miller FA (1959) Homografts of the small bowel. Surg Forum 10:197–199

Monchik GJ, Russell PS (1971) Transplantation of small bowel in the rat: Technical and immunological considerations. Surgery 70:693–702

Powles RL, Clink HM, Spence D (1980) Cyclosporin A to prevent graft-versus-host disease in man after allogeneic bone-marrow transplantation. Lancet 1:327–329

Reznick RK, Craddock GN, Langer B, Gilas T, Cullen JB (1982) Structure and function of small bowel allografts in the dog: Immunosuppression with cyclosporin A. Can J Surg 25:51–55

Schraut WH, Abraham VS, Lee KKW (1985) Portal versus systemic venous drainage for small-bowel allografts. Surgery 98:579–585

Schraut WH, Rosemurgy AS, Riddell RM (1983) Prolongation of intestinal allograft survival without immunosuppressive drug therapy. J Surg Res 34:597–607

Silvers WK, Billingham RE (1969) Studies on the immunotherapy of runt disease in rats. J Exp Med 129:647–661

Slavin RE, Santos (1973) The graft-versus-host reaction in man after bone marrow transplantation: Pathology, pathogenesis, clinical features and implications. Clin Immunol Immunopathol 1:472–498

Graft-vs-Host Reaction After Small-Bowel Transplantation Compared with Graft-vs-Host Reaction After Bone Marrow Transplantation

H. K. MÜLLER-HERMELINK and E. DELTZ

Graft-vs-host (GvH) disease has been considered the reverse situation of transplant rejection. However, in analyzing both situations in individual organs, definite differences with regard to target cells may be found. While MHC class I transplantation antigenic differences are crucial, and although they are expressed, in all the nucleated cells of the body, not all tissue constituents of the host or transplant are at equal risk. Thus, unlike organ transplantation, the blood vessels remain undamaged in graft-vs-host disease. Furthermore, as recently stated, "there is probably no other reaction resulting from the injection of normal tissue into ostensibly normal recipients that produces the diversity of histopathological and functional changes as those seen during GvH-reaction" (LAPP et al. 1986).

Besides the well-known situation in experimental and clinical bone marrow transplantation, small-bowel transplantation is the only other type of organ transplantation in which graft-vs-host reaction (GvHR) plays a significant role. This may be due to the fact that every gram of small-bowel mucosal tissue in man contains 6×10^6 lymphoid cells, and gut-associated lymphoid tissue makes up one-fourth of the gastrointestinal mucosa (GOODACRE et al. 1979). If we compare these values with those of bone marrow transplantation, where 5%–10% of the cell suspension used for transplantation is composed of lymphocytes, equal amounts of lymphoid cells are contained in a small-bowel transplant of about 175 g mucosal tissue and 2×10^8 nucleated bone marrow cells per kg of the recipient. The relationship of the severity of GvHR to the amount of mucosal tissue has been clearly shown in experimental full-length and half-length semiallogeneic small-bowel transplantation (DELTZ 1981).

The following presentation attempts to compare the histopathologic effects of GvHR in bone marrow transplantation to those of one-way experimental small-bowel transplantation in a parent-F_1 hybrid situation.

GvHR in Human Bone Marrow Transplantation

The characteristic lesion of intestinal GvHR consists of necrosis of individual crypt cells localized at the glandular neck region in the stomach and upper intestinal tract mucosa and in the basis of colonic glands (SALE et al. 1979; EPSTEIN et al. 1980; GALLUCCI et al. 1982; SALE and SHULMAN 1984; SNOVER et al. 1985). Some so-called crypt abscesses are usually found (Fig. 1). The more severe degrees of intestinal tract GvHR are caused by a total drop-out of the glands or by denudation of the mucosa by loss of the epithelial glandular layer in large, often macroscopically visible sheets of

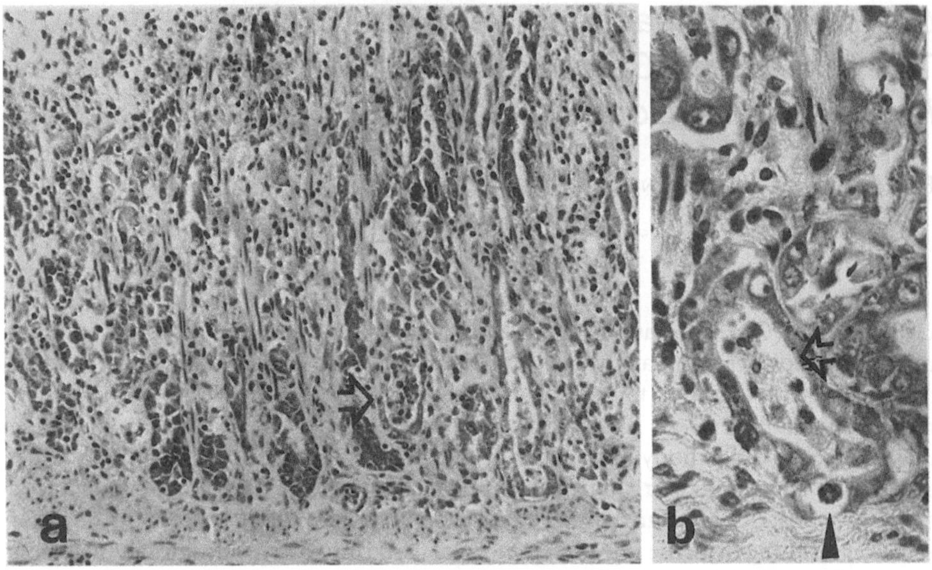

Fig. 1a, b. Acute intestinal graft-vs-host disease in rhesus monkey after allogeneic bone marrow transplantation. Grade II lesion with crypt abscesses *(open arrows)* and single epithelial cell necrosis *(arrow)*. **a** magnification, × 120; **b** magnification, × 400; Giemsa stain

mucosal membrane. Histopathologic gradation of human intestinal graft-vs-host disease (SALE et al. 1979) is listed as follows:

Grade I: Necrosis of individual crypt cells
Grade II: Crypt abscess, dilatation of individual crypts with flattening of epithelial cells
Grade III: Drop-out of entire intestinal glands
Grade IV: Epithelial denudation of mucosa

Characteristic lesions may be diagnosed in endoscopic specimens. They are, however, in themselves not specific, since irradiation damage, as well as viral infection such that produced by cytomegalovirus, may cause identical lesions (SNOVER et al. 1985).

In recent years, histopathologic alterations in biopsy specimens of intestinal GvHR have usually been in the range of grade I and II lesions. Usually, they are focally accentuated, with unaffected mucosal areas between. Recently, LAMPERT et al. (1985) drew attention to the fact that enterochromaffin cells are spared in acute intestinal GvHR in bone marrow transplantation. They found foci of enterochromaffin cells as remnants of largely destroyed intestinal glands.

Fig. 2a–c. Semiallogeneic small-bowel transplantation in rats (BN-F344 x BN). **a** Transplant showing normal height of small-bowel villi and a normal intestinal mucosal pattern (magnification, × 120; **b** Recipient small bowel with loss of intestinal villi and superficial erosions, as well as inflammatory infiltration of lamina propria (magnification, × 64; **c** Portal infiltration of the liver around small portal veins and bile ducts suggestive of GvHR (magnification, × 400), hematoxylin-eosin stain ▷

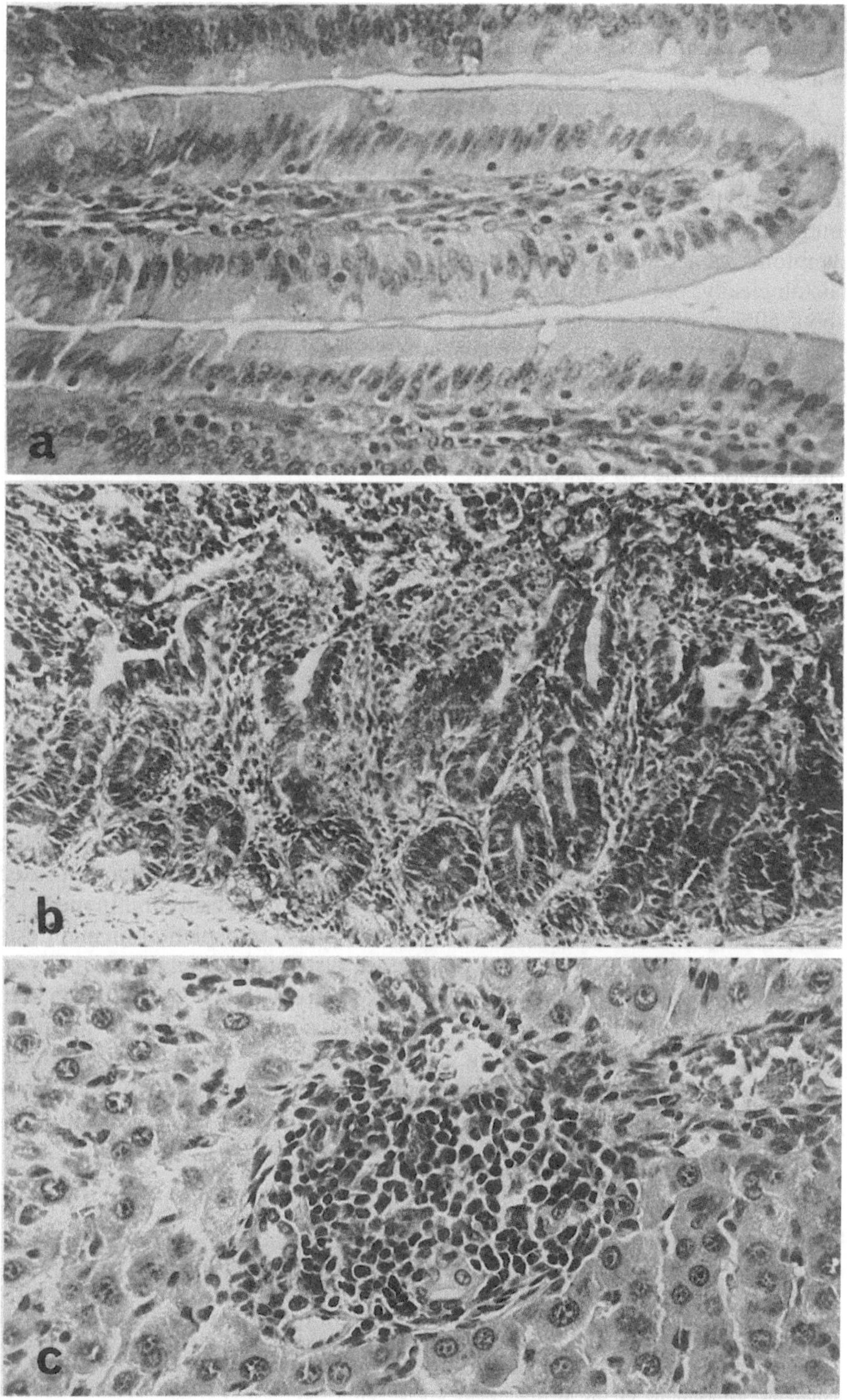

Along with intestinal GvHR, mucosal IgA-mediated immunity is severely impaired, leading to IgA deficiency in the serum as well as in the saliva (BESCHORNER et al. 1981).

A comparison of the degree and extent of GvHR manifestation in different organs and tissues of individual patients is very difficult because of the incomparability of grading systems. In view of the different pathways of circulation and recirculation that transplanted T-lymphocytes take, this comparison would, however, be of great interest. In human bone marrow transplantation, most patients develop intestinal symptoms as a result of irradiation damage, infection, chemotherapy, or GvHR. Histologically, only about 30%–50% of all bone marrow transplanted patients and about 60% of those manifesting GvHR in other organs develop intestinal GvHR. Target organs that are more regularly affected by acute GvHR in human allogeneic bone marrow transplantation are skin, liver, and thymus (MÜLLER-HERMELINK and SALE 1984). Although lymphoid organs are always severely altered at autopsy of bone marrow transplanted patients, no characteristic GvHR lesions have been described in either lymph nodes or spleen.

Histopathological Studies of GvHR in Experimental Small-Bowel Transplantation

The main target of acute GvHR in experimental small-bowel transplantation is the host intestinal mucosa. In a strong semiallogeneic strain combination (BN-F344 x BN), a diffuse loss of intestinal crypts that leads to erosions and villus loss is observed, whereas the transplanted mucosa remains well preserved (Fig. 2). In half-length small-bowel transplantation, loss in intestinal villus height, inflammatory infiltration, and single cell necrosis are observed. These characteristics are similar to those found in full-length small-bowel transplantations in "weak" F_1-hybrid combinations (DELTZ 1981). The systemic effect of GvHR after small-bowel transplantation manifests itself in slight organic changes in the liver that are distributed similarly to those in bone marrow transplantation (Fig. 2c). The most severe effects are seen in the lymphoid tissues. Animals afflicted by GvH disease in small-bowel transplantation show generalized lymphadenopathy (Fig. 3a). Histologically, enlarged paracortical areas with small granulomas, loss of lymphoid follicles, and prominent polyclonal plasmacytosis are observed. Comparable changes can also be detected in splenic white pulp.

Fig. 3a–c. Thymus in GvHR caused by semiallogeneic small-bowel transplantation (BN-F344). **a** ▷ Mediastinal lymphadenopathy *(ln)* with massive enlargement of perithymic lymph nodes, while thymus itself *(t)* is atrophic. Sample taken 15 days after whole-length small-bowel transplant (magnification, × 64). **b** Severe atrophy of thymic cortex *(c)* with increase of plasma cells *(open arrows)* in the epithelial space of the thymic cortex. Sample taken 15 days after whole-length small-bowel transplant. *m*, medulla. Magnification, × 400. **c** Atrophy and fibrosis of the thymus with complete effacement of the thymic structure 20 days after whole-length small-bowel transplant (magnification, × 64)

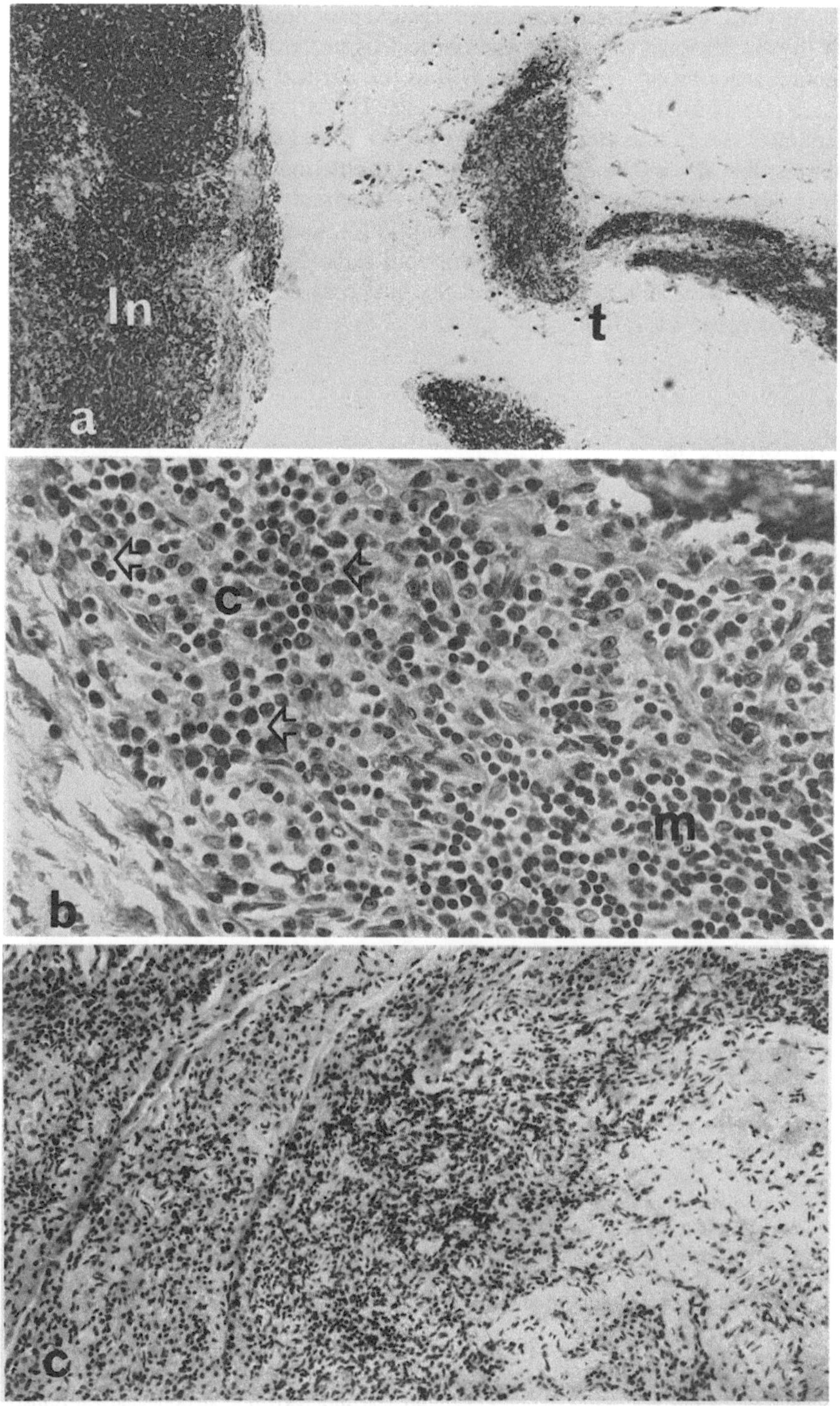
ln
t
a
c
m
b
c

Very interesting findings are the early and profound thymic changes. These consist of thymic atrophy, usually of the cortical tissue, although recent observations also include atrophy of the medulla. Within the cortical area, epithelial cell necrosis is seen, as well as infiltration by plasma cells. The latter changes are seen in the thymic medulla. Here, activated lymphoid cells are found not only within the perivascular spaces, but also in the epithelial space of the thymic medulla itself. Recently, it has been shown that activated T-lymphocytes recirculate to the thymus and may exist there for long periods (Naparstek et al. 1982). One may speculate that recirculation pathways of activated intestinal lymphoid cells (first to the gut, then to peripheral lymphoid tissue, liver, spleen, and thymus) may reflect the distribution of GvHR-induced tissue alterations.

Conclusions

For the follow-up of experimental and clinical small-bowel transplantation, it appears to be important that pathologic effects of GvHR may manifest themselves in the host's own intestinal tissue (where they also may be followed by endoscopy). It is also important to note that severe GvHR may result in an indefinite period of severe immunosuppression, as judged from the degree of thymic GvHR. The slight differences in tissue distribution and frequency of GvHR-induced lesions after bone marrow transplantation compared with results after small-bowel transplantation, may result from the varying pretreatment, as well as from the different tissue affinities of circulating activated lymphoid cells.

References

Beschorner WE, Yardley JH, Tuschka PJ (1981) Deficiency of intestinal immunity with graft-versus-host disease in humans. J Infect Dis 144:38–46

Deltz E (1984) Die allogene Dünndarmtransplantation: Funktionelle und morphologische Untersuchungen der Abstoßungs- und der Transplantat-gegen-Wirt-Reaktion (GVHR) im Rattenmodell. Zuckschwerdt, Munich, pp 1–150

Epstein RJ, McDonald GB, Sale GE, Shulman HM, Thomas ED (1980) The diagnostic accuracy of the rectal biopsy in acute Graft-Versus-Host disease: A prospective study of thirteen patients. Gastroenterology 78:764–771

Gallucci BB, Sale GE, McDonald GB, Epstein R, Shulman HM, Thomas ED (1982) The fine structure of human rectal epithelium in acute graft-versus-host disease. Am J Surg Pathol 6:293–305

Goodacre R, Davidson R, Singal D, Bienenstock J (1979) Morphologic and functional characteristics of human intestinal lymphoid cells isolated by a mechanical technique. Gastroenterology 6:300–308

Lampert IA, Thorpe P, van Noorden S, Marsh J, Goldman JM, Gordon-Smith EC, Evans DJ (1985) Selective sparing of enterochromaffin cells in graft versus host disease affecting the colonic mucosa. Histopathology 9:875–886

Lapp WS, Ghayur T, Mendes M, Seddik M, Seemayer TA (1986) The functional and histological basis for graft-versus-host-induced immunosuppression. Immunol Rev (to be published)

Müller-Hermelink HK, Sale GE (1984) Pathological findings in human bone marrow transplantation. In: Lennert K, Hübner K (eds) Pathology of the bone marrow. Fischer, Stuttgart, pp 255–280

Naparstek Y, Holoshitz J, Eisenstein S, Reshef T, Rappaport S, Chemke J, Ben-Nun A, Cohen IR (1982) Effector T lymphocyte line cells migrate to the thymus and persist there. Nature 300:262
Sale GE, Shulman HM (1984) The pathology of bone marrow transplantation. In: Sternberg SS (ed) Masson monographs in diagnostic pathology. Masson, New York, pp 77–103
Sale GE, Shulman HM, McDonald GB, Thomas ED (1979) Gastrointestinal graft-versus-host disease in man: A clinicopathologic study of the rectal biopsy. Am J Surg Pathol 3:291–299
Snover DC, Weisdorf SA, Vercellotti GM, Rank B, Hutton S, McGlave P (1985) A histopathologic study of gastric and small intestinal graft-versus-host disease following allogeneic bone marrow transplantation. Hum Pathol 16:387–392

Rejection in Heterotopic Small-Bowel Transplantation

P. Liedgens, H. K. Müller-Hermelink, and E. Deltz

Introduction

Management and prevention of rejection by effective immunosupressive therapy are two of the most important problems of small-bowel transplantation. Cyclosporine A, already used in clinical organ grafting with great success, has greatly prolonged the survival times of experimentally transplanted small intestines (Diliz-Perez et al. 1984; Raju et al. 1984). Although the exact identity of the cells causing morphological graft destruction is not yet know, T cells are thought to play a significant role in this process (Loveland and McKenzie 1982; Lowry et al. 1982; Asher et al. 1983; Gurley et al. 1983). With the availability of monoclonal antibodies, an identification of T cell subsets with different functions is now possible.

In the study reported here, we tried to investigate the T cell distribution pattern in the transplant's intestinal wall during rejection and the influence of cyclosporine A on this pattern.

Material and Methods

Animals

Rats in this study were of the BN and (BN-LEW)F_1 strains, weighing between 250 and 350 g.

Experimental Groups

Auxiliary heterotopic bowel transplantation as described by Preissner et al. (see "Microsurgical Techniques of Heterotopic and Orthotopic Small-Bowel Transplantation in the Rat, this volume) was performed on two experimental groups, each consisting of 15 (BN-LEW)F_1 donors to BN recipient rats. In this strain combination, a unidirectional rejection reaction without interference by a graft-versus-host reaction (GvHR) occurs.

The first group (group 1) remained untreated, whereas the second (group 2) was treated with 15 mg cyclosporine A per kg body weight orally during an observation period of 15 days.

In addition, two groups of syngeneically grafted animals without (group 3, $n = 9$) and with (group 4, $n = 9$) cyclosporine A treatment (15 mg/kg body weight for 15 days) served as controls.

Histology

At days 5, 10, and 15 after transplantation, five animals of each group were killed. Specimens of intestine from both the transplant and the recipient were taken and stained with hematoxylin eosin. Special staining for T cell subsets was done using the peroxidase-antiperoxidase technique of STERNBERGER (1979) with the following monoclonal antibodies: MAS41c, directed against cytotoxic and suppressor T cells, and MAS1131c, directed against T helper cells (BRIDEAU et al. 1980; FORBES et al. 1983). Both antibodies were purchased from Sera Lab. (Oxford, England). The peroxidase-stained sections were analyzed under the microscope by counting the positively stained cells in 20 randomized microscopic fields. The percentage of these cells with respect to the overall mononuclear cell population was defined in the lamina propria (LP) and lamina muscularis (LM) of both the transplant and the recipient.

Results

Manifest signs of graft rejection could be maximally observed at day 10 in the untreated group. The histologic examination revealed progressive damage to the

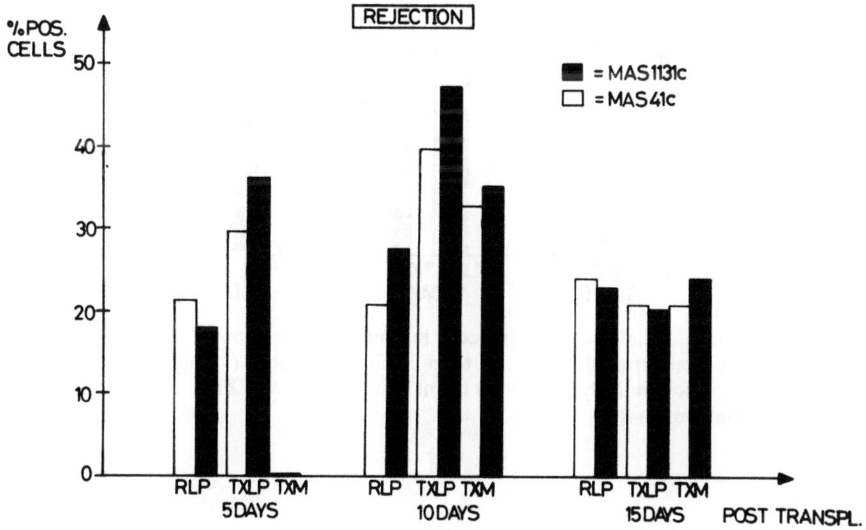

Fig. 1. Percentage of antibody-positive cells in graft and recipient small bowel after heterotopic accessory small-bowel transplantation. Group 1, no treatment. *RLP,* recipient lamina propria; *TXLP,* transplant lamina propria; *TXM,* transplant lamina muscularis

mucosa in the villi region and an infiltration of mononuclear cells inside the whole intestinal wall. Further analysis with monoclonal antibodies demonstrated the involvement of T cells in this process (Fig. 1). In the LP of the graft, a maximum of T helper (48.4%) and of T suppressor and cytotoxic T cells (39.3%) could be determined at day 10, with a decrease in their numbers to day 15 (20.2% and 20.9% respectively), reflecting the almost complete destruction of the tissue at that time.

The T cell counts in the recipient LP, which served as a control, were lower than those in the graft at day 5 (18.6% and 21.3%) and day 10 (27.6% and 21.3%), whereas the LM of the recipient remained T cell free during the whole observation period. The transplant LM was still T cell free on day 5 and maximally infiltrated by T cells on day 10 (35% and 32.6%).

In the cyclosporine-treated group during the observation period of 15 days, only slight morphological alterations consisting of epithelial desquamation in the villi tips could be observed. The kinetics of the T cell distribution pattern in the transplant intestinal wall of the animals receiving cyclosporine therapy is different from that of the untreated group (Fig. 2). In the LP of the graft, the T cell peak shifted to day 5 (40.1% and 28.8%), with a decrease at day 15. In contrast to that of the untreated group, the LM of the graft remained completely T cell free at days 5, 10, and 15.

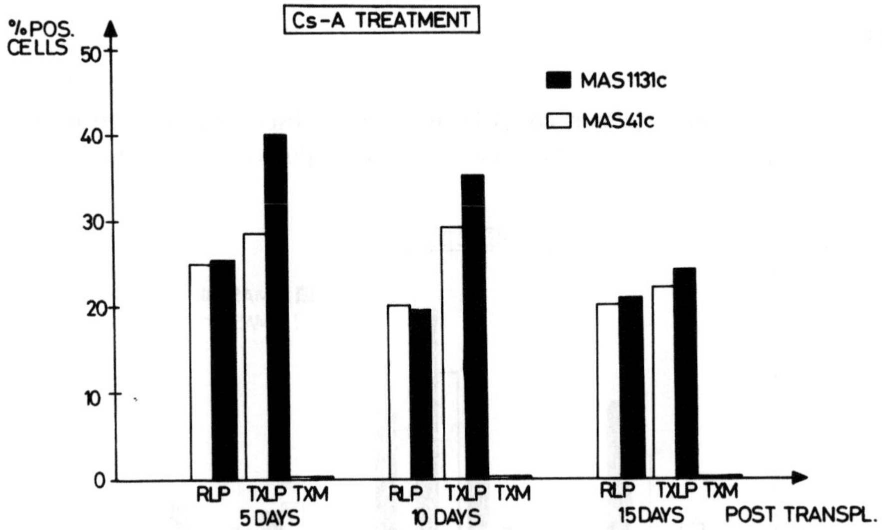

Fig. 2. Percentage of antibody-positive cells in graft and recipient small bowel after heterotopic accessory small-bowel transplantation. Group 2, CsA treatment (15 mg/kg body weight per day orally, 15 days postoperatively). *RLP,* recipient lamina propria; *TXLP,* transplant lamina propria; *TXM,* transplant lamina muscularis

Discussion

Routine histologic staining gives only limited information about the cellular infiltrate in rejected grafts, whereas staining with monoclonal antibodies allows a discrimination of cell subpopulations.

In regard to the value of controls, it is important to mention that syngeneic organ transplantation also leads to an inflammatory response in the transplant, although to a lesser degree (VON WILLEBRAND et al. 1979). In our syngeneic controls, we found about 20% T cells at 5, 10, and 15 days after transplantation in both the treated and untreated control groups, a finding which has to be regarded as unspecific background infiltration.

Almost without exception, graft rejection is preceded by an infiltration of the transplant with lymphocytes from the blood (COX et al. 1984). T cells are thought to be the most important mediators in the rejection process (LOVELAND and MCKENZIE 1982), but the mechanism of graft rejection is not yet known (DALLMAN and MASON 1982).

In the rejection group maximal T cell infiltration in the transplant correlates with morphological evidence of graft destruction. This seems not to be an organ-specific phenomenon because most of the inflammatory cells after allogeneic heart transplantation in the rat model are also T cells (STORM et al. 1977).

Cyclosporine A reduced the surprisingly high percentage of T helper cells on day 5 (40.1% in group 1, Fig. 1) to 24.3% (group 2, Fig. 2) on day 15, which may be interpreted as a further argument for the central role of this cell population in the afferent limb of rejection (DALLMAN and MASON 1982; LOVELAND and MCKENZIE 1982; HALL et al. 1983). The success of cyclosporine A in experimental small-bowel transplantation may be due to its influence on T cell infiltration into the LM of the graft, which is completely suppressed by cyclosporine A treatment.

References

Asher NL, Hoffman R, Hanto DW, Simmons RL (1983) Cellular events within the rejecting allograft. Transplantation 35:193–197

Brideau RJ, Carter PB, McMaster WR, Mason DW, Williams AF (1980) Two subsets of rat T lymphocytes defined with monoclonal antibodies. Eur J Immunol 10:609–615

Cox JH, Forsyth AT, De Villiers JS, Yacoub MH, Chisholm PM (1984) The kinetics and specificity of cardiac allografts in unmodified and cyclosporine-treated rats. Transplantation 38:17–22

Dallman MJ, Mason DW (1982) Role of thymus-derived and thymus-independent cells in murine skin allograft rejection. Transplantation 33:221–223

Diliz-Perez HS, McClure J, Bedetti C, Hong H-Q, De Santibanes E, Shaw BW, Van Thiel D, Iwatsuki S, Starzl TE (1984) Successful small bowel allo-transplantation in dogs with cyclosporine and prednisone. Transplantation 37:126–129

Forbes C, Guttman RD, Gomersall M, Hibberd J (1983) Leucocyte subsets in first-set rat cardiac allograft rejection. Transplantation 36:681–686

Gurley KE, Lowry RP, Forbes RD (1983) Immune mechanisms in organ allograft rejection (II). Transplantation 36:401–405

Hall BM, De Saxe I, Dorsch SE (1983) The cellular basis of allograft rejection in vivo. Transplantation 36:700–705

Loveland BE, McKenzie IFC (1982) Which T-cells cause graft rejection? Transplantation 33:217–219
Lowry RP, Gurley KE, Forbes RD (1983) Immune mechanisms in organ allograft rejection (I). Transplantation 36:391–401
Raju S, Didlake RH, Cayirli M, Turner MD, Grogan JB, Achord J (1984) Experimental small bowel transplantation utilizing cyclosporine. Transplantation 38:561–566
Sternberger LA (1979) Immunochemistry, 2nd edn. Wilney, New York, p 104
Storm TB, Tilney NL, Paradysz JM, Bancewicz J, Carpenter CB (1977) Cellular components of allograft rejection: Identity, specificity and cytotoxic function of cells infiltrating acutely rejecting allografs. J Immunol 118:2020–2029
von Willebrand E, Soots A, Häyry P (1979) In situ effector mechanisms in rat kidney allograft rejection. Cell Immunol 46:309–316

Rejection in Orthotopic Small-Bowel Transplantation and Immunosuppression by Cyclosporine A: Evidence for Development of Tolerance Mechanisms

W. CH. PREISSNER, P. LIEDGENS, M. GUNDLACH, E. SCHRÖDER, H. K. MÜLLER-HERMELINK, and E. DELTZ

Introduction

The immunologic response in small-intestine transplantation is characterized by an interaction between rejection and graft-versus-host reaction (GvHR) (DELTZ 1981). In a fully allogeneic donor-recipient combination, an interaction of both reactions occurs (DELTZ 1984). As has been shown in previous investigations, a GvHR may not develop in the case of strong rejection reactions. In this situation, rejection predominates. Therefore, we investigated rejection after orthotopic small-bowel transplantation and tried to elaborate the patterns of T cell infiltration in the graft in order to characterize the course of rejection without immunosuppression and during administration of cyclosporine A (CsA).

Material and Methods

Orthotopic small-bowel transplantation in the rat was achieved by the so-called "two-step operative technique" (see PREISSNER et al., "Microsurgical Techniques of Heterotopic and Orthotopic Small-Bowel Transplantation in the Rat," this volume). Besides the syngeneic control group 1 (LEW-LEW, n = 20), small-bowel grafts using AS or DA rats were transplanted into LEW recipients. The animals of group 2 [AS ($RT1^{l}$) → LEW ($RT1^{l}$)], [non major histocompatibility complex (non-MHC) different system, $n = 22$], and group 4 [DA ($RT1^{avl}$) → LEW (MHC and non-MHC different system), $n = 20$] got no further treatment. The animals of group 3 (AS → LEW, $n = 20$) and group 5 (DA → LEW, $n = 16$) received oral immunosuppression with CsA at a dose of 10 mg/kg body weight during the first 20 days, then parenterally in a reduced dose (5 mg/kg body weight for 10 days, 2.5 mg/kg body weight for 10 days, 2.5 mg/kg body weight every second day for 10 days) for the next 40 days. CsA treatment was terminated 60 days after the first operation.

The analyses of T cell subsets were performed with the method described by LIEDGENS et al. (see "Rejection in Heterotopic Small-Bowel Transplantation," this volume). T helper cells were stained by the monoclonal antibody MAS 1131c, T cytotoxic and suppressor cells by the monoclonal antibody MAS 41c. The pattern of T cell infiltration was observed in the grafts of group 3 at day 20 ($n = 4$), when the graft was still in heterotopic position, and at day 60 ($n = 4$) after orthotopic interposition, as well as in the grafts of group 1 60 days after transplantation.

Results

Of 20 animals (85%) in group 1 (LEW-LEW), 17 survived more than 180 days after orthotopic small-bowel transplantation (Table 1). All grafts of group 2 and group 4 underwent severe rejection 12.2 ± 2 and 10.3 ± 2 days respectively after transplantation, causing the death of the recipients. During rejection, the animals showed progressive weight loss, and the grafts showed heavy inflammatory alterations macroscopically. The first signs of rejection appeared on the 5th–7th day after small-bowel transplantation, when the graft was still in the heterotopic position. Histologically, there was atrophy of the villi, fibrosis of the lamina propria, and a decreased number of glands. End-stage rejection was observed at day 12 after small-bowel transplantation, with complete necrosis and sloughing of the mucosa.

Table 1. Experimental groups and survival rates after orthotopic small-bowel transplantation

Experimental groups	Strain combination	Surviving animals	
		n	%
1	LEW → LEW	17/20	85
2	AS → LEW (no treatment)	0/22	0
3	AS → LEW (CsA)	12/20	60
4	DA → LEW (no treatment)	0/20	0
5	DA → LEW (CsA)	9/16	56

In group 3, 12 of 20 (60%) animals and nine of 16 animals (56%) in group 5 survived more than 180 days and 100 days respectively after small-bowel transplantation (Table 1).

Death of the animals was caused mainly by pneumonia. The grafts appeared normal macroscopically and histologically 110 days (group 3) and 40 days (group 4) after the cessation of CsA administration. The pattern of T cell infiltration in the graft (Fig. 1) at day 20 after small-bowel transplantation showed a slight increase of T helper and T cytotoxic and suppressor cells in the lamina propria compared with the recipient's lamina propria. By day 60, when the graft was in orthotopic position, cell infiltration had diminished to almost normal, a situation which is apparent from a comparison of the results of the orthotopic graft with the percentage of cell infiltration in syngeneically transplanted small bowels. The lamina muscularis was free of T cells at both 20 and 60 days after transplantation.

Discussion

The results demonstrate that small-bowel transplantation in the rat without CsA treatment leads to rejection reactions beginning on the 5th day after transplantation. This rejection is characterized by heavy inflammatory alterations, atrophy of the villi, fibrosis of the lamina propria, and complete necrosis with sloughing of the mucosa, as

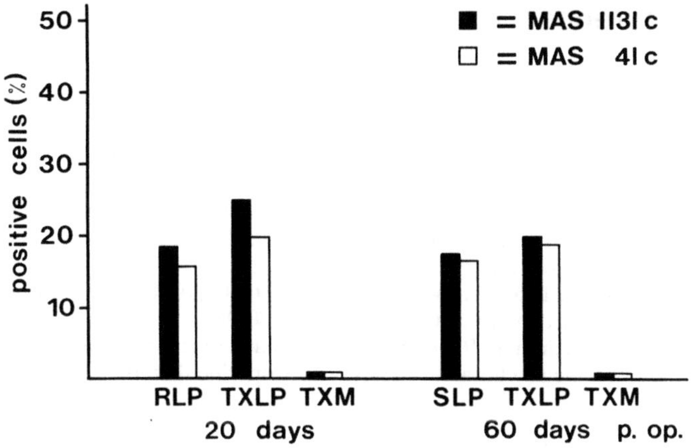

Fig. 1. Percentage of antibody-positive cells within the graft and recipient's small bowel after heterotopic accessory small-bowel transplantation (20 days postoperatively) and orthotopic small-bowel transplantation (60 days postoperatively, group 3). *RLP,* recipient lamina propria; *TXLP,* transplant lamina propria; *TXM,* transplant lamina muscularis; *SLP,* syngeneically transplanted graft lamina propria

has been reported by KIRKMAN et al. (1984), MADARA et al. (1985), and LIEDGENS (see "Rejection in Heterotopic Small-Bowel Transplantation," this volume). CsA treatment markedly enhances survival of an AS or DA small bowel transplanted into a LEW host. CsA is useful in the prevention of both rejection and graft-versus-host reaction (KIRKMAN et al. 1984; MADARA and KIRKMAN 1985; DELTZ et al. 1986).

The analysis of T cell subsets within the graft showed that T cell infiltration leads to a slight increase of T helper and T suppressor cells in the graft at day 20 compared with the recipient's small bowel at this time. By the time the graft is in orthotopic position at day 60, cell infiltration has diminished to almost normal levels as represented by the cell infiltration of syngeneically transplanted small bowels. With CsA treatment, the infiltration can be demonstrated in the lamina propria only; the lamina muscularis remains free of T cells.

This pattern of T cell distribution 20 and 60 days after transplantation in a fully allogeneic combination resembles the T cell infiltration which can be found after suppression of a unidirectional rejection reaction by CsA in a semiallogeneic donor-recipient combination at day 15. This situation has been described by LIEDGENS et al. (see "Rejection in Heterotopic Small-Bowel Transplantation," this volume). As in these experiments, T cell infiltration after CsA treatment does not differ significantly from unspecific cell infiltration and the infiltration of syngeneic grafts. The animals of group 3 and 5 survived until 110 and 40 days after cessation of CsA administration. That means that a certain degree of long-lasting graft acceptance or tolerance was induced by CsA treatment. The underlying mechanisms of this phenomenon and the role which T cells infiltrating small-bowel grafts play in inducing a state of tolerance are unknown and need further investigation. The elucidation of tolerance mechanisms in small-bowel transplantation might have a major impact on immunosuppressive treatment regimens.

References

Deltz E (1984) Die allogene Dünndarmtransplantation. Zuckschwerdt, Munich

Deltz E, Müller-Hermelink HK, Ulrichs K, Thiede A, Müller-Ruchholtz W (1981) Development of graft-versus-host reaction in various target organs after small intestine transplantation. Transplant Proc 13:1215–1216

Deltz E, Ulrichs K, Schack T, Friedrichs B, Müller-Ruchholtz W, Müller-Hermelink HK, Thiede A (1986) Graft versus host reaction in small intestine transplantation and possibilities for its circumvention. Am J Surg 151:379–386

Kirkman RL, Lear PA, Madara JC, Tilney NC (1984) Small intestine transplantation in the rat: Immunology and Function. Surgery 96:280–287

Madara JC, Kirkman RC (1985) Structural and functional evolution of jejunal allograft rejection in rats and the ameliorating effects of cyclosporine therapy. J Clin Invest 75:502–512

Course of Rejection in Pancreaticoduodenal Allografts in the Rat

T. SCHANG, W. TIMMERMANN, G. SCHUBERT, and A. THIEDE

In previous studies of several techniques of pancreas transplantation in the rat, we observed histologic changes in both duct-ligated and duct-occluded segmental grafts that led not only to an expected atrophy of exocrine tissue, but also to deformation and disintegration of islets (SCHANG et al. 1985). In contrast, draining of exocrine secretion led to a situation in which morphologically unaltered isografts were not distinguishable from a normal pancreas 300 days after transplantation. The simplest and most reliable technique of exocrine secretion drainage was revealed to be the pancreaticoduodenal graft described by LEE et al. (1972). Therefore, we used this technique for a rejection study of allogeneic pancreas grafts in the rat. The aim of the study was to describe the course of rejection of allografts in untreated and in temporarily immunosuppressed recipients, with special regard to comparing the rejection of duodenal and pancreactic tissue.

Materials and Methods

Male LEW rats (RT 1^{1}) were rendered diabetic by a single dose of 55 mg/kg body weight streptococin i.v. and served as recipients. All animals had serum glucose levels of above 20 mmol/l within 24 h. DA rats (RT 1^{avl}) served as pancreas donors. A pancreaticoduodenal graft consisted of the whole pancreas and the duodenum. An aortic segment bearing the celiac axis and superior mesenteric artery was anastomosed to the infrarenal aorta of the recipient. The portal vein was anastomosed to the infrarenal vena cava. The oral end of the donor's duodenum was ligated, and its aboral end was anastomosed end to side to the recipient's first jejunal loop.

After transplantation, the serum glucose levels and body weight of the recipients were controlled daily. Isografted recipients were controlled weekly. The day of rejection was defined as the first day of lasting recurrence of hyperglycemia above 11 mmol/l.

For immunosuppression, cyclosporin A (CsA) was dissolved in olive oil, and 15 mg/kg body weight were given orally from day 0 to day 13 after transplantation. Group 1 consisted of 30 LEW-LEW isografts, which were observed for 300 days. Group 2 consisted of ten DA-LEW allografts. Group 3 consisted of 10 DA-LEW allografts in temporarily immunosuppressed recipients. In addition, 40 allogeneic transplantations were performed for histologic follow-up.

Results

All of the isografts functioned well for 300 days. Their morphology was completely unaltered. Untreated allografts were rejected an average of 8.2 days (SD ± 0.632 days) after transplantation (one graft on day 7, six grafts on day 8, three grafts on day 9). Immunosuppressed allograft recipients rejected the graft after a mean time of 25.8 days (SD ± 0.6 days; three grafts on day 25, six on day 26, one on day 27).

Morphological Findings

Both allografts and isografts show slight edema 2 days after transplantation. An unspecific interstitial cellular infiltration can be seen in all the grafts. At 4 days after transplantation, untreated allografts show marked interstitial and perivascular infiltration consisting of lymphocytes and macrophages and incipient destruction of the exocrine tissue. Islets are surrounded but not disrupted by mononuclear cells. The allografted duodenum does not show any alteration except for some mild cellular infiltrations, which can also be found in corresponding isografts. In CsA-treated allografts, some mononuclear infiltrations of the exocrine tissue can also be found, but the graft remains intact.

By 7 days after transplantation, rejection of untreated allografts can be diagnosed macroscopically: The grafts are swollen and of solid consistency. The duodenum appears to be somewhat dilated. The exocrine tissue is totally destroyed and is being replaced by fibrous tissue. However, there are still enough islets within the graft to keep the animal normoglycemic, although these islets are subjected to disruption by mononuclear infiltration and fibrous tissue (Fig. 1).

The duodenum now shows some histologic changes. Mononuclear infiltrations can be found in the submucosa and the muscular wall, but they are relatively mild compared with the severe reactions in the adjacent pancreas. The intestinal villi have become shorter and plumper. On the whole however, the histologic architecture of the duodenum is still intact (Fig. 2).

By day 7, CsA-treated allografts have not changed from their condition on day 4 after transplantation. On day 14 CsA-treated allografts show no further changes except for some discrete shortening of the villi in the duodenum. At 23 and 27 days after transplantation, CsA-treated allografts have the appearance of untreated allografts on day 7. By 33 days after transplantation, the pancreatic tissue of the CsA-treated allografts has become totally fibrotic, and islets can be found. The duodenum is also destroyed. The epithelium has vanished, and the necrotic wall is being replaced by fibrous tissue.

Discussion

The three main tissues of a pancreaticoduodenal allograft are destroyed by rejection successively. Destruction of the exocrine tissue is followed by loss of the islets. The allografted duodenum maintains its histologic architecture for the longest time.

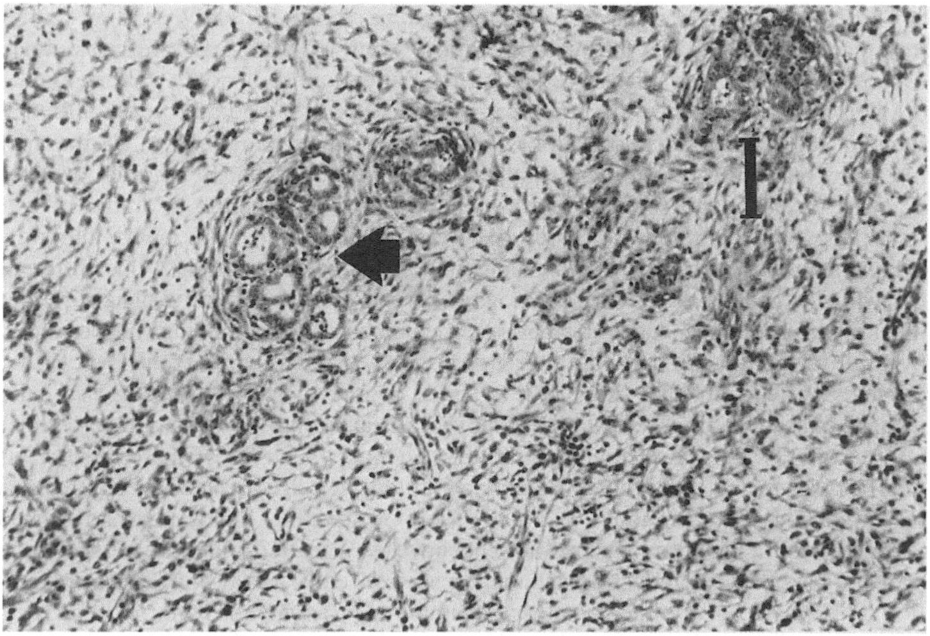

Fig. 1. Untreated DA-LEW allograft 7 days after transplantation: rejected pancreatic tissue. *Arrow* shows remnants of pancreatic ducts. Goldner's trichrome stain; *bar* = 100 μm

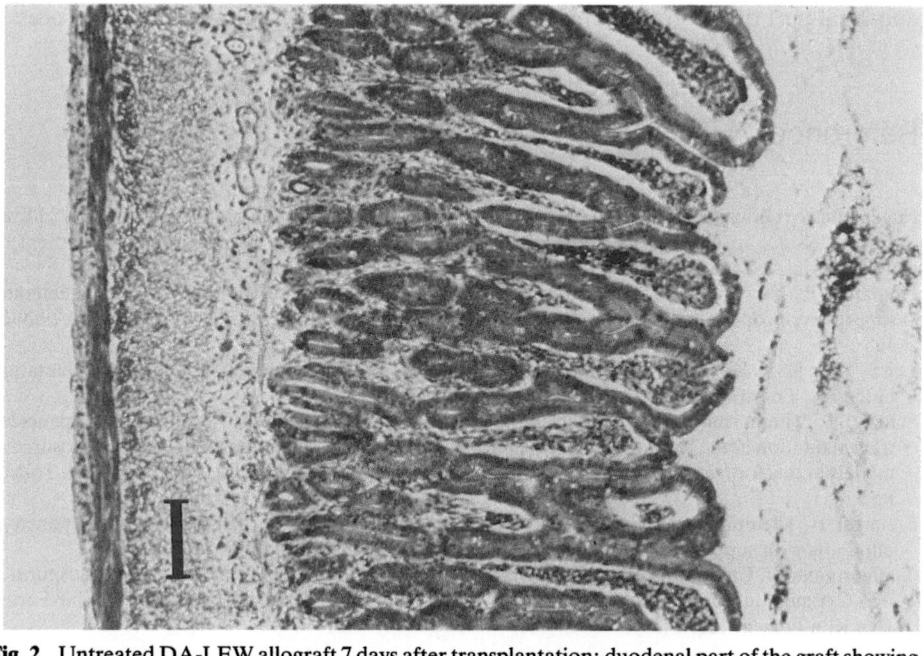

Fig. 2. Untreated DA-LEW allograft 7 days after transplantation: duodenal part of the graft showing mild cellular infiltration of the submucosal layer and shortening of the villi. Goldner's trichrome stain; *bar* = 160 μm

The first histologic signs of rejection can be found as early as day 4 after transplantation in the DA-LEW combination, when mononuclear infiltrates attack exocrine tissue. At this stage of rejection, the duodenum shows only a shortening of the villi. CsA is able to prevent graft destruction as long as it is administered, although some local cellular infiltration can be found. After the termination of CsA therapy, the rejection pattern is similar to that of untreated allografts. In contrast to these findings, the same course of CsA treatment is able to induce graft tolerance in liver (ENGEMANN et al. (1983), kidney (HOMAN et al. 1980), and heart allografts (TIMMERMANN et al. 1980). It remains an open question whether this different behavior is due to a different immunogenicity of pancreas allografts. The different times of morphological destruction of the three main graft components may be caused by differing immunogenicity, but there are no further data to support this hypothesis. It seems more likely that there is a different degree of sensitivity to the vascular damage caused by rejection. Interestingly, islets are relatively resistant to cellular infiltrations, as was also demonstrated by STEINIGER et al. (1984). The reason for this may be mechanical rather than immunologic. Intensive cell contact between islet cells may hinder rapid infiltration of the entire islet. On the other hand, pure handpicked islet allografts in an intraportal position that have been grafted under the renal capsule provoke a lymphocytic reaction around the islets as early as day 4 after transplantation. This may be an argument against an immunologic advantage of unmodified islets (own unpublished data). Whether the successive stages of rejection of a pancreaticoduodenal allograft can be stopped by additional immunosuppression or whether the destruction of exocrine tissue causes irreversible damage that limits the endocrine function of the graft as well is another interesting question. In any case, the duodenal part of the graft seems not to be the main target of the rejection process.

References

Engemann R, Ulrichs K, Thiede A, Müller-Ruchholtz W, Hamelmann H (1983) Induction of liver graft tolerance in a primarily nontolerant rat strain combination with temporary treatment of cyclosporin A. Transplant Proc 15:2983–2991

Homan WP, Fabre JW, Williams KA, Millard PR, Morris PJ (1980) Studies on the immune suppressive properties of cyclosporin A in rats receiving renal allografts. Transplantation 29:361–366

Lee S, Tung KSK, Koopman H, Chandler JG, Orloff MJ (1972) Pancreaticoduodenal transplantation in the rat. Transplantation 13:421–425

Schang T, Timmermann W, Thiede A (1985) Various techniques of experimental pancreas transplantation in the rat. In: Thiede A, Deltz E, Engemann R, Hamelmann H (eds) Microsurgical models in rats for transplantation research. Springer-Verlag, Berlin Heidelberg New York Tokyo, pp 57–63

Steiniger B, Klempnauer J, Brüsch U, Wonigeit K (1984) Histology of rejection in rat pancreas allografts with suppressed or preserved exocrine function. Transplant Proc 16:783

Timmermann W, Calne RY, White DJG, White D, Thiede A (1980) Die Wirkung von Cyclosporin A und Cytimun auf die Überlebenszeit von RT 1 allogenen Rattenherztransplantaten. Chir Forum Exp Klin Forsch: 139–143

*Prevention of Graft-vs-Host Disease Using in Vitro Irradiation of Small-Bowel Grafts**

K. K. W. LEE, W. H. SCHRAUT, and H. G. SUTTON

Introduction

Although the significance of graft-vs-host (GvH) disease in clinical small-bowel transplantation remains undetermined, transplantation of the small bowel between appropriate inbred animal strains has been shown to provoke severe and often fatal GvH reactions (POMPOSELLI et al. 1985; SCHRAUT et al. 1985). These reactions result from the transfer of large numbers of immunologically competent lymphocytes contained within the intestinal graft (DELTZ et al. 1981). In experimental studies, regimens for the control of intestinal allograft rejection have been inconsistently effective for the control of GvH disease (DELTZ et al. 1985; KIRKMAN et al. 1984). If GvH disease proves to be a genuine clinical concern, separate therapeutic methods may be needed which effectively prevent the development of GvH disease and which can be combined with equally effective regimens for preventing graft rejection. Using the rat model of vascularized small-bowel transplantation, in vitro graft irradiation prior to transplantation was evaluated as such a method of preventing GvH disease.

Materials and Methods

Experimental Groups

Small-bowel transplantation was performed in the inbred Lewis (LEW) → Lewis by Brown Norway F_1 (LBN F_1) hybrid strain combination to ensure a unidirectional GvH reaction. In groups 1–4, heterotopic (accessory) transplantation of grafts irradiated in vitro with 0 ($n = 9$), 250 ($n = 6$), 500 ($n = 6$), and 1000 ($n = 6$) rad respectively was performed to determine the effective radiation dose. In groups 5 and 6, grafts were transplanted orthotopically after irradiation with either 0 ($n = 5$) or 1000 ($n = 7$) rad respectively in order to assess the function of small-bowel allografts after irradiation with 1000 rad. Control groups consisted of age-matched normal LEW ($n = 6$) and LEW → LEW orthotopic isograft recipients ($n = 8$).

---

* Supported by The National Institutes of Arthritis, Metabolism, and Digestive Diseases (Grant No. AM27332).

Operative Procedure and Irradiation Technique

Small-bowel transplantation was performed as previously described (Schraut et al. 1983). The donor small bowel was harvested on a vascular pedicle consisting of the superior mesenteric artery and the portal vein. The cold (4°C) allograft was then irradiated in vitro at the dosage specified by the experimental protocol using a GE Maxitron at 250 kV at a dose rate of 100 rad/min. Following irradiation, the graft was revascularized by end-to-side anastomosis of the superior mesenteric artery to the infrarenal aorta and of the portal vein to the inferior vena cava. In groups 1–4, heterotopic transplantation was completed by the formation of two abdominal wall stomas. In groups 5 and 6, orthotopic transplantation was completed by resecting the recipient's own small bowel and placing the bowel graft in intestinal continuity by end-to-end intestinal anastomoses.

Postoperative Course

All animals were allowed a normal laboratory diet, and their general health and appearance were monitored. Body weight, serum protein, albumin, and triglycerides were periodically measured using standard laboratory methods. Postmortem examinations were performed on all animals, and sections from liver, spleen, small bowel (donor and recipient), and lymph nodes (donor and recipient) were prepared for light microscopy. Long-term (> 6 months) surviving graft recipients underwent a laparotomy with small bowel and lymph node biopsies or were killed for histopathologic studies.

Results

Heterotopic Transplantation

Recipients of heterotopically transplanted small-bowel grafts irradiated with 0, 250, or 500 rad (groups 1–3) all succumbed to GvH disease characterized by severe weight loss, diarrhea, dermatitis, and alopecia. Average survival for these three groups was 14.4 ± 3.0, 15.0 ± 1.3, and 14.2 ± 1.9 days respectively. Postmortem findings included splenomegaly and a normal appearance of the transplanted bowel, but enteritis of the native small bowel. Histologically, recipient lymph nodes (Fig. 1) and spleen (Fig. 2) showed marked lymphocytic depletion and loss of normal architecture; the recipient small bowel showed mucosal destruction and enteritis, while the transplanted bowel remained histologically intact. Recipients of grafts irradiated with 1000 rad (group 4) developed none of these changes, and all remained alive and healthy until they were killed. No gross or microscopic abnormalities were present in group 4 graft recipients; specifically, the spleen and lymph nodes showed normal cellularity and architecture (Fig. 1C, 2C) and both donor (with the exception of disuse atrophy) and recipient small bowel were microscopically normal.

Orthotopic Transplantation

Control animals remained alive and healthy throughout the study period. Group 5 animals undergoing orthotopic transplantation of nonirradiated grafts had clinical courses identical to animals in groups 1–3. Mean survival was 14.0 ± 0.7 days.

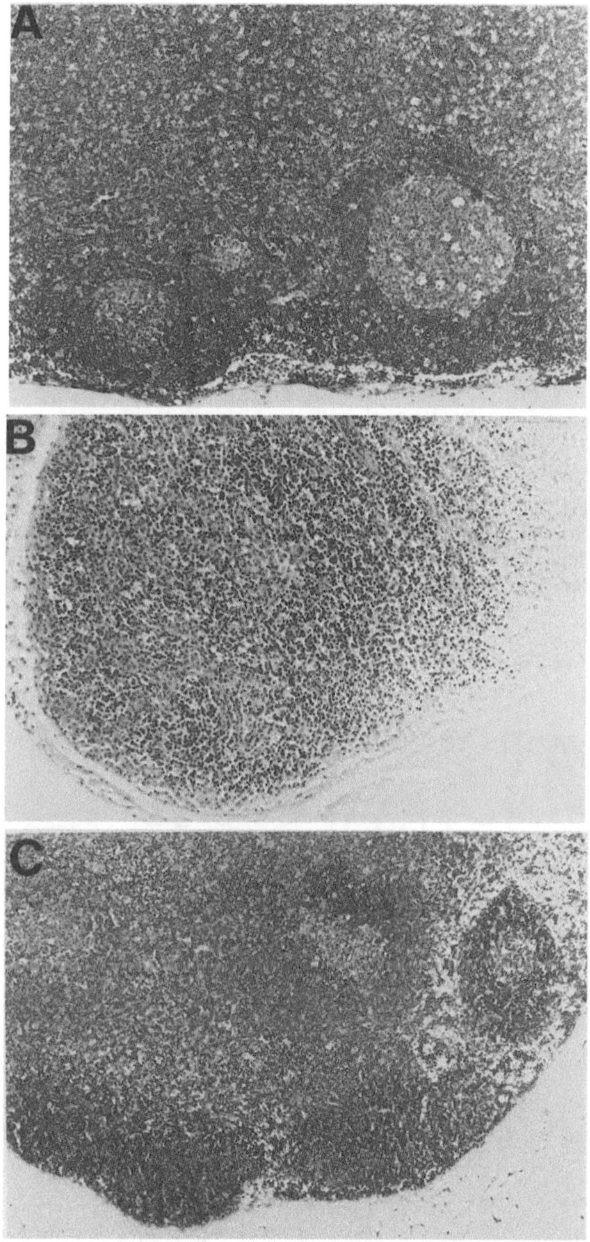

Fig. 1A–C. Histologic changes in the lymph nodes of LBN-F_1 recipients of LEW intestinal allografts. **A** Normal rat lymph node. **B** Lymph node from a recipient of a LEW intestinal allograft irradiated with 500 rad. Lymphocytic depletion and loss of normal follicular architecture are seen. **C** Lymph node from a recipient of a LEW allograft irradiated with 1000 rad. Normal histologic features are seen (hematoxylin-eosin stain; × 100)

Postmortem findings were also similar to the findings in the heterotopic graft recipients in groups 1–3. Group 6 animals undergoing orthotopic transplantation of small-bowel grafts irradiated in vitro with 1000 rad remained alive and healthy for more than 18 months, except for two animals which died of bowel obstruction secondary to adhesions on the 24th and 41st postoperative days; neither of these

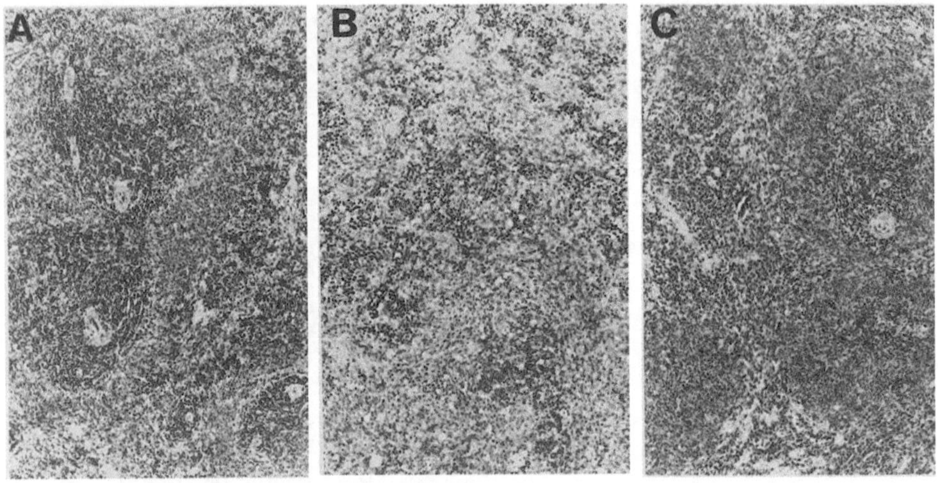

Fig. 2A–C. Histologic changes in the spleen of LBN-F_1 recipients of LEW intestinal allografts. **A** Normal spleen. **B** Spleen from a recipient of a LEW allograft irradiated with 500 rad. Lymphocytic depletion of the white pulp is seen. **C** Spleen from a recipient of a LEW allograft irradiated with 1000 rad. The normal histologic features are preserved (hematoxylin-eosin stain; × 100)

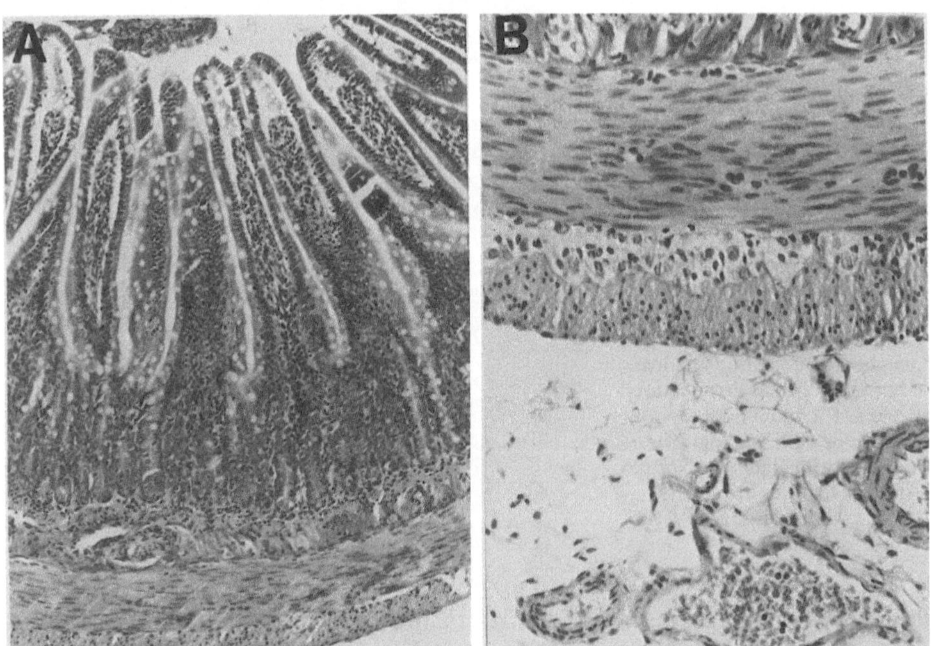

Fig. 3A, B. Histologic appearance of an intestinal graft irradiated with 1000 rad. **A** The mucosa is normal (hematoxylin-eosin stain; × 100). **B** Normal appearance of submucosa and small mesenteric vessels are free of changes suggestive of radiation injury (trichrome; × 200)

animals had gross or microscopic evidence of GvH disease. Lymph node biopsies from group 6 animals demonstrated normal cellularity and architecture, and full-thickness graft biopsies showed a normal intact mucosa (Fig. 3A). Stigmata of radiation injury of the graft such as small-vessel endarteritis or bowel fibrosis were absent (Fig. 3B). The rate of weight gain (51.8% ± 11.7%), serum albumin (3.9 ± 0.7 g/dl), and serum triglycerides (67.0 ± 24.3 mg/dl) for group 6 animals 120 days after transplantation were not significantly different from the values for the age-matched normal LEW rat and LEW rats with isografts.

Discussion

This study confirms that GvH disease may occur following small-bowel transplantation in appropriate rat strain combinations and demonstrates that irradiation of intestinal allografs in vitro prior to transplantation effectively and consistently prevents the development of GvH disease. The effective dose of 1000 rad has been shown to cause pyknotic changes in rat lymphocytes irradiated in vitro (Trowell 1952), suggesting that graft irradiation destroys or functionally impairs the donor lymphocytes which mediate GvH disease.

The long-term, nutritionally healthy survival of animals reciving orthotopic allografts irradiated with 1000 rad and the absence of gross or microscopic evidence of radiation injury support the safety of in vitro allograft irradiation. Irradiation of exteriorized but vascularized rat intestine with 900 rad causes only transient changes in the intestinal epithelium with no residual abnormalities (Sullivan et al. 1959); under hypoxic conditions, no changes in the intestinal epithelium are observed after irradiation with 1050 rad (Forsberg et al. 1978).

In vitro, human lymphocytes are slightly more radiosensitive than rat lymphocytes (Schrek 1958). If GvH disease should occur in human small-bowel transplantation, irradiation with 1000 rad should be sufficient to prevent its development without causing intestinal radiation injury; this is supported in a report by Localio et al. (1969), who found that intestinal radiation injury is unlikely at cumulative doses of less than 3500 rad. The hypoxic conditions under which in vitro irradiation is performed will reduce the potential risk of radiation injury even further. We therefore believe that in vitro irradiation of small-bowel allografts is a safe and effective method of preventing the development of GvH disease.

References

Deltz E, Müller-Hermelink HK, Ulrichs K, Thiede A, Müller-Ruchholtz W (1981) Development of graft-versus-host reaction in various target organs after small intestine transplantation. Transplant Proc 13:1215–1216

Deltz E, Ulrichs K, Schack Th, Friedrichs B, Müller-Ruchholtz W, Thiede A (1985) Distribution and kinetics of anti-host cytotoxicity in a graft-versus-host reaction and after its suppression in small intestine transplantation. Transplant Proc 17:886

Forsberg JO, Jung B, Larsson B (1978) Mucosal protection during irradiation of exteriorized rat ileum. Acta Radiol (Oncol) 17:485–496

Kirkman RL, Lear PA, Madara JL, Tilney NL (1984) Small intestine transplantation in the rat: immunology and function. Surgery 96:280–287

Localio SA, Stone A, Friedman M (1969) Surgical aspects of radiation enteritis. Surg Gynecol Obstet 129:1163–1172.

Pomposelli F, Maki T, Kiyoizumi T, Gaber L, Balogh K, Monaco AP (1985) Induction of graft-versus-host disease by small intestinal allotransplantation in rats. Transplantation 40:343–347

Schraut WH, Rosemurgy AS, Riddell RM (1983) Prolongation of intestinal allograft survival without immunosuppressive drug therapy. Transplantation of small bowel allografts. J Surg Res 34:597–607.

Schraut WH, Abraham VSd, Lee KKW (1985) Portal versus systemic venous drainage for small-bowel allografts. Surgery 98:579–585

Schrek R (1958) In vitro sensitivity of normal human lymphocytes to x-rays and radiomimetic agents. J Lab Clin Med 51:904–915

Sullivan MF, Marks S, Hackett PL, Thompson RC (1959) X-irradiation of the exteriorized or in situ intestine of the rat. Radiat Res 11:653–666

Trowell OA (1952) The sensitivity of lymphocytes to ionising radiation. J Pathol Bacteriol 64:687–704

*Graft Acceptance: Modification of Immunogenicity of the Donor or the Donor Organ with or without Host Immunosuppression**

M. A. Hardy, J. Chabot, G. Tannenbaum, and A. J. Benvenisty

Introduction

Failure of the few reported clinical attempts at small-intestinal transplantation and the greatly improved efficacy and safety of total parenteral nutrition, bringing with it a much greater financial cost, have resulted in a general decrease in interest in small-intestinal transplantation. The use of contemporary immunosuppressive regimens has not yet sufficiently improved the results of intestinal transplantation to the extent that extensive clinical trials are warrented. The purpose of this discussion is to elaborate on approaches and methods which may permit avoidance of chronic immunosuppression of the host and allow for induction of specific donor allograft unresponsiveness. The development of such approaches may eventually permit clinical intestinal transplantation.

Models of specific unresponsiveness can be divided into two major groups as suggested by Hall (1984). One category of immunologic unresponsiveness focuses on the manipulation of the natural process of self- and nonself-recognition which occurs in early development and which has as its classical demonstration neonatal tolerance, (creation of bone marrow chimeras), as well as the use of total immunologic ablation of the adult host with total lymphoid irradiation (TLI) and/or selective lymphoid irradiation (SLI) (Hardy et al. 1979). The other major effort is directed at manipulating the response of mature immune systems, i.e., in adults, to prevent specific responses and includes enhancement models, suppressor cell systems, and anti-idiotype antibody manipulations. Yet another approach in adults, which has not been sufficiently emphasized in the manipulation of immediately vascularized organ allografts, consists of the modification of the donor or donor organ so as to favorably influence its acceptance by the host. Such donor or donor organ manipulations may considerably facilitate the manipulation of the mature immune system, as well as influence the recovery of the immunologic system made transiently immature. Although more is known about the mechanisms of unresponsiveness in the nonchimeric states where allogeneic grafts are markedly prolonged, more reliable achievements of complete tolerance are attained in the chimeric forms of immunologic unresponsiveness. Chimeras characteristically exhibit tolerance, defined by acceptance of a second-set, donor-specific graft and a lack of mixed lymphocyte reactivity (MLR) between the donor and host lymphocytes; nonchimeric

* Supported in part by NIH grants HL14799, AM34232, and AM30468 and Irvington House Institute Fellowship.

unresponsive hosts are generally able to reject a second-set graft and retain donor-host alloreactivity in MLR and in graft-vs-host (GvH) assays. Immunologic unresponsiveness is induced as listed below:

1) Chimera
   - neonatal tolerance
   - TLI
   - bone marrow chimera (in adults)
2) Nonchimera
   a) Host
      - enhancement
      - blood transfusion
      - peritransplant cyclosporine
      - peritransplant antilymphoid serum (ALS)
      - anti-Ia antibody
      - irradiation
   b) Donor
      - antigen
      - concanavalin A
      - steroids
      - cyclophosphamide
      - irradiation
      - UV light

We intend to consider models of immunologic unresponsiveness in the adult which avoid chronic immunosuppression and which may have special clinical applicability to intestinal transplantation. We will initially discuss the approaches to immunologic manipulation of the host and then concentrate on the issue of manipulation of the donor or the donor organ that may be synergistic with brief, peritransplant manipulation of the host.

Manipulation of the Host

Chimerism

Chimeras are created by implantation of appropriate allogeneic bone marrow cells into the host during the neonatal period or by TLI followed by restoration with allogeneic immunocompetent cells, as has been recently suggested by RAPAPORT et al. (1982). Mechanisms proposed to explain such models of tolerance include deletion of alloreactive clones and proliferation of donor-specific suppressor cells. BURNET (1959) originally concluded on the basis of his work with chimeras that tolerance is mediated by clonal deletion, while WOOD et al. (1985) more recently concluded that neonatal tolerance is mediated by deletion of specific alloreactive helper T cell clones. DORSCH and ROSER (1982a, b), by transferring tolerance via lymphocytes from neonatally tolerant rats into sublethally irradiated syngeneic hosts, emphasized the importance of suppressor cells in the maintenance of neonatal tolerance.

Although fully allogeneic and stable bone marrow chimeras can now be created in many animal models using whole-body irradiation and reconstitution with T cell depleted bone marrow, this approach is hampered by numerous technical and theoretical disadvantages. Such chimeras are often chronically ill and unable to mount strong immune responses against antigens presented in association with donor major histocompatibility (MHC) antigens, probably because of inadequate "education" of T cells within the host thymus (SPRENT 1978). It is well known that fully allogeneic bone marrow transplantation remains extremely difficult clinically and in itself has many complex, unsolved, and clinically dangerous problems. Thus, allogeneic bone marrow transplantation in an attempt to achieve chimerism is probably not a suitable alternative for transplantation of organs other than bone marrow. However, allogeneic bone marrow transplantation in modified form and with a minimal amount of bone marrow cells as described by MONACO and WOOD (1982) and THOMAS et al. (1983), may be useful in the manipulation of the host immune responses by other mechanisms than chimerism (perhaps microchimerism) and should be studied further.

Nonchimeric States

Manipulation of the host immune response prior to transplantation by administration of immunologic, as opposed to pharmacologic reagents, is relatively new in clinical medicine. This type of approach needs to be explored further in relation to intestinal transplantation, particularly since small-bowel allografts have large numbers of reactive lymphocytes. Intestinal transplantation, therefore, requires not only the abolition of rejection, but the elimination of GvH reaction to be successful. In other organ transplants, allogeneic unresponsiveness has been induced by a variety of methods that do not involve the induction of chimerism. Some of these include enhancement (BATCHELOR and WELSH 1976; HALL 1984; WILSON et al. 1969); the use of anti-Ia antibodies (PERRY and WILLIAMS 1985); donor-specific transfusions (LENHARD et al. 1985; BURLINGHAM et al. 1985; MARQUET and HEYSTEK 1981; REED et al. 1985; WOOD KJ et al. 1985); and short-term treatments with cyclosporine (NAGAO et al. 1982; WHITE et al. 1983; YOSHIMURA and KAHAN 1985), antilymphocyte globulins (MJORNSTEDT et al. 1983), and a variety of antilymphocyte monoclonal antibodies (COBBOLD et al. 1984).

The various methods of host pretreatment and treatment that do not involve induction of chimerism can be viewed as variants of enhancement (HALL 1984). Such approaches involve initially either the introduction of specific alloantigens during the pretransplant phase and/or a period of protective immunosuppression until the maintenance phase of enhancement is achieved. Reviews of this subject (BATCHELOR and WELSH 1976; HALL 1984) describe four mechanisms of graft acceptance in such situations: graft mediation, immune paralysis by soluble antigen, anti-idiotypic antibodies, and suppressor cells. We have previously demonstrated the feasibility of regularly inducing unresponsiveness to cardiac allografts in rats by the use of SLI and antithymocyte globulin (ATG), by the occasional addition of small doses of donor-type bone marrow (Hardy et al. 1979; Oluwole et al. 1979; Hardy et al. 1981; Oluwole et al. 1980), and by the use of UV-irradiated donor-type blood transfusions (Lau et al. 1983; Hardy et al. 1984). In the strongly histocompatible strain combinations, these approaches have usually required a brief peritransplant treatment, with either ATG or cyclosporine as part of the therapeutic protocol. Monaco and Wood (1982), in a continuing series of murine experiments, have observed that antilymphocyte antibody therapy appears to be particularly effective in facilitating the induction of unresponsiveness. In a series of elegant studies, these investigators demonstrated induction of immunologic unresponsiveness in mice to skin allografs, using appropriate doses of selected bone marrow cell inocula following transplantation in animals briefly treated with ATG. The mechanism of induction of such immunologic unresponsiveness appeared to rely primarily on development of donor-specific suppressor T cells (Monaco et al. 1985). Thomas et al. (1983) have recently shown long-term renal allograft survival in monkeys without the requirement of chronic immunosuppression using a similar approach. In this model, they were able to demonstrate the appearance of donor-specific suppressor cells in the renal allografts themselves. Their regimen, including a brief course of post-transplant ATG therapy, donor bone marrow infusion, and no further therapy, clearly demonstrated the possibility of effective immunologic manipulation of the recipient, which might be particularly useful in clinical intestinal transplantation and appears to rely primarily on development of donor-specific suppressor cells.

Another approach which deserves further intensive evaluation in intestinal transplantation is based on the usefulness of some form of TLI as part of the immunosuppressive regimen which permits induction of an immunologically unresponsive state (Slavin et al. 1977). Initial studies by Strober et al. (1984), which were recently extended to clinical renal transplantation (Sampson et al. 1985), offer an approach to immunologic manipulation of the patient that results in immunologic unresponsiveness. It carries, however, significant morbidity regarding radiation and is somewhat impractical in relation to donor organ procurement. Our development of SLI and the introduction of short peritransplant treatment with ATG (Hardy et al. 1979), is analogous to the use of TLI and may be easier to apply clinically. Both of these approaches, TLI or SLI, with brief peritransplant courses of ATG, led to specific immunologic unresponsiveness, which in the case of SLI was clearly shown to be suppressor cell dependent by appropriate transfer experiments (Hardy et al. 1981). It is possible, but unlikely, that the brief peritransplant immunosuppression that has been found to be so effective in induction of immunologic unresponsiveness when combined with host irradiation may affect the donor antigen-present cells (APC) carried over in the graft, as suggested by studies of Batchelor et al. (1979), Fabre and Morris (1972), and others (Bowen et al. 1981; Stuart et al. 1971). Proposals suggesting that systemic release of graft antigen paralyzes the immune response do not adequately explain active inhibition of graft rejection in the host animal. A much more likely explanation for the specific immunologic unresponsiveness in the nonchimeric animal may be found in the development of anti-idiotypic antibodies and/or donor-specific suppressor cells.

Wood et al. (1985), using a single leukocyte-depleted blood transfusion, produced indefinite survival of renal allografts in the rat. No antibody-mediated effect was detected as an explanation for this phenomenon. Utilizing multiple blood transfusion protocols in the rat, LENHARD et al. (1985) were able to demonstrate the appearance of suppressor cells by the transfer of spleen cells from the tolerant rats to syngeneic animals. In our own studies of cardiac allograft survival in animals receiving donor-specific blood transfusions with and without UV irradiation, we were able to demonstrate suppressor cell mechanisms only intermittently (OLUWOLE et al. 1985), while in the experiments utilizing SLI and ATG, the suppressor cell mechanism was clearly shown by appropriate transfer experiments (HARDY et al. 1981). In clinical situations, we have shown the presence of anti-idiotypic antibodies after donor-specific transfusions in renal transplant recipients (REED et al. 1985), while others have suggested the appearance of specific suppressor cells. It is thus unclear whether anti-idiotypic antibodies or suppressor cells form the primary basis for the effectiveness of donor-specific transfusions in prolonging allograft survival. Although the presence of anti-idiotypic antibodies has been demonstrated in animal models with long-standing allografts (McKEARN et al. 1974), it is likely that both anti-idiotypic antibodies and suppressor cells play an important role in the induction of specific allograft unresponsiveness by various types of enhancement protocols. It is further possible that a better understanding of the mechanisms involved in the induction of immunologic unresponsiveness by such enhancement protocols will permit us to manipulate the host directly by the use of appropriate anti-idiotypic antibodies, which is already beginning at the experimental level.

It is possible that in an approach to the regulation of transplantation immunity in vivo, antibodies directed against host la molecules may alter the course of host immunity (PERRY et al. 1979; PERRY and WILLIAMS 1985; WALDOR et al. 1983) and thus convert a potential immune response into a tolerant response. This would be most important in induction of donor-specific unresponsiveness in the host. The usefulness of this approach will be further explored in the discussion on the treatment of the donor and particularly of the donor organ, where the primary aim will be the elimination or alteration of the Ia-bearing donor APC cells or dendritic cells. It should be remembered that Ia-equivalent glycoproteins in the mouse and other species have been categorized as class II antigens to distinguish them from the structurally and functionally distinct class I antigens. The mechanisms by which antibodies directed against class II gene products influence the pattern of immunity are twofold. The first exists at the level of T cell-APC interactions required for antigen presentation (SCHWARTZ et al. 1976). Antibody-induced blockade and redistribution of cell surface Ia antigens directly inhibit T cell-APC binding (ZIEGLER and UNANUE 1979) and thus prevent the induction of recognition. This may have obvious applicability not only in the treatment of the host, as is being explored presently, but particularly in the modification of the donor organ. Re-expression of class II molecules 72 h after a single antibody injection correlates with the return of APC function in one study (KRUISBEEK et al. 1985) and therefore may be more applicable to the treatment of the donor or the donor organ than that of the recipient, unless it is used on a repetitive basis. Several studies have revealed that anti-Ia antibody-mediated inhibition of transplant rejection (WILLIAMS and PERRY 1985) and of tumor immunity (PERRY and GREENEE 1982) are due not only to the effects of antibody and antigen presentation, but also to the activation of antigen-specific suppressor T cells that serve to maintain a state of specific unresponsiveness in the absence of continued treatment. It is obvious, therefore, that there is a close interrelationship between the use of anti-Ia antibodies, the development of anti-Ia antibodies in the host, antigen presentation, and, most importantly, suppressor cell activation, which is important in the maintenance of an immunologically unresponsive state. Thus, even with successful manipulation of the donor or the donor organ so that its presence is not readily recognized by the host initially, approaches must be found to manipulate the host in such a way as to allow the graft to adapt without the use of chronic immunosuppression.

Cyclosporine is the only pharmacologic agent currently available with selective toxicity towards helper and cytotoxic lymphocytes that may logically be considered for use concomitant with anti-Ia therapy and other specific immunologic manipulation of the host. Peritransplant treatment of allograft recipients with cyclosporine alone has already produced extended graft survival in dogs and in rats. Yoshimura and Kahan (1985) have recently demonstrated the appearance of a donor-specific T suppressor cell population, 10 days after heart allografts of rats which received a single dose of a solubilized donor antigen and three doses of cyclosporine. Since it is presently thought that treatment of recipients with anti-Ia antibodies results in eventual development of donor-specific suppressor T cells, it is likely that a combination of immunologic as well as pharmacologic treatments using cyclosporine may be synergistic and eventually most effective in inducing specific donor unresponsiveness to an allograft.

The consideration of this or any other experimental therapy for clinical application, particularly of an organ that is not in the category of life-saving replacement, depends upon its relative merits and drawbacks when compared with available and proven treatment protocols. Immunosuppression of the transplant recipient using pharmacologic agents with broad toxicity against all dividing cells and nonspecific immunologic effects, as well as the more recent use of cyclosporine has resulted in many different, undesirable toxic side effects which are detrimental to the patient's well-being and which have been ineffective for intestinal transplantation. In a continuing effort to develop more specific immunosuppression of the recipient, which would be particularly important in the so far impractical transplantation of small bowel, the advantage of anticlass II immunotherapy, when compared with any drug therapy, lies in its immunologic specificity in inducing long-term unresponsiveness to donor alloantigens without affecting normal recognition of environmental pathogens and in the lack of a requirement for prolonged antibody treatment. In addition, this might prove to be extremely useful in the treatment of the donor organ (vide infra) and may prove to be most beneficial when the approaches are combined. The use of other monoclonal antibodies is probably impractical except for treatment of rejection. These would include in particular those reactive with T cell idiotypes, which would require individual tailoring, as well as anti-T cell subset monoclonal antibodies, such as anti-OKT3 and anti-T12, which are being clinically evaluated. This is because antibody efficacy is gradually reduced by host recognition of the injected mouse immunoglobulins, while prolonged treatment may be necessary to induce long-term acceptance of an allograft. It is hoped that eventually the use of anti-Ia antibodies in the treatment of the host in clinical transplantation (anti-DR) will lead to the induction of donor alloantigen-specific suppressor cells and thus results in no further need for treatment of the transplant recipient.

Donor and Donor Organ Pretreatment

Dramatic strides have been made in the last 5 years regarding the knowledge of the molecular basis of human T cell differentiation and recognition. T Cell surface molecules have been identified by the use of monoclonal antibodies and divided into three major classes: (a) differentiation, (b) activation, and (c) antigen receptor (idiotype) molecules. In dealing with the host, our attention was turned to differentiation markers and most recently to antigen receptor molecules, while in discussing donor and donor organ pretreatment, we need to concentrate on the activation markers. These fall into two categories: molecules with a restricted distribution and those widely found on dividing cells. While the IL-2 receptor is in the restricted category, the HLA-DR marker is one of those found on most dividing cells. Obviously, the specific markers are more suitable as therapeutic targets. Since the activation markers appear in an overlapping sequence, it is possible that, eventually, elimination of cells carrying such markers will depend on the use of a family of monoclonal antibodies in order to delay or prevent the eventual modulation of the target cells. Meanwhile, this must be considered only as a complementary approach in conjunction with immunologic modification of the host. The small bowel a high lymphoid cell content, which not only stimulates rapid rejection by the host, but also responds in a GvH graft reaction as described elsewhere in this workshop. Therefore, the elimination of the appropriate lymphoid cells may decrease the incidence of its rejection and prevent or decrease the incidence of GvH reaction.

Studies using endocrine, skin, kidney, and heart grafts pretreated with cytotoxic agents (Corry et al. 1980; Guttman et al. 1975; Guttman and Lindquist 1969; McCabe et al. 1980; McKenzie et al. 1984a, b; Zincke et al. 1978), ALS (Freeman et al. 1971), irradiation (McKenzie et al. 1984a, b; Steinmuller et al. 1971; Wolf and Hume 1966), tissue culture (Lacy et al. 1979; Sollinger et al. 1977; White et al. 1983; Yasunami et al. 1983), and UVB irradiation (Hardy et al. 1984; Lau et al. 1984a, b) have all led to a relative decrease in organ immunogenicity. The original work of Elkins and Gutman (1968) demonstrated that "passenger leukocytes" are primarily responsible for allograft immunogenicity. They induced a local GvH reaction with Lewis rat lymphocytes inplanted in a Lewis kidney which was originally transplanted into a (Lewis x BN) F_1 hybrid. The work of Steinmuller (1967) subsequently showed that skin grafts from mouse chimeras (A × B) were rejected by the original A strain mouse and that this must have been induced by cells from the B strain carried by the skin graft. Since these important experiments, interest in APC manipulation has persisted. We have recently reviewed this subject; the reader is referred to that review for further discussion (Hardy and Lau 1986) and to Snell's original article (Snell 1957).

It is well known that cell-mediated immune response depends on interaction between the T cell and an antigen-presenting cell which results in T cell activation. Experimental evidence supports the hypothesis that the APC stimulates the T cell with two signals (Lafferty et al. 1983). One signal involves the foreign antigen in association with the MHC antigen, while the second signal includes the T cell activation factor, which induces T cell growth factor (IL-2) receptors and IL-2 production by the T cell. According to Lafferty et al. (1983), graft APC, stimulator cells (S+), are unique in that they not only present foreign antigens, but they are capable of production of the second signal – the activation factor – necessary for specific T cell activation. The cell type responsible for such antigen presentation appears to be a morphologically unique cell found within the spleen, which is described as a dendritic cell that has been found in the stroma of most organs and tissues examined (STEINMAN and WILMER 1978; STEINMAN et al. 1979).

Allograft rejection is primarily a cell-mediated immune response. Small-intestinal and pancreatic islet allografts are rejected rapidly if transplanted across MHC or even minor histocompatibility barriers. It is already well known that dendritic cells are present in the pancreatic islets, and our own preliminary evidence strongly suggests that such dendritic cells are also present in small-intestinal allografts in Peyer's patches. We have now postulated that, analogous to the situation in pancreatic islets, the APC cells in MHC-incompatible allografts present their MHC antigen directly to the recipient immune system. Since the MHC being recognized is of the class I type in both small-bowel transplantation and in pancreatic islets, cytotoxic T cells are generated and kill the graft in a specific manner. If such a mechanism of T cell activation applies in small-bowel allograft rejection, and if such activated T cells are primarily responsible for graft rejection, then elimination of the APC from the donor organ, either by vigorous pretreatment of the donor and/or pretreatment of the donor organ in vitro, should lead to reduced immunogenicity of the organ.

Donor Pretreatment

Modulation of the afferent limb of immune response has obvious and distinct advantages over techniques of recipient immunosuppression. Previous reports (NOWYGROD et al. 1979; TODD et al. 1978) have shown hat prolongation of allograft survival by donor treatment prior to donor organ removal is experimentally possible both for renal and cardiac allografts. The suggested mechanism of this prolongation is thought to be depletion of passenger leukocytes. Early clinical results were also promising (GUTTMAN et al. 1975; ZINCKE et al. 1978), but were never confirmed in randomized clinical studies. Because of unimproved and sometimes conflicting results in the use of donor pretreatment protocols in clinical renal transplantation, the subject never regained the interest that it deserves. Our own interest in this area included experiments in rodents where donors were treated with cyclophosphamide, ALG, and total body irradiation and where the hearts of Fisher donors were transplanted to Lewis recipients which were either unmodified or mildly immunosuppressed (NOWYGROD et al. 1978, 1979; TODD et al. 1978). The results of these studies, in terms of cardiac allograft survival, were correlated with the newly developed quantitative assay of graft passenger leukocyte in the heart using Indium-111 oxine-labeled cells (NOWYGROD et al. 1979) prior to, during, and following donor pretreatment. In vivo treatment of the donor with ALG 24 h prior to obtaining the donor heart led to doubling of the cardiac allograft survival with effective Indium-111-labeled leukocyte depletion from the cardiac allograft. Pretreatment of the donor with cyclophosphamide, on the other hand, resulted in no decrease in Indium-111-labeled cells in the cardiac allograft and yet led to identical prolongation of cardiac allograft survival in the nonimmunosuppressed host. Thus, it appears either that the appropriate cells were not labeled, which is possible since these experiments were done prior to our ability to identify dendritic cells with appropriate monoclonal antibodies, or less likely, that donor pretreatment does not result in subsequent allograft prolongation because of alteration in graft parenchymal cells. It is possible that the conflicting positive and negative results of donor pretreatment reported from a number of laboratories are due to variable and incomplete depletion of donor passenger leukocytes or to the depletion of inappropriate cells.

Donor Organ Pretreatment

The problems of rejection and GvH reaction remains the greatest obstacle to successful intestinal transplantation. Although the whole small intestine is strongly immunogenic, its stimulatory ability probably derives primarily from the cells in the accompanying lymph nodes in the mesentery and from the cells present in Peyer's patches. Whether the accompanying endothelial cells and intestinal mucosal cells are equally stimulatory is uncertain. Studies by LECHLER and BATCHELOR (1982a, b) in rat kidney transplantation suggest that the elimination of donor APC may be most important in immediately vascularized organ transplantation. It appears that, for both isolated cell and vascularized organ allografts, the stimulatory cell is the dendritic cell. FAUSTMAN et al. (1981) treated pancreatic islets from the mouse with antidendritic cell monoclonal antibodies and complement and produced extended survival of the islets without host immunosuppression after a clear demonstration of elimination of Ia+ dendritic cells. In short, it appears that in all systems where allograft prolongation was achieved by either graft and/or donor organ pretreatment, the major reason for such accomplishment depended on selective destruction or inactivation of passenger leukocytes or dendritic cells.

It is beyond the scope of this discussion to review in detail past work in this area summarized by BILLINGHAM (1971) and recently reviewed (HARDY and LAU 1986). Briefly, organ culture, especially in a high oxygen environment, has been shown to allow thyroid allografts (LAFFERTY et al. 1976) and xenografts (SOLLINGER et al. 1977) and pancreatic allografts (LACY and DAVIE 1984) to survive for extended periods in rodents. High oxygen or low temperature in such cultures has been shown to be selectively toxic for lymphoreticular cells. Although there are no established systems for the culture of solid organs, BATCHELOR and his colleagues developed a somewhat analogous process for kidney allograft pretreatment (BATCHELOR et al. 1979; LECHLER and BATCHELOR 1982a, b). Allogeneic rat kidneys were passaged through rats which had been treated with an enhancement protocol, and subsequently these passaged kidneys were successfully retransplanted into secondary hosts which had not been enhanced. Of particular interest was that exposure of such passaged kidneys to allogeneic lymphoid cells prior to transplantation abrogated the protective effect of such intermediate hosts. SOLLINGER et al. (1985) used the "nude" mouse to passage both human parathyroids and fetal pancreata in order to deplete them of APC. That the prolongation in such systems depends on the almost complete elimination of intragraft passenger cells has been strongly suggested by the experiments of TALMADGE et al. (1976), who showed that established endocrine allografts will be promptly rejected when exposed to as few as 1000 cells bearing donor-type class II antigens. Our own experiments (HARDY et al. 1984), using UV irradiation as a treatment method for donor pancreatic islets or donor-type blood transfusions, suggested that it is inactivation, not necessarily elimination, of the passenger leukocytes that increases graft viability. We have shown that with appropriate doses of UVB irradiation, the antigen-presenting function of the lymphoreticular cells is altered so as to render them ineffective as stimulator cells, as previously shown by LINDAHL-KIESSLING and SAFWENBERG (1971). Furthermore, when three-way MLR is performed by mixing UV-treated lymphocyte stimulators with responders differing at class I and class II antigens, in the presence of gamma-irradiated cells that differ from responders only at the Ia region, a marked proliferative response occurs (TOMINAGA et al. 1983). Thus, UVB irradiation abrogates the effect of the class II antigen-presenting cells apparently without affecting class I presentation, which may be tolerogenic under some circumstances. In our own experiments, where UVB treatment of rat islets resulted in prolonged survival of allografts and xenografts without host immunosuppression, such prolongation was easily abolished by injection of small numbers of donor strain rat dendritic cells, administered either at the time of transplantation or 250 days after transplantation (LAU et al. 1984a). Thus, with this type of donor organ modification, allograft acceptance does not represent true tolerance of the neonatal type. Other methods of graft pretreatment which result in long-term survival of allografts without host immunosuppression have included the demonstration of the effect of anticlass II antisera with complement in the mouse system (FAUSTMAN et al. 1981). It is important to know that a mouse anti-Ia monoclonal antibody has recently been shown to inhibit the stimulatory capacity of rat spleen cells in an MLR (NAKAHARA et al. 1985). It has been suggested, therefore, that such monoclonal antibodies may be effective for graft pretreatment of immediately vascularized organs, particularly if they can penetrate adequately into the various tissues.

Although we have considered the use of anticlass II monoclonal antibodies in the section concerned with host manipulation, additional considerations which are critically important for the clinical use of such antibodies will be mentioned here. Firstly, the nature of the antibody to be used, with regard to isotype, specificity, and affinity, must be carefully selected for maximal efficiency in vivo, when appropriate, or in vitro, when treating an organ directly. Antibodies of the IgG_1 subclass may prove most useful in treatment of the donor organ, since they penetrate tissues more readily than IgM molecules but do not fix complement. On the other hand, reagents of the IgG_2 subclass and most IgG isotypes have been used extensively in mice, dogs, and primates, and their their lack of toxicity is well known. MCKENZIE et al. (1984a), using monoclonal antibodies against class I and class II antigens and immunofluorescence, demonstrated a marked reduction of dendritic cells in kidney and cardiac allografts pretreated by cyclophosphamide and irradiation. More importantly, subsequent graft survival correlated directly with the degree of dendritic cell depletion in this model. Our preliminary studies suggest that similar events may occur in intestinal transplantation, but that they are more complex because of the heavy lymphoid burden in the small bowel and its mesentery.

Other methods of direct organ pretreatment utilize direct irradiation of the graft, which leads to prolongation of allograft survival of heart and kidneys in rat models (STEINMULLER et al. 1971) and in dogs (WOLF and HUME 1966). GUTTMAN et al.

(1969, 1975) and others (CORRY et al. 1980; MCCABE et al. 1980; RUCKER et al. 1982) have shown that pretreatment of the organ with various pharmacologic agents, which included cyclophosphamide, methylprednisolone, methotrexate, and most recently cyclosporine A, resulted in what appeared to be improved graft survival in allogeneic hosts. Some of these experiments were difficult to interpret, since agents like cyclophosphamide need to be metabolized prior to their use, which was not the case in the experiments presented (MCCABE et al. 1980) but may be the case with cyclosporine. Initial efforts at donor pretreatment or treatment of isolated perfused organs utilized primarily nonspecific cytotoxic or cytolytic agents.

In an attempt to be more specific in the treatment of donor organs, we have previously used a phytomitogen, namely concanavalin A (Con A), to perfuse donor grafts ex vivo. While Con A can act as a nonspecific cellular and humoral immunosuppressant, the observation that it can attach to and interfere with the recognition of histocompatibility receptor sites led others to the hypothesis that it might mask graft antigens by binding to cell surfaces and thus interfere with recipient sensitization. Despite initial encouraging results obtained in experiments with canine renal allografts (LEON and SCHWARTZ 1969; STEINMULLER and COLEMAN 1970; TOLEDO-PEREYRA et al. 1974a), the initial hypothesis of simple antigen masking was incorrect, since surface-bound Con A was shown to disappear 7–24 h post perfusion (DE WOLF et al. 1976). In our own studies, we found that Con A heart-graft perfusion under conditions previously reported by others to be successful in dog and rat kidney allografts did not prolong cardiac allograft survival in the rat (NOWYGROD et al. 1978). Despite such discouraging results in the past, the availability of modern technology, particularly the availability of new series of monoclonal and polyclonal antibodies which have specific targets, makes the idea of ex vivo organ pretreatment most attractive as a method that may lead to effective allograft prolongation with minimal host immunosuppression.

Small Intestine

The usefulness of donor pretreatment and organ treatment in small-intestinal transplantation needs to be determined. This is especially true, since the small intestine has a high lymphocyte content, and intragraft cellularity can now be precisely identified in regard to lymphocyte subsets, dendritic cells, and Ia-positive cells by newly available libraries of monoclonal antibodies. Such antibodies can be used not only for identification of specific cells, but also for their selective depletion in vivo. Pretreatment of the donor organ should be more easily accomplished after donor pretreatment, if one views this approach in a mechanical fashion. It should be realized that some agents require in vivo processing before they can take effect. For example, cyclophosphamide is ineffective in organ perfusion unless it passes through the liver and is converted to its active form, while ATG and most monoclonal antibodies directed against lymphocyte subsets will not be cytotoxic without complement. One must be very careful in designing experimental or clinical protocols that utilize commonly effective agents in vivo in isolated perfusions that are performed in vitro. Some donor pretreatments may therefore be more effective than isolated donor organ treatment; usually, the two methods will be complementary.

Very few reports have been published about donor pretreatment or graft manipulation in regard to small-intestinal transplantation. Existing reports are difficult to interpret, because only animal survival has been used as the end point of experiments which may be confused by technical problems, rejection, infection, or GvH disease. Toledo-Pereyra et al. (1974b) noted that canine small-intestinal allografts that were preserved for 24 h prior to transplantation survived considerably longer than allografts transplanted immediatley. The median survival time of dogs was 16 days for those transplanted immediately, as compared with 28 days in the group whose allografts were perfused with cold canine cryoprecipitated plasma and 50 days in the group perfused with cold human Plasmanate. It is important to note that in both groups whose allografts were preserved for 24 h, the perfusates included methylprednisolone (500 mg/liter), while the immediately transplanted dogs received intestinal allografts that were not exposed to the high dose of steroids.

Another form of modification of donor graft immunogenicity that has important historical precedent (Wolf and Hume 1966) consists of direct irradiation of canine small-bowel allografts, as performed by Cohen et al. (1976). Small-bowel allografts treated in vitro with 150 R led to no increase in recipient survival and were rejected in a standard fashion. On the other hand, animals transplanted with small-intestinal allografts irradiated with only 50 R showed prolonged allograft survival (mean survival time of 28 days) and on direct examination displayed relatively little evidence of cell-mediated rejection. It was assumed by the authors that the animals died of GvH disease. It appears from this study that at lower doses of radiation, the cells involved in rejection are modified while those involved in GvH reaction are spared. The opposite is true when the graft is irradiated with 150 R. This type of speculation leads to the idea that the presence of a low-grade GvH reaction may be immunosuppressive in itself and results in prolonged allograft survival. This study also suggests that the lymphoreticular elements responsible for GvH reaction are more sensitive to irradiation than those cells responsible for allostimulatory reaction and subsequent rejection. With the present availability of various types of monoclonal antibodies against subsets of lymphoreticular cells, more precise definition of the mechanisms involved in high-dose and low-dose irradiation of the allograft may be achieved.

The dynamics of migration of small-intestinal isograft and allograft passenger leukocytes has been previously studied in our laboratory (Hardy et al. 1985). Using Indium-111 oxine-labeled cells, we demonstrated that passenger leukocytes migrate from the intestinal allograft to host lymphoid organs, particularly the spleen, more slowly than passenger leukocytes from cardiac allografts in the rat. Since intestinal allografts have a large quantity of lymphoid tissue associated with them, it is possible that the slow migration pattern of small-intestinal passenger leukocytes enables this organ to be allostimulatory for prolonged periods of time and thus continue to maintain a persistent rejection. Theoretically, it would be advantageous to deplete intestinal allografts of as many allostimulatory cells as possible prior to grafting. This could be accomplished by direct perfusion of the organ with appropriate antibodies and complement, by pharmacologic agents, by direct organ irradiation, and/or by carrying out perfusion with radioactive isotopes that home to lymphoid organs. It may be further advantageous initially to pretreat the donor in such a fashion as to deplete the organ of the APC to a maximal degree.

We have initiated studies in this direction using a rat intestinal allograft model to study the effect of external manipulation on the total amount of lymphoid tissue that is transplanted through intestinal allografts. Our initial efforts were directed primarily to pretreatment of the donor by total body irradiation 48 h prior to transplantation, by abdominal lymphadenectomy 6–8 weeks prior to transplantation, and by thoracic duct drainage 48 h prior to retrieving the donor organ. Only the combination of all these modalities had a significant influence on subsequent intestinal allograft survival when the host was briefly treated with cyclosporine. Extension of these studies are in progress, and LIEDGENS has presented some of these data at this workshop (see P. LIEDGENS et al., this volume).

Combined Approach

Immunomodulatory protocols previously described for direct treatment of allografts and xenografts, particularly pancreatic islets, not only reduced the immunostimulatory properties of the allografts, but also induced a state of antigen-specific tolerance in the recipient, usually based on the development of specific suppressor cell mechanisms. Other approaches to the development of immunologic unresponsiveness have included infusion of whole blood that has been treated either with anti-Ia serum and complement or with UVB irradiation into future allograft recipients. Cyclosporine A, a relatively new immunosuppressive drug, has been used in a few studies to induce specific allogeneic unresponsiveness. Certainly in organs other than the small intestine, all of the methods of graft pretreatment described above produced a range of allograft prolongation, depending on the strains of the experimental animals used and on the organs being transplanted. In islet allograft transplantation in the rat, the use of UVB irradiation was very effective when ACI rats served as recipients but was less effective when "high responder" W/F rats served as recipients. Brief peritransplant immunosuppression of the W/F host with cyclosporine was required for successful allograft acceptance. Similarly, in xenograft experiments, B10/BR mice readily accepted UVB-treated rat islets, while Balb/C mice required brief peritransplant immunosuppression with cyclosporine to accept rat islets indefinitely. It is now well known that cyclosporine A prevents allograft rejection by interfering with the initial T cell activation process. It inhibits the synthesis of IL-2, while sparing the generation of antigen-specific suppressor cells and allowing the development of an active mechanism of suppression. This was elegantly shown in a short-term study of cyclosporine A by WHILE et al. (1983), who demonstrated that heart allografts in rats established for 6 weeks or longer were retained, along with a subsequently transplanted donor-specific skin allograft. They further showed that this type of protection is mediated by a cellular rather than a humoral mechanism. A recent report by ALEJANDRO et al. (1985) confirms the above findings in a higher mammal. This report shows that dogs exposed to short-term treatment with cyclosporine A maintain prolonged survival of highly purified islet allografts, to which they develop a state of immune unresponsiveness. It is thus possible that a combination of vigorous donor organ treatment will be synergistic with brief peritransplant manipulation of the host.

Total small-intestinal transplantation without chronic immunosuppression will undoubtedly require both direct treatment of the organ allograft and brief peritransplant manipulation of the host. These types of treatments are expected to be synergistic, as we have noted in pancreatic-islet transplantation. Although the use of cyclosporine as a major immunosuppressive agent in experimental intestinal transplantation has been fairly effective, it has required chronic administration (CRADDOCK et al. 1983 ; RICOUR et al. 1983) which would undoubtedly have detrimental effects similar to those found when cyclosporine is used for transplantation of other organs. Total elimination of the lymphoid tissue in intestinal allografts appears to be extremely difficult to achieve and may in fact be undesirable. On the other hand, selective depletion of the APC from the allograft and of the proliferating cells involved GvH reaction may be accomplished with appropriate use of biologic, pharmacologic, and physical methods of direct graft treatment in vitro, with or without perfusion. These types of approaches must be carefully evaluated individually, so as to maximize their donor lymphocyte depletion capability without significant toxicity to the cells of the intestinal mucosa and to other structural elements necessary for the proper function of an intestinal allograft. In that regard, establishment of donor pretreatment protocols and donor organ treatment protocols are expected to be complementary to each other and more effective than each one alone. There are already many lines of evidence that suggest that direct treatment of intestinal allografts may be much more complex than that effectively used for pancreatic islets. There is already sufficient evidence to suggest that Ia-bearing vascular endothelium from human umbilical cord vein can express immunostimulatory functions in mixed lymphocyte-endothelial cultures. It is thus quite possible that in vivo the immunostimulatory role of Ia-bearing endothelium will substitute for APC of lymphoreticular origin and may require other specific approaches which wll either mask it or alter it transiently, so as to decrease the initial antigen recognition.

In conclusion, the problems engendered by chronic immunosuppression of the recipient are well known. A logical and promising alternative that we are actively studying in relation to pancreatic islet transplantation and, more recently, in relation to intestinal allografts is modulation of graft immunogenicity before transplantation by a combination of donor pretreatment and direct treatment of the donor organ. We have briefly reviewed the available in vivo and in vitro methods that have been used for prolongation of allograft survival without recipient immunosuppression. Many of the methods described have been utilized for organs other than the small intestine, and some need to be appropriately adapted to the treatment of this unusual organ, which is highly allostimulatory, thus leading frequently to GvH reaction. The methods previously described for donor pretreatment or direct organ treatment are of particular relevance and importance to small-intestinal transplantation with its high lymphoid content. It is probable that depletion of APC cells alone will prevent neither allograft rejection nor GvH reaction; thus, further objective assessments of the effects of pretreatment on mobile and fixed lymphoid cell populations in the intestinal allograft are needed. Based on studies involving other immediately vascularized organs, it appears that modification of the donor organ alone will be insufficient to permit its complete acceptance. Continued studies on the induction of donor-specific immunologic unresponsiveness in the host must continue in relation to intestinal allografts with the goal of making intestinal allografts a safe and effective clinical modality.

References

Alejandro R, Cutfeld RG, Shienwold FL, Latif Z, Mintz DH (1985) Successful long-term survival of pancreatic islet allografts in spontaneous or pancreatectomy-induced diabetes in dogs. Cyclosporine induced unresponsiveness. Diabetes (in press)

Batchelor JR, Welsh KI (1976) Mechanisms of enhancement of kidney allograft survival. Br Med Bull 32:113–117

Batchelor JR, Welsh KI, Maynard A (1979) Failure of long surviving passively enhanced allografts to provoke T-dependent alloimmunity. I. Retransplantation of (AS × Aug) F_1 kidneys into secondary AS recipients. J Exp Med 155:31–44

Billingham RE (1971) The passenger cell concept in transplantation immunology. Cell Immunol 2:1–12

Bowen KM, Prowse SJ, Lafferty KJ (1981) Reversal of diabetes by islet transplantation: vulnerability of the established allograft. Science 213:1261–1262

Burlingham WJ, Sparks EMF, Sondel PM, Glass NR, Belzer FO, Sollinger HW (1985) Improved renal allograft survival following donor-specific transfusions. Transplantation 39:12–17

Burnet FM (1959) The clonal selection theory of acquired immunity. Cambridge University Press, Cambridge, pp 87

Cobbold SP, Jayasuriya A, Nash A, Prospero TD (1984) Therapy with monoclonal antibodies by Elimination of T-cell subsets in vivo. Nature 312: 548–551

Cohen Z, MacGregor AB, Moore KTH, Falk RE, Langer B, Cullen JB (1976) Canine small bowel transplantation. Arch Surg 111:248–253

Corry RJ, Patel NP, West JC, Schanbacher BA (1980) Pretreatment of cadaver donors with cyclophosphamide and methylprednisolone: Effect of renal transplant outcome. Transplant Proc 12:348–351

Craddock GN, Nordren SR, Reznick RK, Gilas T, Lossing AG, Cohen Z, Stiller CR, Cullen JB, Langer B (1983) Small bowel transplantation in the dog using cyclosporine. Transplantation 35:284–288

DeWolf WC, Bentley M, Staley NA (1976) The effect of concanavalin A on canine renal allograft survival. Transplantation 22:406–411

Dorsch S, Roser B (1982a) Suppressor cells in transplantation tolerance. I. Analysis of the suppressor status of neonatally and adoptively tolerized rats. Transplantation 33:518–524

Dorsch S, Roser B (1982b) Suppressor cells in transplantation tolerance. II. Identification and probable mode of action of chimeric suppressor T-cells. Transplantation 33:525–529

Elkins WL, Guttman RD (1968) Pathogenesis of a local graft versus host reaction: Immunogenicity of circulating leucocytes. Science 159:1250–1251

Fabre JW, Morris PJ (1972) The mechanism of specific immunosuppression of renal allograft rejection by donor strain blood. Transplantation 14:634–640

Faustman D, Hauptfeld B, Lacy PE (1981) Prolongation of murine islet allograft survival by pretreatment of islets with antibody directed to Ia determinants. Proc Natl Acad Sci (USA) 78:5156

Freeman JS, Chamberlain EC, Reemtsma K, Steinmuller D (1971) Prolongation of rat heart allografts by donor pretreatment with immunosuppressive agents. Transplant Proc 3:580–582

Guttman RD, Lindquist RR (1969) Renal transplantation in the inbred rat: XI. Reduction of allograft immunogenicity by cytotoxic drug pretreatment of the donors. Transplantation 8:490

Guttman RD, Beaudoin JG, Morehouse DD et al (1975) Donor pretreatment as adjunct to cadaver renal allotransplantation. Transplant Proc 7:117–121

Hall BM (1984) Mechanisms of specific unresponsiveness to allografts. Transplant Proc 16:938–943

Hardy MA, Lau H (1986) Graft modification. In: Flye W (ed) Organ transplantation. Saunders, New York (in press)

Hardy MA, Fawwaz R, Oluwole S, Todd G, Nowygrod R, Reemtsma K (1979) Selective Lymphoid irradiation. I. An approach to transplantation. Surgery 86:194–202

Hardy MA, Oluwole S, Fawwaz R, Reemtsma K (1981) Induction of specific unresponsiveness in adult rats: Role of serum blocking factors and suppressor cells. Transplant Proc 13:629–632

Hardy MA, Lau H, Weber C, Reemtsma K (1984) Pancreatic islet transplantation. Induction of graft acceptance by ultraviolet irradiation of donor tissue. Ann Surg 200:441–450

Hardy MA, Iga C, Satake K, Kuromoto N, Oluwole S (1985) Migration of donor passenger cells during rat cardiac and intestinal allograft rejection. In: Microsurgical Models in Rats for Transplantation Research. Thiede A, Deltz E, Engemann R, Hamelmann H eds.; Springer, Berlin Heidelberg New York 1985, pp 135–144

Kruisbeek AM, Titus JA, Stephany DA, Gause BL, Longo DL (1985) In vivo treatment with monoclonal anti-I-A antibodies: Disappearance of splenic antigen-presenting cell function concomitant with modulation of splenic cell surface I-A and I-E antigens. J Immunol 134:3605–3614

Lacy PE, Davie JM (1984) Transplantation of pancreatic islets. Ann Rev Immunol 2:183–198

Lacy PE, Davie JM, Finke EH (1979) Prolongation of islet allograft survival following in vitro culture (24°C) and a single injection of ALS. Science 204:312–313

Lafferty KJ, Bootes A, Dart G, Talmage DW (1976) Effect of organ culture on the survival of thyroid allografts in mice. Transplantation 22:138–149

Lafferty KJ, Prowse SJ, Simeonovic CJ, Warren H (1983) Immunobiology of tissue transplantation: A return to the passenger leukocyte concept. Ann Rev Immun 1:143

Lau H, Reemtsma K, Hardy MA (1983) Pancreatic islet allograft prolongation with donor specific blood transfusions treated with ultraviolet irradiation. Science 221:754–756

Lau H, Reemtsma K, Hardy MA (1984a) Prolongation of rat islet allograft survival by direct ultraviolet irradiation of the graft. Science 223:607–609

Lau H, Reemtsma K, Hardy MA (1984b) The use of direct ultraviolet irradiation and cyclosporine A in facilitating indefinite pancreatic islet allograft acceptance. Transplantation 36:566

Lechler RI, Batchelor JR (1982a) Restoration of immunogenicity to passenger cell depleted kidney allografts by addition of donor strain dendritic cells. J Exp Med 155:31–44

Lechler RI, Batchelor JR (1982b) Immunogenicity of retransplanted rat kidney allografts effect of inducing chimerism in the first recipient and quantitative studies on immunosuppression of the second recipient. J Exp Med 156:1835–1841

Lenhard V, Dieter R, Hansen B, Opelz G (1985) Suppression of antibody response and prolongation of skin graft survival by multiple blood transfusions in the rat. Transplantation 39:424–429

Leon M, Schwartz H (1969) Inhibition of delayed hypersensitivity to tuberculin by concanavalin A. Proc Soc Exp Biol Med 131:735

Lindahl-Kiessling K, Safwenberg J (1971) Inability of UV-irradiated lymphocytes to stimulate allogeneic cells in mixed lymphocyte culture. Int Arch Allergy 41:670–678

Marquet RL, Heystek GA (1981) Induction of suppressor cells by donor specific blood transfusions and heart transplantation in rats. Transplantation 31:272

McCabe R, Swistel A, Lorico D, Fitzpatrick HF (1980) Prolongation of canine renal allografts in the immunosuppressed host by donor pretreatment with cytolytic agents. Transplant Proc 12:355–357

McKearn TJ, Stuart FP, Fitch FW (1974) Anti-idiotypic antibody in rat transplantation immunity. J Immunol 113:1876–1882

McKenzie JL, Beard ME, Hart DN (1984a) The effect of donor pretreatment on interstitial dendritic cell content and rat cardiac allograft survival. Transplantation 38:371–376

McKenzie JL, Beard ME, Hart DN (1984b) Depletion of donor kidney dendritic cells prolongs graft survival. Transplant Proc 16:948–951

Mjornstedt L, Olausson M, Lindholm L et al (1983) Appearance of suppressor cells and importance of graft presence in ATG-induced transplantation tolerance in the adult rat. Transplant 15:748

Monaco AP, Wood ML (1982) The potential for induction of specific unresponsiveness to organ allografts in clinical transplantation. Heart Transplant 1:257–284

Monaco AP, Wood ML, Maki T, Madras PN, Sakyoun AI, Simpson MA (1985) Attempt to induce unresponsiveness to human renal allografts with ATG and donor specific bone marrow. Transplant Proc 17:1312–1314

Nagao T, White DJG, Calne RY (1982) Kinetics of unresponsiveness induced by a short course of cyclosporine A. Transplantation 33:31–35

Nakahara K, Kaplan D, Bjorn M, Fathman CG (1985) The effectiveness of anti-Ia-immunotoxins in the suppression of MLR. Transplantation 40:62–67

Nowygrod R, Todd G, Katz S et al (1978) Failure of concanavalin A graft perfusion to prolong rat cardiac allograft survival. Transplantation 25:341

Nowygrod R, Hardy MA, Todd G, Oluwole S, Reemtsma K (1979) Donor pretreatment in cardiac allografts. Transplant Proc 11:1462–1464

Oluwole S, Hardy MA, Fawwaz R, Todd G, Nowygrod R, Reemtsma K (1979) Selective lymphoid irratiation (SLI). II. Comparison with total body irradiation on cardiac allograft survival in rats. Transplantation 28:492–495

Oluwole S, Hardy MA, Fawwaz R, Satake K, Nowygrod R, Reemtsma K (1980) The effect of bone marrow cells on induction of tolerance with selective lymphoid irradiation and ALG in ACI to Lewis rats. Surg Forum 31:382–384

Oluwole S, Iga C, Lau H, Hardy MA (1985) Prolongation of rat heart allografts by donor-specific blood transfusion treated with ultraviolet irradiation. Heart Transplant (in press)

Perry LL, Greene MI (1982) Conversion of immunity to suppression by in vivo administration of I-A subregion-specific antibodies. J Exp Med 156:480–491

Perry LL, Williams IR (1985) Regulation of transplantation immunity in vivo by monoclonal antibodies recognizing host class II restriction elements. J Immunol 134:2935–2941

Perry LL, Dorf ME, Benacerraf B, Greene MI (1979) Regulation of immune response to tumor antigen: Interference with syngeneic tumor immunity by anti-IA alloantisera. Proc Natl Acad Sci (USA) 76:920–924

Rapaport F, Bachvaroff R, Waltzer W, Sato T, Asari H, Chanana A, Cronkite E (1982) Further progress in the induction of allogeneic unresponsiveness in the adult host. Transplant Proc 14:531–534

Reed E, Hardy M, Lattes C, Brensilver J, McCabe R, Reemtsma K, Suciu-Foca N (1985) Anti-idiotypic antibodies and their relevance to transplantation. Transplant Proc 17:735–738

Ricour C, Revillon Y, Arnaud-Battandier F, Ghnassia D, Weyne P, Lauffenburger A, Jos J, Fontaine JL, Gallix P, Vaiman M (1983) Successful small bowel allografts in piglets using cyclosporine. Transplant Proc 15:3019–3026

Rucker J, Toledo-Pereyra LH, MacKenzie GH, Gordon DA (1982) Improvement of kidney transplant survival after graft pretreatment with cyclosporine A. Transplantation 34:356–359

Sampson D, Levin BS, Hoppe RT, Bieber CP, Miller E, Waer M, Kaplan HS, Collins G, Strober S (1985) Preliminary observations on the use of TLI, rabbit ATG and low dose prednisone in human cadaver renal transplantation. Transplant Proc 17:1299–1303

Schwartz RH, David CS, Sachs DH, Paul WE (1976) T Lymphocyte enriched urine peritoneal exudate cells. III. Inibition of antigen-induced T lymphocyte proliferation with anti-Ia-antisera. J Immunol 117: 531–540

Slavin S, Strober S, Fuks Z, Kaplan S (1977) Induction of specific tissue transplantation tolerance using fractionated total lymphoid irradiation in adult mice: Long-term survival of allogeneic bone marrow and skin grafts. J Exp Med 146:34–48

Snell GD (1957) The homograft reaction. Ann Rev Microbiol 2:439–459

Sollinger HW, Burkholder PM, Rasmus WR, Bach FH (1977) Prolonged survival of Xenografts after organ culture. Surgery 81:74–79

Sollinger HW, Mack E, Cook K et al (1983) Allotransplantation of human parathyroid tissue without immunosuppression. Transplantation 36:599–602

Sprent J (1978) Role of H-2 gene products in the function of T-helper cells from normal and chimeric mice measured in vivo. Immunol Rev 42:108

Steinman RM, Witmer MD (1978) Lymphoid dendritic cells are potent stimulators of the primary mixed leukocyte reaction in mice. Proc Natl Acad Sci (USA) 75:5132

Steinman RM, Kaplan G, Witmer MD, Cohn ZA (1979) Identification of a novel cell type in peripheral lymphoid organs of mice. J Exp Med 146:1–16

Steinmuller D (1967) Immunization with skin isografts taken from tolerant mice. Science 158:127–129

Steinmuller D, Coleman DA (1970) Prolonged survival of rats receiving kidney allografts perfused with concanavalin A. Transplantation 21:430–433

Steinmuller D, Warden G, Coleman M, Lofgreen J, Reemtsma K, Stuart F, Garrick T, Holter A, Lynch A (1971) Prolonged survival of rat heart and kidney allografts irradiated in vitro. Transplantation 12:153–155

Strober S, Modry DL, Hoppe RT, Pennock JL, Bieber CP, Hohn BI, Jamieson SW, Stinson EB, Schroder J, Suomalainen H, Kaplan HS (1984) Induction of specific unresponsiveness to heart allografts in mongrel dogs treated with TLI and ATG. J Immunol 132:1013–1018

Stuart FP, Fitch FW, Rowley DA, Biesecker JL, Hellstrom KE, Hellstrom I (1971) Presence of both cell-mediated immunity and serum-blocking factors in rat renal allografts "enhanced" by passive immunization. Transplantation 12:331–333

Talmadge DW, Dart GA, Radovich J et al (1976) Activation of transplant immunity: Effect of donor leukocytes on thyroid allograft rejection. Science 191:385

Thomas FT, Carver FM, Foil MB, Pryor WH, Larkin EW, Hall WR, Haisch CE, Thomas JM (1983)

Long-term incompatible kidney survival in outbred higher primates without chronic immunosuppression. Ann Surg 198:370–378

Thomas JM, Carver FM, Foil MB, Hall WR, Adams C, Fahrenbruch GB, Thomas FT (1983) Renal allograft induced with ATG and donor bone marrow in outbred rhesus monkeys. Transplantation 36:104–106

Todd G, Nowygrod R, Hardy MA, Reemtsma K (1978) Donor and donor organ pretreatment in cardiac allografts. Surg Forum 29:362–364

Toledo-Pereyra L, Ray P, Callender C et al (1974a) Renal allograft prolongation using phytomitogens to mask graft antigens. Surgery 76:121

Toledo-Pereyra LH, Simmons RL, Najarian JS (1974b) Prolonged survival of canine orthotopic small intestinal allografts preserved for 24 hours by hypothermic bloodless perfusion. Surgery 75:368–376

Tominaga A, Lefort S, Mizel SB, Dambrauskas JT, Granstein R, Lowy A, Benacerrat B, Greene MI (1983) Molecular signals in antigen presentation. Clin Immunol Immunopathol 29:282–293

Waldor MK, Srivam S, McDevitt HO, Steinman L (1983) In vivo therapy with monoclonal anti-I-A antibody suppresses immune responses to acetylcholine receptor. Proc Natl Acad Sci (USA) 80:2713–2717

White D, Davies H, Kamada N, Nagao T (1983) Potential for tolerance induction with cyclosporine. Transplant Proc 15:2278–2284

Williams IR, Perry LL (1985) Regulation of transplantation immunity in vivo by monoclonal antibodies recognizing host class II restriction elements. Effects of anti-Ia immunotherapy on host T-cell responses to graft alloantigens. J Immunol 134:2942–2947

Wilson RE, Rippin A, Dagher RK, Kinneart P, Busch GJ (1969) Prolonged canine renal allograft survival after pretreatment with solubilized antigen. Transplantation 7:360–371

Wolf JS, Hume DM (1966) Transplant immunity in animals with lymphocytopenia induced by indwelling beta irradiation. Surg Forum 16:202–204

Wood KJ, Evins J, Morris PS (1985) Suppression of renal allograft rejection in the rat by class I antigens on purified erythrocytes. Transplantation 39:56–62

Wood PJ, Strome P, Streilein JW (1985) Immunological tolerance clonal frequency of alloreactive cells in mice tolerant of H-2. Transplant Proc 17:1137–1139

Yasunami Y, Lacy PE, Davie JM, Finke EH (1983) Prolongation of islet Xenograft survival (rat to mouse) by in vitro culture at 37° C. Transplantation 33:281–283

Yoshimura N, Kahan BD (1985) Nature of the suppressor cells mediating prolonged graft survival after administration of extracted histocompatibility antigen and cyclosporine. Transplantation 39:162–168

Ziegler HK, Unanue ER (1979) The specific binding of listeria monocytogenes Immune T lymphocytes to macrophages. I. Quantitation and role of H-2 gene products. J Exp Med 150:1143–1160

Zincke H, Woods JE, Khan AU, Holley KE, Leary FJ (1978) Immunological donor pretreatment in combination with pulsatile preservation in cadaveric renal transplantation. Transplantation 26:207–211

Session 4: Summary

W. MÜLLER-RUCHHOLTZ

This session comprised 13 papers with an emphasis on morphological studies, various specific aspects of graft-versus-host reactions (GVHR), and some approaches toward immunologic manipulation of graft survival. Fortunately, though this is still not self-evident, all of them dealt with rodent (rat) models, thus allowing adequante immunologic analyses. Seven of the more elaborate studies are presented in this volume.

FERGUSON and CUMMINS report on damage to intestinal tissue in GVHR and host-versus-graft reaction (HVGR), which they studied using quantitative histologic techniques. Among other things, they analyze crypt hyperplasia and interpret this as being due to factors secreted by infiltrating T_{DTH} cells; furthermore, they describe greatly accentuated mucosal effects of GVHR in irradiated recipients and, in a subsequent short paper (FERGUSON et al.), mucosal mast cell features. SCHRAUT and LEE start from the fact, well established in the meantime, that in small-bowel transplantation, unlike other organ transplantation, HVGR and GVHR may even arise at the same time – unless particular $P \rightleftarrows F_1$ experimental models are devised. They concentrate on morphological criteria that will allow us to differentiate between these reactions, and they conclude that the triad of diarrhea, diffuse dermatitis, and lymphoid hypertrophy points toward GVHR inman as well. The paper by MÜLLER-HERMELINK and DELTZ provides a very valuable extension of these morphological studies, in that it compares the GVHR found in small-bowel transplantation with that seen in bone marrow transplantation. These authors point out that the different tissue constituents of the host are at quite different risks, since, e.g., blood vessels remain undamaged in GVHR (unlike in HVGR), while the thymus is subject to early and profound changes.

The short contribution by LIEDGENS et al. deals with successful attempts to manipulate various immunologic reactions. It reports on a $F_1 \rightarrow P$ model in which HVGR, expressed as T cell infiltration into the lamina muscularis of the graft, was completely suppressed by a 15-day treatment with cyclosporine A. In a $P \rightarrow F_1$ model, on the other side, LEE et al. observed GVHR prevention by in vitro irradiation of the graft. Finally, HARDY et al. provide an impressive overview of approaches toward manipulation of graft immunogenicity, which is too substantial to lend itself to a brief summary. I may add that the elimination of cells (expressing major transplantation antigens) that are not required for the function of a graft, or at least the suppression of their immunogenicity, and the prevention of an increase in the immunogenicity of cells that are required for graft function are now becoming "hot issues" in transplantation immunology research. In concluding this summary, it may be stated that this session offered a fascinating view of various facets of the state of the art in small-bowel transplantation immunology, though obviously not all aspects could be covered.

Session 5
Immunosuppression

*Long-Term Survival of Orthotopic Small-Bowel Allografts Using Cyclosporin A**

W. H. SCHRAUT and K. K. W. LEE

Introduction

Although small-bowel transplantation was first described by LILLIHEI nearly 30 years ago (LILLIHEI et al. 1959), clinical small-bowel transplantation has to date been limited to fewer than ten reported cases. The major obstacle to successful human small-bowel transplantation has been the lack of an effective immunosuppressive regimen for control of graft rejection. Early experimental and clinical attempts at intestinal transplantation using corticosteroids, azathioprine, and antilymphocyte serum failed to achieve long-term graft and recipient survival (PRESTON et al. 1966; ALICAN et al. 1971; HARDY et al. 1970). The recent successful use of cyclosporine A (CsA) in transplantation of other vascularized organ grafts has led to its use in small-bowel transplantation as well. With CsA, long-term survival of accessory, defunctionalized intestinal allografts has been achieved (KIRKMAN et al. 1984). However, long-term healthy survival of graft recipients who are entirely dependent upon the transplanted small intestine for nutritional intake has yet to be demonstrated consistently. A rat model of small-bowel transplantation was therefore used to determine if rejection can be satisfactorily controlled using CsA so as to permit normal recipient growth and maintenance of a normal nutritional state.

Materials and Methods

Experimental Groups

As described in Table 1, Male Lewis (LEW) and Brown Norway (BN) hybrid rats weighing between 200 and 300 g were used. In groups 1–3, transplantation was performed in the BN → LEW combination. Group 1 received no immunosuppressive therapy, group 2 received CsA 15 mg/kg on postoperative days 0, 1, 2, 4, and 6 (short course), and group 3 received CsA on postoperative days 0, 1, 2, 4, and 6 and then every other day until day 28. Control groups consisted of age-matched normal LEW rats and age-matched LEW isograft recipients.

* Supported by The National Institutes of Arthritis, Metabolism, and Digestive Diseases (Grant No. AM27332).

Table 1. Effect of CsA therapy on recipient survival after BN → LEW orthotopic intestinal transplantation

Group	Strain combination	Treatment	Survival (days)
1	BN → LEW (n = 6)	None	8, 9, 9, 10, 10, 11
2	BN → LEW (n = 5)	CsA days 0, 1, 2, 4, 6	23, 32, 39, 44, > 500
3	BN → LEW (n = 7)	CsA days 0, 1, 2, 4, 6 and q to day 28	All > 500
Controls:	LEW → LEW (n = 9)	None	All > 500
	Normal LEW (n = 6)	None	All > 500

CsA Administration and Monitoring

CsA and CsA radioimmunoassay kits were generously provided by Sandoz Inc., East Hanover, New Jersey, U.S.A. CsA was suspended in 10% Intralipid at a concentration of 3 mg/cc and was injected intramuscularly. The first dose was given immediately after surgery. Whole blood CsA levels measured 24 and 48 h after dosing were between 600 and 1500 ng/ml and were considered to be therapeutic.

Operative Procedures

Orthotopic small-bowel transplantation was performed using standard microsurgical techniques as described by SCHRAUT et al. (1983). Animals surviving for fewer than 4 days after transplantation were considered technical failures and were excluded from further analysis.

Postoperative Care

Graft recipients were given a regular laboratory diet ad libitum beginning on the 2nd postoperative day. Their general health (appearance, posture, food consumption, bowel function) and weight were monitored, and serum protein, albumin, and triglyceride levels were periodically measured using standard laboratory methods. Long-term surviving graft recipients underwent laparotomy to permit gross inspection and full-thickness biopsy of the grafts. At laparotomy, absorption of maltose from the transplanted bowel was also studied using the technique of BILLIAR et al. (1984). Postmortem examinations were performed on all animals, and graft, lymph node, and other tissue specimens were prepared for light microscopy using hematoxylin and eosin stains.

Results

Clinical Course and Survival

Without immunosuppressive therapy, LEW recipients of BN (group 1) allografts all died of acute rejection with an average survival of 9.5 ± 1.0 days (Table 1). Following transplantation, these animals initially exhibited normal food intake, passage of solidly formed feces, and maintenance of total body weight, but then developed severe diarrhea and weight loss leading to death. Treatment with short courses of CsA therapy resulted in significantly prolonged survival times for the BN (group 2) allograft recipients in comparison with the untreated animals. In this group, there were occasional long-term survivors; the remaining animals had courses consistent with subacute or chronic rejection in which they remained healthy (weight gain, normal bowel function) for periods ranging from 3 to 7 weeks before succumbing to progressive inanition and diarrhea. With continuation of CsA therapy until post-operative day 28, all BN allograft recipients in group 3 have remained healthy and free of clinical signs of graft rejections for 17 months. All have gained weight and maintained clinically normal bowel function.

Pathohistologic Findings

At postmortem examination, all vascular and intestinal anastomoses were patent. Allografts taken from group 1 showed evidence of acute rejection consisting of thinning and distention of the bowel wall, mucosal hemorrhage, injection of the graft mesentery, and liquid intraluminal contents (Fig. 1A). Microscopic findings of acute rejection included extensive mucosal destruction with a prominent cellular infiltrate (Fig. 2A). Allografts taken from group 2 exhibited changes indicate of chronic rejection. These grafts had stenotic segments with fibrosis and thickening. Microscopically, widespread loss of mucosa and marked submucosal fibrosis and bowel wall thickening (Fig. 2B) were observed.

At laparotomy, allografts in group 3 appeared grossly normal with patent anastomoses, good vascularization, and semisolid intraluminal contents (Fig. 1B).

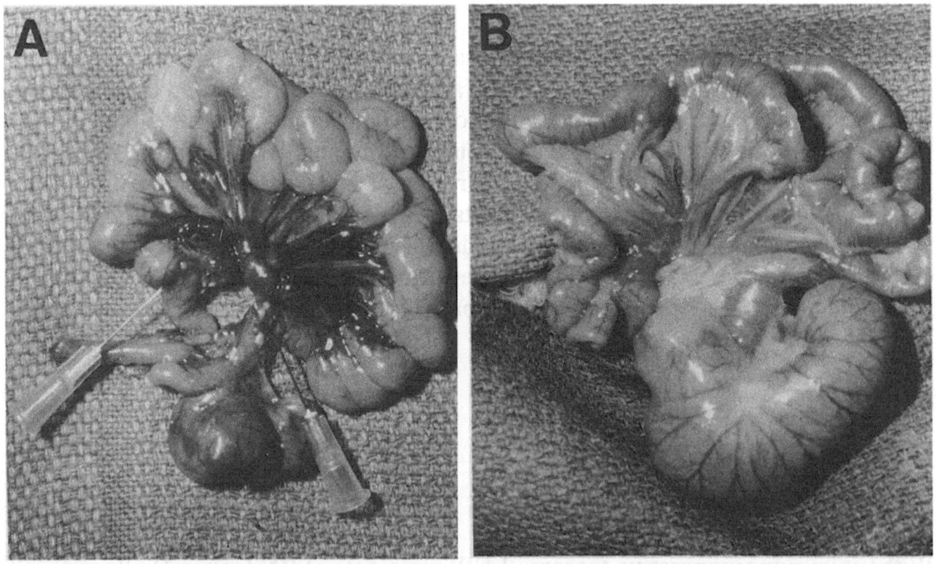

Fig. 1A, B. Macroscopic changes of BN intestinal allografts transplanted into LEW recipients. **A** Allograft from a recipient given no immunosuppressive therapy showing signs of acute rejection. Liquid intraluminal contents, thinning and distention of the bowel wall, and injection of the graft mesentery are evident. The patent intestinal anastomoses are indicated by the *markers*. **B** Normal appearance of an allograft from a recipient treated with extended CsA therapy (group 3)

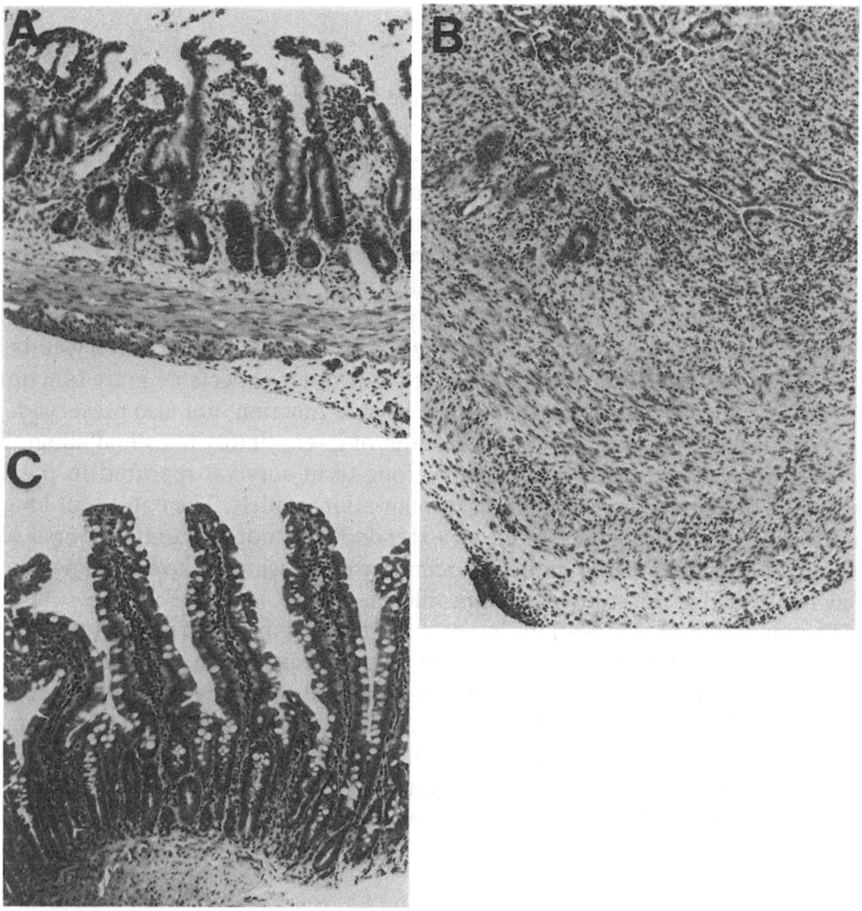

Fig. 2A–C. Histologic appearance of BN intestinal allografts transplanted into LEW recipients. **A** Allograft from a recipient given no immunosuppressive therapy. The acutely rejected graft is thin with extensive mucosal destruction and a marked cellular infiltrate. **B** Allograft from a recipient given a short course of CsA therapy. The chronically rejected graft shows thickening of the bowel wall with mucosal destruction and submucosal fibrosis. **C** Full-thickness biopsy of allograft from a recipient treated with an extended course of CsA. The normal histologic features are preserved. (hematoxylin and eosin stain; × 100)

Full-thickness allograft biopsies showed an intact morphology without cellular infiltrate, fibrosis, or wall thickening (Fig. 2C).

Nutritional Observations

Group 3 graft recipients initially gained weight at rates slower than the control animals. However, after 5 months, their net increase in total body weight (37%) did not differ significantly from control values, nor did serum protein (5.5 ± 0.4 g/dl), serum albumin (3.4 ± 0.15 g/dl), or serum triglycerides (82 ± 10.7 mg/dl). Maltose absorption from the intestinal allografts also did not differ significantly from control animals.

Discussion

These results demonstrate that in this rat model of small-bowel transplantation, CsA therapy significantly prolongs graft and recipient survival. With short courses of treatment, rejection in some instances is permanently prevented and in others is delayed and follows a chronic course. With longer duration of treatment, a tolerant state is achieved in which rejection does not occur despite discontinuation of immunosuppressive therapy. With successful prevention of graft rejection, the intestinal allograft remains morphologically intact and unaltered. Most importantly, allograft absorptive function is sufficiently preserved to maintain normal nutritional parameters and to support normal healthy recipient growth. The overall well-being of these allograft recipients further suggests that other aspects of graft function and physiology, such as motility and mucosal barrier function, are also preserved.

Structural and functional characterization of in-continuity intestinal allografts has been hampered by the very infrequent long-term survival reported in previously described orthotopic intestinal allotransplantation models. The consistent long-term survival of group 3 animals given an extended, but not indefinite, course of CsA therapy suggests that this model of immunosuppression following transplantation may be useful for the study of such problems.

Extrapolation of observations in one experimental model to other strain combinations or species, including humans, must be undertaken with caution. For example, the long-term graft survival after cessation of immunosuppressive therapy seen in this study is unlikely to be found in larger animal models or clinical transplantation. Nevertheless, the success achieved with this model offers encouragement that successful clinical small-bowel transplantation using CsA alone or in combination with other immunosuppressive agents may be possible.

References

Alican F, Hardy JD, Cayirli M, Varner JE, Moynihan PC, Turner MD, Anas P (1971) Intestinal transplantation: Laboratory experience and report of a clinical case. Am J Surg 121:150–159

Billiar TR, Garberoglio C, Schraut WH (1984) Maltose absorption as an indicator of small-intestinal allograft rejection. J Surg Res 37:75–82

Hardy MA, Quint J, State D (1970) Effect of anti-lymphocyte serum and other immunosuppressive agents on canine jejunal allografts. Ann Surg 171:51–60

Kirkman RL, Lear PA, Madara JL, Tilney NL (1984) Small intestine transplantation in the rat: Immunology and function. Surgery 96:280–287

Lillihei RC, Goott B, Miller FA (1959) Homografts of the small bowel. Surg Forum 10:197–201

Preston FW, Macalalad F, Wachowski TJ, Randolph DA, Apostol JV (1966) Survival of homografts of the intestine with and without immunosuppression. Surgery 60:1203–1210

Schraut WH, Rosemurgy AS, Riddell RM (1983) Prolongation of intestinal allograft survival without immunosuppressive drug therapy: Transplantation of small bowel allografts. J Surg Res 34:597–607

Influence of Cyclosporine A on Small-Bowel Grafts and Subsequent in Vitro Immune Reactions

K. Ulrichs, E. Deltz, B. Friedrichs, G. Leimenstoll, A. Thiede, and W. Müller-Ruchholtz

Introduction

Having previously reported on clinical and morphological features of graft-versus-host (GvH) reaction in correlation to basic cell-mediated immune reactions involved in GvH disease after heterotopic small-bowel (SB) transplantation in the rat (Ulrichs and Deltz 1985; Deltz et al. 1985; Müller-Hermelink and Deltz, this volume), it was the aim of this study to investigate various administration protocols for cyclosporine A (CsA) in order to prevent lethal GvH disease and prolong animal survival.

Materials and Methods

Technique of SB Transplantation
The technique of heterotopic SB transplantation has been previously described in detail by Deltz and Thiede (1985).

Experimental Groups
Four experimental groups were set up using the parental strain/F_1 hybrid model BN (LEW × BN) F_1 with a full-lenght SB graft. Group 1 was a control group without cyclosporine A CsA treatment; group 2 received 15 mg/kg body weight per day CsA from day 0–13 post-operatively; group 3 received 15 mg/kg body weight per day CsA from day 0–2 post-operatively; group 4 received 15 mg/kg body weight per day CsA from day −2–0 preoperatively. CsA was soluted in olive oil and administered per os.

Test for Cell-Mediated in Vitro Reactivity
Cell-mediated in vitro reactivity of the various lymphatic compartments of the recipient (blood, spleen, peripheral lymph nodes, mesenteric lymph nodes, Peyer's patches) and of the graft (mesenteric lymph nodes, Peyer's patches) was tested at different times (14–33, 87–181 days) postoperatively using the microcytotoxicity assay (Takasugi and Klein 1970). Embryonic fibroblasts of the parental strains and of third-party strain served as target cells: GvH reactivity was tested against LEW fibroblasts, GvH-dependent cell-mediated autoreactivity (CAR) against BN fibroblasts, and specificity of reactivity against DA fibroblasts.

Results

Mortality Rates

GvH reaction-induced mortality of semiallogeneic SB recipients in the four experimental groups is documented in Table 1. In contrast to the dramatic situation in the control group 1, where none of the graft recipients survived beyond day 22, each of the three different CsA protocols, however variant, prolonged survival significantly. Even a short-term application of the drug before grafting exerts a strong immunosuppressive effect on the resulting GvH disease.

Table 1. Graft survival after different protocols of CsA treatment

Experimental groups	CsA treatment	Surviving animals *n*	%
1	none	0/26	0
2	day 0–13 postoperatively	14/19	74
3	day 0–2 postoperatively	12/24	50
4	day −2–0 preoperatively	13/20	65

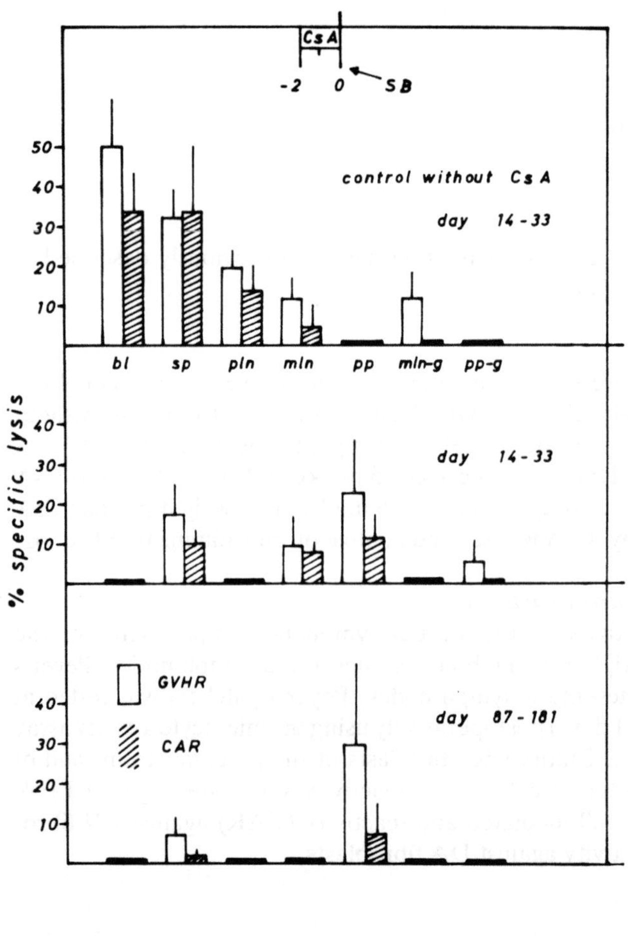

Fig. 1. Cell-mediated in vitro reactivity after CsA treatment from day −2 to day 0 (day of grafting) (group 4) of the various lymphatic compartments of the recipient (*bl*, blood; *sp*, spleen; *pln*, peripheral lymph nodes; *mln*, mesenteric lymph nodes; *pp*, Peyer's patches) and of the graft (*mln-g*, mesenteric lymph nodes; *pp-g*, Peyer's patches). CsA administration scheme and reactivity of the untreated control animals are indicated in the *top panel*

Cell-Mediated in Vitro Reactivity

As can be seen from Figs. 1–3, cell-mediated in vitro reactivities, such as GvHR and GvH-dependent CAR, obviously correlate well with the above in vivo data, thus indicating a less severe course of the disease. However, a closer look at the reactivities of the various lymphatic compartments reveals a certain reaction pattern:

Figure 1 presents the results of the short-term preoperative CsA administration, bringing out three striking points concerning the kinetics of reactivity:

1) As an immediate effect of CsA treatment, reactivities in the blood, peripheral lymph nodes, and graft mesenteric lymph nodes decrease to zero.
2) Reactivity in the spleen also decreases slightly but is somewhat less susceptible to the drug treatment.
3) Instead of persistent nonreactivity, reactivity in the Peyer's patches increases with prolonged survival time.

The situation is somewhat different using the second treatment protocol (short-term postoperative CsA application, Fig. 2):

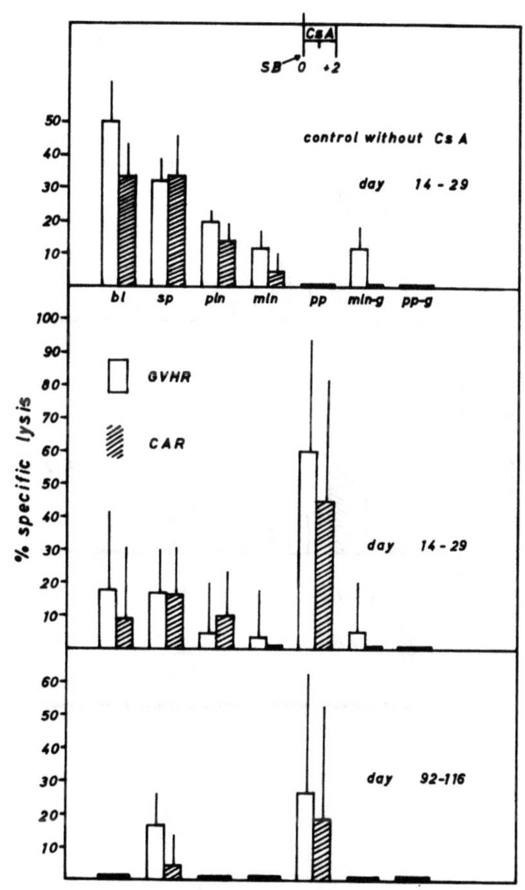

Fig. 2. Cell-mediated in vitro reactivity after CsA treatment from day 0 (day of grafting) to day +2 (group 3) of the various lymphatic compartments of the recipient (*bl*, blood; *sp*, spleen; *pln*, peripheral lymph nodes; *mln*, mesenteric lymph nodes; *pp*, Peyer's patches) and of the graft (*mln-g*, mesenteric lymph nodes; *pp-g*, Peyer's patches). CsA administration scheme and reactivity of the untreated control animals are indicated in the *top panel*

1) Compared with the previous protocol, lymphocytes in the blood, peripheral lymph nodes, and graft mesenteric lymph nodes are slightly less susceptible to the drug treatment, as their reactivities only decrease in the late stage of observation.
2) The reaction in the spleen is similar to that in the previous protocol.
3) Similar but more pronounced reactivity in the Peyer's patches increases with prolonged animal survival.

The best long-term effects, however, are observed with the classical rat CsA protocol (Fig. 3):

1) Similar if not identical to the first protocol, reactivities in the blood and lymph nodes and the mesenteric lymph nodes of the graft decrease to zero in the early stage of testing.
2) Only after as much as a 14-day course of CsA, reactivity in the spleen, which has so far been difficult to suppress, also decreases to zero.
3) Even the comparatively longer administration of the drug cannot prevent the increase in Peyer's patch reactivity.

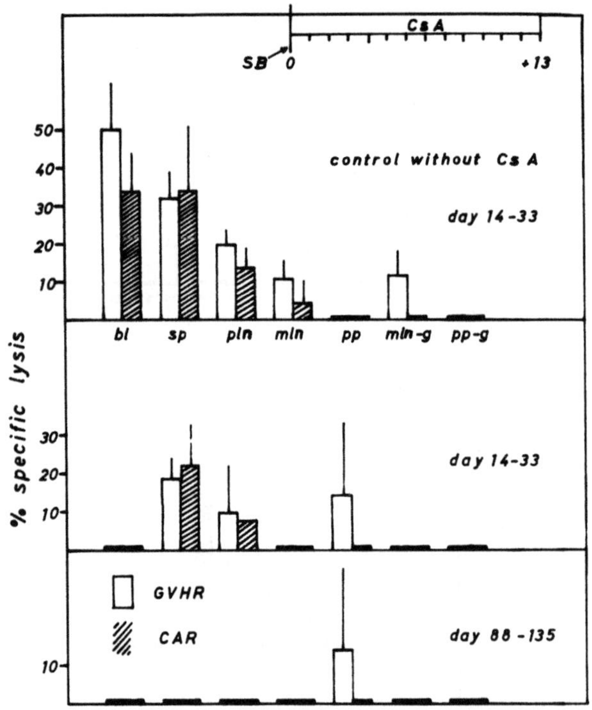

Fig. 3. Cell-mediated in vitro reactivity after CsA treatment from day 0 (day of grafting) to day +13 (group 2) of the various lymphatic compartments of the recipient (*bl,* blood; *sp,* spleen; *pln,* peripheral lymph nodes; *mln,* mesenteric lymph nodes; *pp,* Peyer's patches) and of the graft (*mln-g,* mesenteric lymph nodes; *pp-g,* Peyer's patches). CsA administration scheme and reactivity of the untreated control animals are indicated in the *top panel*

Discussion

Of the three different CsA administration protocols studied here, the short-term treatment initiated before the day of graft performance results in animal survival significantly prolonged by over 50%, thus indicating that CsA also appears to be an effective drug for SB recipients. Concerning the resulting cell-mediated in vitro reactivities, such as GvHR and GvH-dependent CAR, the various lymphatic compartments investigated apparently react differently to CsA treatment, mostly with a decrease in reactivity, but surprisingly, in the case of Peyer's patches, with an increase in reactivity as well. Thus, prolonged animal survival may be the cause of a shift of reactivity from one compartment to another, rather than a decrease in reactivity. Similar "locking-in" phenomena have already been observed in SB recipients (Ulrichs and Deltz 1985), as well as in a different experimental rat transplantation model (Bröcker et al. 1975), and always result in improved animal and graft survival. The specific behavior of Peyer's patch lymphocytes and their biological function, e.g., their IgA secretion, should be carefully investigated in detail in the more physiologic orthotopic model to assure their impaired in vivo function.

References

Bröcker EB, Schienle W, Müller-Ruchholtz W (1975) Time- and compartment-dependent variation of lymphocytotoxicity in sensitized animals. Pathol Microbiol 38:35

Deltz E, Thiede A (1985) Microsurgical technique for small-intestine transplantation. In: Thiede A, Deltz E, Engemann R, Hamelmann H (eds) Microsurgical models in rats for transplantation research. Springer-Verlag, Berlin Heidelberg New York Tokyo, pp 51–55

Deltz E, Ulrichs K, Thiede A (1985) Rejection and graft-versus-host reaction following small-bowel transplantation and methods of circumventing them. In: Thiede A, Deltz E, Engemann R, Hamelmann H (eds) Microsurgical models in rats for transplantation research. Springer-Verlag, Berlin Heidelberg New York Tokyo, pp 145–152

Takasugi M, Klein E (1970) A microassay for cell-mediated immunity. Transplantation 9:219–227

Ulrichs K, Deltz E (1958) Immunological reactions induced by graft-versus-host reaction following small-bowel transplantation. In: Thiede A, Deltz E, Engemann R, Hamelmann H (eds) Microsurgical models in rats for transplantation research. Springer-Verlag, Berlin Heidelberg New York Tokyo, pp 153–156

Different Modes of Cyclosporine A Administration in Experimental Small-Bowel Transplantation

G. LEIMENSTOLL, W. CH. PREISSNER, G. LOSKE, W. TIMMERMANN,
P. SCHROEDER, E. DELTZ, and W. NIEDERMAYER

According to GIBALDI and PERRIER (1975), a two-compartment model can be used to describe the pharmacokinetics of drugs metabolized in the liver, such as cyclosporine A (CsA). Compartment 1 refers to the central compartment (blood or plasma) and compartment 2 refers to the hepatoportal system.

The bioavailability of the drug is greater when administered in the central compartment, the so-called peripheral routes (intravenous, intramuscular), than when it is administered in the hepatoportal compartment. Using the hepatic routes (oral or intraperitoneal), a significant fraction of the dose is metabolized during the first passage. According to WASSEF et al. (1985), CsA is also transported via lymphatic routes, which run peripherally. They have not been considered in this model.

The purpose of this study was to define the optimal trough levels necessary to prevent rejection and then to study how these levels can be achieved.

Methods

The small bowels of eight DA rats were transplanted to Lewis rats in a heterotopic position see PREISSNER et al., this volume). CsA was first administered orally at 10 mg/kg per 24 h for 15 days, at 5 mg/kg per day for the next 15 days, and at 2.5 mg/kg every 48 h thereafter. The trough levels were measured by radioimmunoassay (Sandoz Ltd., Basel, Switzerland) after 14, 29, and 38 days.

Four groups of five Lewis rats received CsA as a single dose of 15 mg/kg orally, intramuscularly, and intraperitoneally and 5 mg/kg intravenously. Blood levels were measured after 1, 2, 4, 6, 8, 12, 24, and 48 h. After anesthesia with ether, blood was collected from the tail vein (500 μl blood in a heparinized tube).

CsA was given orally by stomach tube (750 mg CsA dissolved in 22.5 ml olive oil). For the intravenous and intramuscular routes, we used the CsA solution provided by Sandoz Ltd. (Basel). The desired amount was dissolved in physiologic saline solution. To administer CsA intraperitoneally, 400 mg of the drug was dissolved in 90 ml Intralipid.

Pharmacokinetic parameters were calculated using a one-compartment model. For calculation of the total areas under the blood concentration-vs-time curves, the trapezoidal rule was used (GIBALDI and PERRIER 1975). Streptocotocin was administered intravenously (55 mg/kg).

Results

After transplanting the small bowels of eight DA rats to Lewis rats, six animals survived. The rats were given CsA orally, as described above, and after 50 days, no signs of rejection were observed. Trough levels rose to 1850 ± 327 ng/ml after 14 days, dropped to 707 ± 166 ng/ml after 29 days, and after 38 days dropped to 65.6 ± 8.1 ng/ml (Fig. 1). Another five animals treated with 15 mg/kg per day died from infections. We concluded from this experiment that trough levels ranging between 1800 ng/ml and 700 ng/ml ensure sufficient immunosuppression.

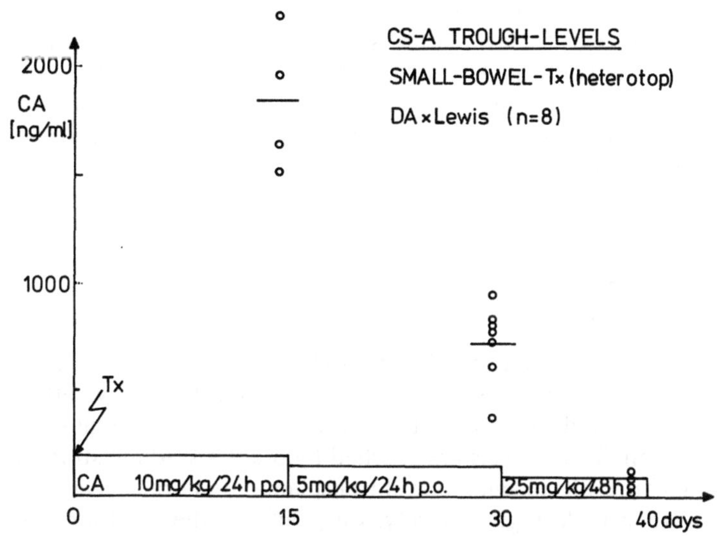

Fig. 1. CsA trough levels (ng/ml) after small-bowel transplantation (*DA* rats to Lewis rats) in a heterotopic position (values for eight animals). CsA was administered orally *(po)*

Table 1. Areas of blood concentration-vs-time curves calculated after a single dose of 15 mg/kg CsA administered intramuscularly, intraperitoneally, and orally and 5 mg/kg administered intravenously (mean of five Lewis rats)

Administration route	AUC_T (in μg · h/ml)		
i.v.	187.478 ± 25.1		i.v./i.m., $p < 0.5$
i.m.	157.492 ± 21.9		
p.o.	50.33 ± 10.7	$\frac{AUC_{p.o.}}{AUC_{i.m.}} = 0.32$	
i.p.	138.718 ± 9.8	$\frac{AUC_{i.p.}}{AUC_{i.m.}} = 0.88$	i.m./i.p., $p < 0.025$

AUC_T, area of blood concentration-vs-time curve

From a theoretical point of view, these levels can be achieved by the hepatic or peripheral routes. This prompted us to measure the blood concentration-vs-time curves of five Lewis rats after a single dose of CsA. A dose of 15 mg/kg were administered intraperitoneally, orally, and intramusculary, and 5 mg/kg were given intravenously. The total areas of the blood concentration-vs-time curves (AUC_T) are shown in Table 1. The AUC_T after intravenous and intramuscular application did not differ. When the drug was given orally, only 30% of the total amount reached the central circulation, whereas 88% of the intraperitoneal dose appeared in the central circulation.

To prove the influence of disturbed enteral absorption, groups of two Lewis rats were treated with streptocotocin. CsA was administered orally and intraperitoneally (15 mg/kg) at 5 and 11 days after this treatment and 5 mg/kg were administered intravenously 5 days) after streptocotocin treatment. Liver function remained normal, as confirmed by the fact that the areas of the AUC_T and the elimination rate constant were identical. The AUC_T were altered after oral administration as well as after intraperitoneal application, so that no results could be obtained from this experiment.

Discussion

In human kidney transplantation (Kahan et al. 1982; Fidelus et al. 1982), CsA trough levels correlate well with the immunosuppressive effect. As our experiment demonstrated, trough levels between 1800 and 700 ng/ml ensure good immunosuppression. These levels are reached by oral CsA administration. To our knowledge, simular results in small-bowel transplantation in rats have not been published.

When CsA is given orally, only 30% of the total amount reaches the central circulation, while intraperitoneal administration allows 80%–90% of the drug to reach the central blood circulation. Thus, the hepatic first-pass effect amounts to 10%–20%, whereas 50% of the oral dose is likely to be metabolized or may not be absorbed in the intestine.

When anastomosing the vena mesenterica superior to the vena cava, bioavailability will increase by 15% when the drug is administered by hepatic routes. On the other hand, disturbances of the lymphatic drainage may equalize this effect. Rejection or graft-vs-host disease, as well as altered hepatic blood flow or metabolism, may also influence the drug disposition. No exact data are available on these subjects. Consequently, in this situation the intramuscular route should be preferred as long as these factors cannot be calculated. As an example, to achieve an "average" blood concentration at steady state of 1500 ng/ml, 3.4 mg/kg CsA should be administered intramuscularly as a maintenance dose.

References

Fidelus RK, Ferguson RM, Widmer MB, Wee S, Bade FH, Orosz C (1982) Effect of cyclosporin A on murine and human T-helper-cell clones. Transplantation 34/5:308–311
Gibaldi M, Perrier D (1975) Pharmacokinetics. Deccer, New York
Kahan BD, van Buren CT, Lin SN, Ono Y, Agostino G, Le Grue SJ, Boihan M, Payne WD, Kerman RH (1982) Immunopharmacological monitoring of cyclosporin A-treated recipients of cadaveric kidney allografts. Transplantation 34/1:36–46
Wassef R, Cohen Z, Nordgren S, Langer B (1985) Cyclosporine absorption in intestinal transplantation. Transplantation 39/5:496–499

Session 5: Summary

Z. COHEN

The study of intestinal structure and function following small-intestinal transplantation has been hindered in the large-animal model by the fact that there have been infrequent long-term survivors in both dog and pig models. The most recent work in a rat model, both orthotopic and heterotopic, has allowed for isolation of rejection and graft-versus-host responses and more detailed immunologic assessment. In transplantation from Lewis-to-Brown Norway rats, there was more consistent long-term survival when cyclosporine was given over an extended, but not indefinite, period, suggesting that this model of immunosuppression following small-bowel transplantation may be useful for such studies. Extrapolation to humans or to larger animals is difficult however, and it is unlikely that cessation of cyclosporine medication will result in long-term graft survivals. Nevertheless, the success of the experiment described by Schraut's group provides some encouragement that successful clinical small-bowel transplantation using cyclosporine alone or in combination with other immunosuppressive agents may be possible.

One must also examine the effects of cyclosporine given to the recipient before transplantation, and in the studies described in this section, there seemed to be significantly prolonged animal survival of over 50% with short-term treatment prior to the dady of grafting. Pretreatment of the donor, along with further studies of techniques of preserving the small intestine will be important to successful small-bowel transplantation in humans.

Comparing the routes of administration is somewhat more difficult, and again, one can not easily extrapolate from small-animal experiments to the human situation. Cyclosporine has been administered orally, intraperitoneally, and intravenously. Obviously, following clinical transplantation, the cyclosporine must be given parenterally. It is difficult at this time to state categorically whether it should be by the intravenous or the intramuscular route. Intramuscular injection of cyclosporine can be painful, whereas intravenous injection of cyclosporine can be unpredictable and rather dangerous, with anaphylactoid reactions having been reported. In our own experience with a clinical intestinal transplant, we feel that cyclosporine given intravenously either as a slow bolus infusion or continuously played a large part in the failure of the graft and subsequent death of the recipient.

Cyclosporine has been used with increasing success in transplant situations, but it is a difficult drug to utilize and control. It has rekindled interest in intestinal transplantation because of its dual effect in both graft-versus-host disease and rejection, but it is possible that we might have to use this drug in combination with other agents, such as prednisolone or antilymphocyte globulin, or even utilize more conventional therapy in the early post-transplantation period prior to instituting cyclosporine therapy.

Session 6

Surgical Techniques in Animals and Man

Intestinal Transplantation: Surgical Techniques in Animals and Man

S. NORDGREN and Z. COHEN

Introduction

The physiologic and surgical basis for a successful experimental small-intestinal transplantation was first investigated by Richard LILLEHEI and coworkers (1959). Work at that time focused on the effects of intestinal ischemia on body hemodynamics, as well as on problems related to intestinal in vitro preservation and subsequent reimplantation. It was demonstrated that the small bowel could be removed from a dog, stored outside the body for 2 h, and then reimplanted. It was also demonstrated that the autotransplanted small intestine could sustain life in the experimental animal and that after an initial period of diarrhea these dogs gained weight. During the following decade, a large number of experimental reports were presented. Despite the fact that long-term survival in allotransplanted experimental animals was not consistantly achieved, a small number of cases of intestinal transplantation in man were attempted. However, these clinical attempts were universally unsuccessful, with the longest survival being only 79 days, and experimental research activity diminished.

With the discovery of cyclosporine A (BOREL et al. 1976), interest in small-intestinal transplantation was rekindled, and research activity increased again. The two major questions in current research have centered on how to characterize and avert the immunologic response and elucidate the mechanisms by which an intestinal allotransplant can sustain long-term life of the recipient. Immunologic problems have been in the foreground, but today it appears necessary to widen the scope of research and to focus on technical surgical aspects, as these have a profound impact on results.

The aim of this report is to review the surgical techniques employed in small-intestinal transplantation, with emphasis on surgical techniques which influence the specific immunologic situation unique to intestinal allotransplantation and on technical aspects of relevance to specific experimental protocols.

Graft Preservation

The small intestine contains tissue that is highly sensitive to hypoxia and has therefore been used in an experimental model for the investigation of ischemic damage (LILLEHEI 1957). Different preservation techniques to prolong ischemic tolerance of the small intestine have been studied in dogs (Table 1). Short segments of the terminal

Table 1. Preservation of small bowel: experimental results (excerpt)

Method	Tolerance (h)	Reference
Cooling to room temperature	2	LILLEHEI et al. 1959
Cooling to 5°C	5	LILLEHEI et al. 1959
Blood perfusion at 37°C	5	IIJIMA and SALERNO 1967
Pulsatile blood perfusion	18	AUSTEN and MCLAUGHLIN 1965
Collins' solution at 4°C	20	RICOUR et al. 1981
O_2 at 7.9 atm, 4°C, chlorpromazine	48	MANAX et al. 1965

ileum were exposed to ischemia for various lengths of time, and the macroscopic and microscopic appearance after revascularization was examined. It was demonstrated that cooling of the bowel to 5°C by cold perfusion resulted in no microscopic damage for up to 5 h after blood flow was interrupted (LILLEHEI et al. 1959). Increasing the oxygen tension to 3 atm increased the ischemic tolerance to 24 h and with the combination of oxygen at 7 atm and chlorpromazine, ischemic tolerance in a nonperfusion system was increased to 48 h (MANAX et al. 1965). Ischemic tolerance exceeding 48 h has not been reported.

It is of interest to note that preservation techniques may change the immunologic response to the small intestine in the allotransplant situation. TOLEDO-PEREYRA et al. (1974a) have demonstrated that perfusion of canine intestinal allografts for 24 h with cryoprecipitated canine plasma or xenogeneic plasma preparations significantly prolonged survival of whole orthotopic small-intestinal allotransplants in moderately immunosuppressed dogs. The reason for this increase in immunologic tolerance remains unknown. Perfusion of the vascular bed of the intestinal graft with Ringer's lactate or saline at 4°C, as used by most laboratories, appears adequate for experimental work in the rat, pig and dog. Collins' solution at 4°C was used by RICOUR et al. (1981) similarly to its routine use in kidney transplantation, and successful preservation for 20 h was achieved. A nonperfusion technique using Collins' solution and a pulsatile perfusion system were compared by TOLEDO-PEREYRA and NAJARIAN (1973). It was concluded that pulsatile perfusion may be the most satisfactory method for preservation of intestinal grafts. The importance of antibiotics and steroids in the preservation solution of the small intestine has been investigated in a dog model. The survival times of dogs following total small-intestinal allotransplantation using perfusates with and without the addition of an antibiotic were compared by TOLEDO-PEREYRA et al. (1974b). Endotoxemia and bacteremia were more common in recipient dogs with unprepared bowels, and survival was prolonged in dogs transplanted with intestines prepared with neomycin, kanamycin and steroids.

NonVascularized Grafts

The possibility of studying intestinal transplants without doing time-consuming vascular anastomoses appears attractive, but there are definite limitations in the nonvascularized techniques that should be kept in mind. Few reports have been published. The histology and time course of rejection of nonvascularized fetal intestinal grafts were studied in the mouse by FERGUSON and PARROTT (1973). Small fragments, 0.5–1.0 cm long, of fetal mouse small intestine were implanted under the kidney capsule in adult mice and subsequently examined histologically. Of 214 grafts, 173 were available for histologic examination, indicating an 80% technical success rate. Segmental heterotopic transplantation of rat fetal small intestine in a subcutaneous position was performed by LEAPMAN et al. (1974). In this series of experiments, transplanted segments of bowel were also cannulated and used for perfusion studies. Of 160 segments thus transplanted, 120 were acceptable for further experimentation – a 75% success rate, comparable to vascularized techniques. Subcutaneously transplanted fetal rat small intestine has also been brought into intestinal continuity by the same group (DEUTSCH et al. 1973), but with limited success. Only five of 86 operated rats survived transection of the native intestine previously bypassed by the graft. Attempts have also been made to transplant 5-cm lengths of newborn piglet small intestine avascularly (KLOS 1977). These segments were wrapped in the omentum as free transplants, but considerable structural damage was noted in most of these transplants.

The technique employing nonvascularized grafts appears adequate for comparative immunologic studies, but it is not clear to what extent the heterotopic position of the graft changes bowel architecture and function. Furthermore, allogeneic properties of the small intestine that differ from the fetal to the adult stage render the technique less important for clinically oriented research.

Significance of the Volume of the Transplanted Tissue

The length of small intestine necessary to sustain life in a recipient has not been determined. This question is of importance, because there are observations indicating that the volume of the transplanted intestine and mesentery has a bearing on the subsequent immunologic response. To illustrate this point, we note that RUIZ and LILLEHEI (1972) report that ten dogs, after intestinal allotransplantation of the entire small intestine, died in a characteristically precipitous fashion, and at autopsy no satisfactory explanation for the cause of death was found. The intestinal allografts appeared viable, although the lymph nodes in the allograft mesentery were enlarged. In contrast, short segments of allotransplanted nonimmunosuppressed small intestine invariably develop severe structural damage compatible with rejection (HARDY et al. 1970). Since a bidirectional immunologic response is known to occur in small-intestinal transplantation (MONCHIK and RUSSELL 1971), it is hypothesized that graft-vs-host reaction (GvHR) dominates over rejection in animals with total small-intestinal allografts, and particularly in dogs after splenectomy (RUIZ and LILLEHEI 1972). The importance of the length of the transplanted intestine appears to be less pronounced in the rat, although indirect evidence for an impact on the balance between rejection and GvHR by varying the length of the graft was presented by DELTZ (1981).

Aspects of Techniques for Vascular Anastomoses

In contrast to the surgical techniques necessary for hepatic and cardiac transplantation, small-bowel transplantation is not technically demanding. In the dog and the pig, mesenteric vessels are large enough for standard surgical techniques, and in the rat a microscope or other means of magnification are sufficient for satisfactory results. The vascular dissection for harvesting the small intestine in the dog is simple, and the middle colic artery must only occasionally be severed. Therefore, the harvest per se does not preclude survival of the donor, and autotransplantation can easily be performed in the dog.

In the rat, harvest of the mesenteric artery with an aortic cuff is generally utilized. This procedure allows for an arterial anastomosis of convenient size (MONCHIK and RUSSELL 1971), but precludes donor survival. Techniques for intestinal harvesting in the rat with donor survival appear to be unnecessary.

Systemic venous return through a vascular anastomosis between the superior mesenteric vein and the inferior vena cava is the predominant technique, although serious concern with respect to the possible deleterious effect of shortcircuiting the liver has been raised (DILIZ-PEREZ et al. 1984). There is to date no report suggesting encephalopathy in experimental animals after intestinal transplantation with systemic venous return, although this has not been the target of specific research. However, there is evidence suggesting that the immunologic response to an intestinal allograft is mitigated when the venous return from the graft is directed by way of portal circulation (SCHRAUT et al. 1983). Similar observations in kidney transplantation have been presented earlier (SAKAI 1970). These findings will most likely have clinical significance, although it is doubtful whether the portal vein is always patent in patients requiring small-intestinal allografts.

Surgical Techniques in Various Species

Rat

Except for the subcutaneous placement of avascular intestinal grafts mentioned above (LEAPMAN et al. 1974), the abdominal heterotopic position has been the prevalent site in the rat (Table 2). Orthotopic nonauxiliary grafting is hazardous in the rat owing to the pronounced loss of water in the early postoperative period, but has been successfully performed by KORT et al. (1973). As the significance of functional survival studies in rats is questionable, present use of the orthotopic nonauxiliary technique in this animal is not usually justified. In using the auxiliary graft with a distal end-to-side anastomosis (DELTZ 1981) or the heterotopic Thiry-Vella loop (SCHRAUT et al. 1983; KIRKMAN et al. 1984) first presented by MONCHIK and RUSSELL (1971), variable lengths of small intestine can be transplanted and allowed to drain into the distal small bowel or drain externally via a cutaneous enterostomy. The Thiry-Vella loop provides an opportunity to obtain sequential biopsies from the graft, and this can also be easily accessed for physiologic studies. When intestinal function is of less

Table 2. Surgical techniques for intestinal transplantation in the rat

Center	Graft site	Drainage	Type of investigation	Reference
Massachusetts General Hospital, Boston, Massachusetts, U.S.A.	Heterotopic Auxiliary	Thiry-Vella	Immunologic Histologic	MONCHIK and RUSSELL 1971
Rotterdam, Netherlands	Orthotopic Non-auxiliary	In continuity	Survival Histological	KORT et al. 1973
Kiel, Federal Republic of Germany	Heterotopic Auxiliary	Distal Anastomosis End-to-side	Immunologic Histologic	DELTZ 1981
Chicago, Illinois, U.S.A.	Heterotopic Auxiliary	Thiry-Vella	Survival Histologic	SCHRAUT et al. 1983
Brigham and Women's, Boston, Massachusetts, U.S.A.	Heterotopic Auxiliary	Thiry-Vella	Immunologic	KIRKMAN et al. 1984

concern, as in immunologic studies, internal drainage by means of an end-to-side anastomosis to the native intestine is adequate.

The problem of creating an appropriate control situation for physiologic studies of the transplanted intestine in the rat can be overcome with a slight modification of the heterotopic auxiliary technique. To avoid structural changes in the graft or changes in graft function induced by the out-of-continuity position of the graft, we suggest an orthotopic auxiliary graft which is brought into continuity by means of a distal and a proximal end-to-side anastomosis, as shown in Fig. 1. This technique has been used in a preliminary series of experiments on rats in our laboratory, and there have been no technical problems related to the intestinal anastomoses. At laparotomy, 2–3 weeks after isotransplantation, the contents of both small intestinal loops looks normal. Possible structural and physiologic changes induced when the graft is out of continuity with the remaining alimentary tract (LEVINE et al. 1974) are avoided by this technique. At a second laparotomy, both sets of small intestine can be used for comparative morphological or physiologic investigations, as the native small intestine serves as an excellent control for the transplanted intestine.

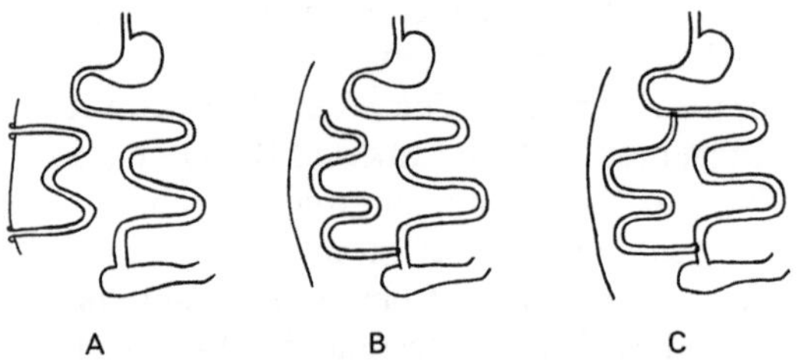

Fig. 1A–C. Three possible types of drainage of the intestinal graft. **A** Thiry-Vella; **B** heterotopic, internal drainage; **C** orthotopic auxiliary

Dog

In the initial experiments in the dog by LILLEHEI et al. (1959), the surgical technique was chosen so as to anticipate the actual clinical situation of small-intestinal transplantation. There, the entire small intestine was removed from the recipient before implantation of the graft. This technique was later adopted by several other laboratories (ALICAN et al. 1971; KUNLIN et al. 1971; GARRIDO et al. 1975; COHEN et al. 1976; DILIZ-PEREZ et al. 1984). The orthotopic nonauxiliary experimental model in the dog is extremely complex and produces a number of technical problems and complications. This, in combination with increased pressures from lay organizations, as well as increasing costs for the experimental animals, has reduced the number of dogs used for the orthotopic technique. Heterotopic, abdominal segmental grafting with a Thiry-Vella loop was used by HOLMES (1973), but even in this situation, disintegration of the graft at rejection may jeopardize recipient survival, causing similar arguments to arise.

Heterotopic cervical transplantation of intestinal segments was first described by MANAX et al. (1965). This technique allows for immunologic, morphological, and functional studies and has been employed by several groups of investigators (PRESTON et al. 1966; STATE 1969; GRENIER et al. 1970; HARDY et al. 1970; WESTBROEK et al. 1970; SCHILLER et al. 1973). Cervical allograft rejection is less harmful for the recipient than small-intestinal allograft rejection, and if necessary, the graft can be removed and the dog salvaged. Possible disadvantages of this technique are those normally connected with grafts that are out of continuity as well as hypothetical changes induced by the heterotopic position of the graft in the neck.

A combination of abdominal small-intestinal transplantations in the dog both in and out of continuity was suggested by KUNLIN et al. (1971). In this study, an isolated pouch was created from the graft and brought to the skin as a mucous fistula. Biopsies from these isolated pouches were compared histologically with biopsies from an open Y loop from the graft in continuity, and congruence was documented. Similar results were reached by other workers comparing histologic studies of isolated pouches and open intestinal biopsies (LOSSING et al. 1982). This technique, including an isolated pouch of the graft brought to the skin, was used for monitoring purposes by FORTNER et al. (1972) in a case of clinical transplantation.

Pig

The pig is biologically more like the human than the dog, but use of this animal in experimental surgery brings with it major disadvantages. Laboratory handling in general, and administration of anesthesia in particular, is hazardous in the adult pig, which makes it less suitable for experimental work (STAUFFER et al. 1974). Although piglets are easier to manage, they have not been widely used in experimental intestinal transplantation. Orthotopic nonauxiliary transplantation of porcine small intestine was used in a survival study by KEAVENY et al. (1970) to investigate the feasibility of intestinal transplantation in this species and to determine whether intestinal allograft tolerance would develop consistent with that which has been observed in porcine allogeneic liver transplants. Heterotopic positioning of the graft as a Thiry-Vella loop is the predominant technique utilized (Stauffer et al. 1974; Ricour et al. 1981). The pig model has been used for morphological and functional studies, as well as for more clinically oriented research. Stauffer et al. (1978) used piglets for studying the possibility of safe explantation of a rejected graft. This is a very important aspect of experimental intestinal transplantation to which little attention has been paid.

Surgical Techniques in Clinical Intestinal Transplantation

Five cases of human intestinal transplantation were reported before 1972 (Lillehei et al. 1967; Olivier et al. 1969; Alican et al. 1971; Ruiz and Llehei 1972; Fortner et al. 1972). In all reported clinical cases, the transplant was brought to the body surface with at least one of its ends as a stoma or an isolated pouch. This method has been adopted in the clinical intestinal transplantation that has been performed in 1985 in Toronto (Table 3). The purpose for construction of a "window" to the graft is obvious: Vascular complications can be diagnosed early, before life-threatening peritonitis develops. Cutaneous access to the graft also allows for sequential biopsies of the graft considered important for monitoring possible rejection. However, in the current literature on intestinal transplantation, the intestinal anastomosis has presented no particular problems, and there are no safety factors that preclude its use. Furthermore, in patients with a colonic remnant, an anastomosis to this organ should be carried out immediately, or at a second operation to make use of the colonic water absorption capacity (Debonguie and Phillips 1978). The general experience has been that experimental animals suffer severe diarrhea for several weeks after

Table 3. Surgical techniques employed in clinical intestinal transplantation

Team	Year	Length of transplant	Venous drainage	Intestinal Drainage
Lillehei et al.	1967	Total small intestine and proximal colon	Inferior vena cava	Thiry-Vella
Okumura et al. (See Ruiz and Lillehei 1972)	1968	170 cm	Left iliac vein	Thiry-Vella
Oliver et al.	1969	Total small intestine and proximal colon	Portal vein	Proximal anastamosis, distal stoma
Alican and Hardy (See Alican et al. 1971)	1969	100 cm	Left renal vein	Thiry-Vella
Fortner et al. (See Fortner et al. 1972)	1970	150 cm	Right iliac vein	Proximal and distal anastamosis and pouch
Cohen et al. (Unpublished experience)	1985	Total small intestine	Inferior vena cava	Thiry-Vella

intestinal transplantation. It is believed that this diarrhea is caused by a reduced capacity for absorption of the transplanted small intestine. This assumption is supported by preliminary observations in the rat (own unpublished observations). Experience in the treatment of patients with Crohn's disease shows that, in patients with short bowel, every inch of remaining colon is useful and can reduce the number and volume of the stools (ANDERSSON et al. 1982).

Based on results of experimental work, no particular technique for human intestinal transplantation can be advised. For reasons mentioned above, a proximal stoma and a distal anastomosis in patients with functioning parts of the colon may be advantageous. Closure of the proximal stoma with a proximal anastomosis, possibly in conjunction with the construction of an isolated pouch, can be performed at a later date. However, there are several questions of a technical nature that remain unanswered. The length of the bowel necessary for sufficient function has not been established. Furthermore, it is known that cyclosporine is absorbed by the allotransplanted small bowel (MACKENZIE et al. 1982), but the question of whether the systemic venous return commonly used in experimental intestinal transplantation has any impact on metabolism and hence on the immunosuppressive properties of this drug has not been investigated. Another question related to cyclosporine is whether enterally and parenterally administered cyclosporine is more rapidly cleared in patients with continuous drainage of the stomach and duodenum (e.g., external biliary drainage) in a nonenteric state. These and other questions will have to be addressed in future experimental work.

Conclusion

Although the basic surgical technique for intestinal transplantation is simple, a great variety of surgical techniques and experimental situations of varying complexity are possible. It is important to scrutinize carefully the aims and objectives of the research in order to select an adequate animal model and experimental technique allowing relevant and maximal information at a reasonable cost. Secondly, technical aspects are important, because the threat of immunologic problems can be mitigated by surgical manipulation of the graft, e.g., by pretreatment of the graft or by performing a portoportal venous return. Finally, questions related to the harvesting of the small intestine in man remain unclear, particularly when one considers the multiorgan donor and the priority of organs to be harvested.

References

Alican F, Hardy JD, Cayirli M, Varner JE, Moynihan PC, Turner MD, Anas P (1971) Intestinal transplantation: Laboratory experience and report of a clinical case. Am J Surg 121:150–159

Andersson H, Bosaeus I, Hellberg R, Hultén L (1982) Effect of a low fat diet and antidiarrhoeal agents on bowel habits after excisional surgery for classical Crohn's disease. Acta Chir Scand 148:285–290

Austen WG, McLaughlin ED (1965) In-vitro small bowel perfusion. Surg Forum 16:359
Borel JF, Feurer C, Gubler HU, Stähelin H (1976) Biological effects of cyclosporin A: A new antilymphocytic agent. Agents Actions 6/4:468–475
Cohen Z, MacGregor AB, Moore TH, Falk RE, Langer B, Cullen JB (1976) Canine small bowel transplantation. Arch Surg 111:248–253
Debonguie JC, Phillips SC (1978) Capacity of the human colon to absorb fluid. Gastroenterology 74:698–703
Deltz E (1981) Die allogene Dünndarmtransplantation. Zuckschwerdt, Munich (Thesis)
Deutsch AA, Leapman SB, Arensman R, Folkman J (1973) Anastomosis of transplanted fetal rat intestine to the normal intestine of the host. J Surg Res 15:176–181
Diliz-Perez HS, McClure J, Bedetti C, Hong HQ, de Santibanes E, Shaw BW, van Thiel D, Iwatsuki S, Starzl T (1984) Successful small bowel allotransplantation in dogs with cyclosporine and prednisone. Transplantation 37:126–129
Ferguson A, Parrott MV (1973) Histopathology and time course of rejection of allografts of mouse small intestine. Transplantation 15:546–554
Fortner JG, Sichuk G, Litwin SD, Beattie ED Jr (1972) Immunological responses to an intestinal allograft with HL-A-identical donor-recipient. Transplantation 14:531–535
Garrido H, de Diego JA, Cano MC, Lucea C, Escribano PM, Manzanos A (1975) Homograft of the small intestine. Metabolic and functional changes causing irreversible shock. Int Surg 60:251–254
Grenier J-F, Doremieux J, Wong P, Bötescu V (1970) Transplantations d'intestin grêle chez le chien: Enseignements tirés d'une statistique de 100 cas. Chirurgie 96:958–968
Hardy MA, Quint J, State D (1970) Effect of antilymphocyte serum and other immunosuppressive agents on canine jejunal allografts. Ann Surg 171:51–60
Holmes JT (1973) Small-bowel transplantation: An experimental study. Ann R Coll Surg Engl 52:165–181
Jijima K, Salermo RA (1967) Survival of small intestine following excision, perfusion and autotransplantation. Ann Surg 166:968
Keaveny TV, Aglubat F, Belzer FO (1970) Porcine small bowel, allotransplantation. Ir J Med Sc 3:483–487
Kirkman RL, Lear PA, Madara JL, Tilney NL (1984) Small intestine transplantation in the rat: Immunology and function. Surgery 96:280–287
Klos I (1977) Avascular transplantation of small bowel in newborn piglets. J Pediatr Surg 12:43–48
Kort WJ, Westbroek DL, MacDicken I, Lameijer LDF (1973) Orthotopic total small bowel transplantation in the rat. Eur Surg Res 5:81–89
Kunlin A, Gaston JP, Shiu MH, Winawer SJ, Fortner JG (1971) The isolated allograft pouch: A useful method for monitoring small bowel allografts. Surg Forum 22:237–239
Leapman SB, Deutsch AA, Grand RJ, Folkman J (1974) Transplantation of fetal intestine: Survival function in a subcutaneous location in adult animals. Ann Surg 179:109–114
Levine GM, Deren JJ, Steiger E, et al (1974) Role of oral intake in maintenance of gut mass and disacharidase activity. Gastroenterology 67:975
Lillehei R (1957) The intestinal factor in irreversible hemorrhagic shock. Surgery 42:1043
Lillehei RC, Goott B, Miller FA (1959) The physiological response of the small bowel of the dog to ischemia including prolonged in vitro preservation of the bowel with successful replacement and survival. Ann Surg 150:543–560
Lillehei RC, Idezuki Y, Feemster JA, Dietzman RH, Merkel FK, Goetz FC (1967) Transplantation of stomach, intestine and pancreas: Experimental and clinical observations. Surgery 62:721
Lossing A, Nordgren S, Cohen Z, Craddock CG, Langer B (1982) Histologic monitoring of rejection in small intestinal transplantation. Transplant Proc 14:643–645
Mackenzie R, Nordgren S, Lossing A, Craddock G, Cohen Z, Stiller C, Langer B (1982) Cyclosporin A absorption in canine small intestinal transplantation. Transplant Proc 14:646–648
Manax WG, Bloch JH, Eyal Z, Lillehei RC (1965) Experimental preservation of the small bowel. Am J Surg 109:26–31
Monchik GJ, Russell PS (1971) Transplantation of small bowel in the rat: Technical and immunological considerations. Surgery 70:693–702
Olivier G, Rettori F, Olivier C (1969) Homotransplantation orthotopique de l'intestin grêle et des côlons droit et transverse chez l'homme. J Chir 98:323

Preston FW, Macalalad F, Wachowski TJ, Randolph DA, Apostol JV (1966) Survival of homografts of the intestine with and without immunosuppression. Surgery 60:1203–1210
Ricour C, Revillon Y, Pletyncx M, Laufenburger A, Jehannin B, Ghnassia D, Duval C, Ghnassia J-C, Jos J, Fontaine J-L, Navarro J, Schmitz J, Gallix P (1981) Conservation hypothermique et autotransplantation du grêle chez le porcelet. Gastroenterol Clin Biol 5:977–986
Ruiz JO, Lillehei RC (1972) Intestinal transplantation. Am J Proct 23:379–393
Ruiz JO, Lillehei RC (1972) Intestinal transplantation. Surg Clin North Am 52:1075–1091
Sakai A (1970) Role of the liver in kidney allograft rejection in the rat. Transplantation 9:333
Schiller WR, Suriyapa C, Mutchler JHW, Gohara SF, Anderson MC (1973) Motility changes associated with canine intestinal allografting. J Surg Res 15:379–384
Schraut WH, Rosemurgy AS, Riddell RM (1983) Prolongation of intestinal allograft survival without immunosuppressive drug therapy. J Surg Res 34:597–607
State D (1969) Experimental studies in intestinal allografts. Surg Clin North Am 49:547–552
Stauffer UG, Becker M, Karamehmedovic O, Gessendorfer H, Rickham PP (1974) Transplantations of small intestines. J Pediatr Surg 9:21–28
Stauffer UG, Becker M, Hirsig J, Meier HP, Kara O (1978) The risks of small intestinal transplantation for the recipient: Experimental results in young minipigs. J Pediatr Surg 13:465–487
Toledo-Pereyra LH, Najarian JS (1973) Small bowel preservation. Arch Surg 107:875–877
Toledo-Pereyra LH, Simmons RL, Najarian JS (1974a) Prolonged survival of canine orthotopic small intestinal allografts preserved for 24 hours by hypothermic bloodless perfusion. Surgery 75:368–376
Toledo-Pereyra LH, Raij L, Simmons RL, Najarian JS (1974b) Role of endotoxin and bacteria in long-term survival of preserved small-bowel allografts. Surgery 73:474–481
Westbroek DL, Rothengatter C, Vriesendorp HM, van Rood JJ (1970) Histocompatibility and heterotopic segmental small bowel allograft survival in dogs. Eur Surg Res 2:401–407

*Stoma or No Stoma in Intestinal Transplantation**

G. TANNENBAUM, A. I. BENVENISTY, J. CHABOT**, and M. A. HARDY

Introduction

More effective methods of host and donor organ immunosuppression and improved microvascular techniques have led to increased interest in small-bowel transplantation in various experimental models. Prior to this decade, intestinal graft loss was frequently the result of technical problems of vascular thrombosis or hemorrhage and in some studies approached 40%–50%. Recently, the reported early graft failure from arterial or venous thrombosis has been less than 10% (DILEZ-PEREZ et al. 1984; PRITCHARD et al. 1985). The use of cyclosporine as an immunosuppressive has resulted in prolonged intestinal allograft survival (CRADDOCK et al. 1983; DILEZ-PEREZ et al. 1984). Although interest in clinical trials is being rekindled by the improvement in experimental results, it is clear that there are still many unanswered questions about the technical aspects of small-bowel transplantation.

An important issue that requires further studies relates to the management of the intestinal ends of the graft. Should the graft be placed in continuity with the recipient's native bowel or should it be left excluded? The surgeon has several options to consider (Table 1, Fig. 1). In experimental models, the native bowel is acutely removed prior to implantation and anastomosis, while in clinical practice most of the small intestine is resected prior to consideration of transplantation. In this more difficult surgical and

Table 1. Options in management of the intestinal ends in intestinal allograft

No stoma: graft entirely in continuity
Stoma
Two stomas: graft entirely excluded from continuity
One stoma
Proximal jejunostomy, distal anastomosis
Proximal anastomosis, distal ileostomy
Combinations
Blind proximal and/or distal pouch with rest of graft in continuity
Roux-en-Y type mucous fistula

* Supported in part by NIH grants AM34232 and AM30468.
** Irvington House Institute Fellow, 1985.

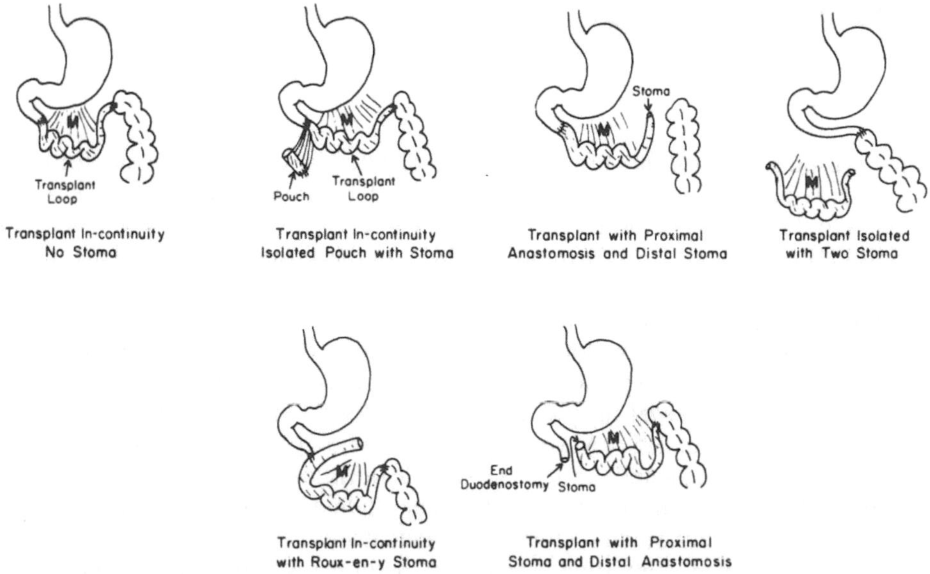

Fig. 1. Intestinal transplantation: options in management of intestinal end

nutritional setting, any existing enteroenterostomy or enterocolostomy would require division prior to the insertion of the transplant, with proximal and distal anastomoses of the graft to the host's remaining intestine. The required dissection might be formidable.

Alternatively, the bowel graft could be kept entirely excluded from the host's gastrointestinal tract by attaching both ends of the transplant to the skin as stomas. Thus, the operative procedure would entail only the vascular anastomoses, and the surgical field would not be exposed to bowel contamination. Intestinal continuity could be established secondarily at another time, after graft viability and function have been assured.

Other options include the establishment of only partial intestinal continuity. Choices include a proximal stoma with distal graft-to-colon anastomosis or proximal gastro- or enteroenterostomy and distal graft enterostomy. Such procedures would also require extensive dissection of the host's bowel and risk contamination of the operative field.

Another option described by KUNLIN et al. (1971) places the graft in continuity with the host's bowel while a short segment of the proximal and/or distal end of the transplant, isolated with its vasculature intact, is closed at one end and brought to the skin as a blind pouch that can be used as a stoma. This also includes the risk of contamination and the risks involved with two intestinal anastomoses. A variation of this method is reconnection of the isolated segment to the transplant as a Roux-en-Y type enterostomy.

Historical Perspectives

Experimental

The decision to use a stoma has in part been dictated by the choice of site for graft placement. Transplanted bowel has been placed heterotopically in the necks of animals to study allograft motility (SCHILLER et al. 1973) and to evaluate function and survival (HARDY et al. 1970; RAJU et al. 1984). In this position, proximal and distal stomas permit gross inspection of mucosal viability and serve as an access for biopsies and functional studies of the transplanted intestine.

Graft placement in the peritoneal cavity demands a decision on how best to deal with two ends of the transplant. When the gastrointestinal tract remains intact, an auxiliary heterotopic bowel allograft is usually placed so that rejection (HOLMES et al. 1971; KIRKMAN et al. 1984; MADARA and KIRKMAN 1985), graft-vs-host disease (DELTZ et al. 1983; LEE and SCHRAUT 1985; MONCHICK and RUSSEL 1971), or graft absorptive function (HOLMES et al. 1970) can be studied in an otherwise nutritionally intact animal. For such studies, stomas are mandatory.

When the recipient's intestine is removed, as in many experimental studies (by choice) and in all clinical cases (by necessity), the question of whether or not to establish partial or complete autograft or allograft intestinal continuity becomes important. The answer to this question may influence the possible complications of the procedure, the function of the graft, and ultimately the well-being of the transplant recipient.

Clinical

In the few reported cases of human intestinal transplantation, several of the proposed options for management of the allograft ends have been employed. LILLEHEI et al. (1967) transplanted the entire jejunoileum and ascending colon of a cadaver donor with two stomas: a proximal jejunostomy and a distal transverse colostomy. An orthotopic transplant was performed by OLIVIER et al. (1969) with a proximal duodenum-to-graft jejunal anastomosis and distal colostomy. The patient lived 26 days, and the distal graft stoma provided access for serial mucosal biopsies. ALICAN et al. (1971) transplanted a segment of ileum from a living donor into the peritoneal cavity of a related 10-year-old recipient without any intestinal continuity and with two stomas. On the 3rd postoperative day, the stomas were noted to be necrotic, and the graft was removed. FORTNER et al. (1972), in transplanting 170 cm of jejunoileum from a living related donor, placed the graft in continuity with the host's remaining bowel. A short segment of the allograft's proximal end was used as an isolated pouch with a stoma on the anterior abdominal wall. The pouch provided access for mucosal biopsies until the patient's death on the 76th day after transplantation.

Stomas in Intestinal Transplantation

Advantages

Most importantly, a proximal or distal stoma can be used for obtaining mucosal biopsies from the allograft. The biopsy continues to be the most reliable indication of early graft rejection (KIRKMAN et al. 1984; LOSSING et al. 1983; RICOUR et al. 1983) and thus serves as a guide to management of immunosuppressive therapy. Histologic evidence for rejection, which includes blunting of mucosal villi, mononuclear cell infiltration of the intestinal wall, and epithelial cell attenuation and vacuolization have also been noted in biopsies from isolated allograft pouches (COHEN et al. 1984). The findings were the same in both the allograft pouch and the transplant placed in continuity with the host's intestine when the effect of cyclosporine was evaluated.

Monitoring of the grafts physiologic function as a means of detecting rejection has not been uniformly reliable. Studies of radioactively labeled glucose in rejecting jejunal autograft and allograft segments revealed gradually decreased absorption as histologic rejection progressed (COHEN et al. 1969; HARDY et al. 1968, 1970). Similar findings were reported by RUIZ et al. (1972) using D-xylose absorption studies and by MACKENZIE et al. (1982), who measured blood levels of orally administered cyclosporine. HOLMES et al. (1970), on the other hand, found increased glucose absorption during progressive intestinal rejection. More recently, the Toronto group (NORDGREN et al. 1984) confirmed the original observations in a proximal blind jejunal pouch by evaluating serial [^{14}C]glucose absorption as a test of graft function. They found a gradual decrease in both the rate and the absolute amount of absorption in a rejecting graft. These findings suggest that the earlier conflicting results might be related to problems inherent in the feeding of experimental animals. Reports on the absorptive capabilities of isolated bowel autografts and allografts suggest that function can return promptly if rejection is controlled (HARDY et al. 1970; STANFORD and HARDY 1974). It appears, therefore, that in either the isolated pouch or through the stomas of the entire graft, absorptive studies performed can be reliably correlated with other findings of rejection.

Other studies of graft function can be carried out through accessible stomas. Motility studies of isolated intestinal segments placed in the neck (SCHILLER et al. 1973) demonstrated changes in muscular activity that correlate with impending rejection and graft necrosis. Monitoring of changes in the differences in mucosal potential of an intestinal allograft has been shown to be valuable in predicting rejection (MADARA and KIRKMAN 1985; RAJU et al. 1984) and requires a stoma. Another important benefit of a stoma is that it allows direct visual inspection of the bowel mucosa and aids in the early diagnosis of any vascular complications which may be nonimmunologic.

Disadvantages

Complications which occur in patients undergoing total protocolectomy for inflammatory bowel disease, familial polyposis, and other neoplastic diseases can also be expected to occur in recipients of small-bowel allografts if stomas are used. Such complications would be amplified in patients receiving immunosuppressive medications and in those who are chronically nutritionally depleted.

Although the risk of stomal necrosis from impaired circulation to the bowel (Cassidy and Verdenheimer 1985) decreases after the immediate postoperative period, the effect of rejection on mesenteric blood flow might be such as to lead to stomal ischemia in an intestinal allograft. In animals which have survived with intestinal allografts for prolonged periods, there is obliteration of small arterioles by intimal thickening (Craddock et al. 1983; Kort et al. 1973). Similar findings in the vasculature of other transplanted organs are seen with rejection. The complications of allograft necrosis leading to local or systemic infection are lessened by placing the end of the bowel at skin level, as compared with placing it intraperitoneally as part of an intestinal anastomosis. Stomal necrosis was reported by Alican et al. (1971) on the 3rd postoperative dady, and although blood flow to the midportion of the graft was found to be intact, the entire graft was excised.

Stenosis of an ileostomy or a jejunostomy is another complication related to diminished blood flow to the stoma or to fibrotic healing of the peristomal skin. Proximal stagnation and bowel dilatation can result in bacterial overgrowth, a potentially disastrous complication in an immunosuppressed patient. Additionally, bacterial infection in allografted loops has been shown to lead to decreased nutrient absorption from the graft (Holmes et al. 1970). Intestinal disease of any kind reduces cyclosporine absorption (Atkinson et al. 1983), which could further complicate the function of an obstructed and infected graft segment. Parastomal infections can occur and are often caused by improper construction or an ill-fitting appliance. Ileostomy drainage is irritating and can cause skin breakdown leading to infection.

Stomal retraction and prolapse and parastomal herniation are other potential problems. Obstruction of the bowel proximal to an ostomy can occur from adhesions or twisting of the intestine about the point where bowel exits from the peritoneal cavity. This occurs in 10%–30% of patients with ileostomies and often requires operative correction (Morowitz and Kirsner 1981). Furthermore, ileostomies can lead to various metabolic derangements by allowing excessive water and electrolyte loss. These problems are accentuated when large segments of ileum are removed and especially when the terminal ileum is resected (Gallagher et al. 1962). If only a proximal anastomosis is used in an intestinal transplant, the patient will certainly have large fluid losses from the distal stoma. This would be especially true if only a short segment of bowel were transplanted. No excessive fluid losses have occurred from isolated pouches or from segments which are not in continuity with the host's gastrointestinal tract.

Intestinal Allograft in Continuity (Anastomosis)

Healing of Anastomoses

Placing the intestinal graft in-continuity requires special considerations of the healing process in intestinal anastomosis under the influence of immunosuppressive drugs.

Healing of intestinal anastomoses proceeds rapidly in man and in experimental animals. At 2 weeks, in the rat model, jejunal anastomoses have reached the strength of uninjured bowel (JONSSON et al. 1983). Ileal anastomoses never reach the strength of nonoperated ileum, but here, too, healing proceeds rapidly after an initial lag period in the production of wound collagen. The effects on wound healing brought about by some immunosuppressive drugs are well known (EHRLICH and HUNT 1969), but specific information on changes in the healing of intestinal anastomoses is limited. In one study (ASZODI and PONSKY 1984), rats were treated with injections of hydrocortisone for 2 weeks prior to division and reanastomosis of a small-bowel segment. Animals receiving 20 mg/kg steriod per day all developed anastomotic leaks and intra-abdominal collections; those receiving only 5 mg/kg per day had no leaks. This study clearly shows that there is a direct relationship between the dose of steroids and efficiency of healing and tensile strength of the anastomosis.

Cyclosporine does not appear to affect the formation of granulation tissue in the rat (AHONEN et al. 1983). No studies have been published yet which evaluate cyclosporine's effect on bursting strength of intestinal anastomoses.

Effects of Gastrointestinal Continuity

If bowel allograft is placed in continuity with the host's gastrointestinal (GI) tract, problems from fluid and electrolyte losses in the form of diarrhea can be expected in clinical intestinal transplantation. In experimental animals, diarrhea persists for many weeks after an auto- or an allotransplant. This appears to be related to intestinal denervation-induced hypermotility (SCHILLER et al. 1973) and to fat malabsorption from transected lymphatics (COHEN et al. 1983). Return to normal bowel habit coincides with spontaneous reconnection of intestinal lymphatics after approximately 4 weeks (REZNICK et al. 1982), but oral fat feeding, including the administration of cyclosporine in olive oil, continues to cause diarrhea in transplanted dogs at 10 weeks after operation (COHEN et al. 1983). Separation of the graft segment loop from the host's GI tract until reconnection of lymphatics and resolution of postoperative malabsorption have occurred may be beneficial in minimizing fluid and electrolyte disturbances in the recipient. It is presently anticipated that all potential recipients of small-bowel allografts will be maintained on intravenous alimentation and thus at risk of metabolic complications associated with this therapy. A decrease in graft-related fluid and electrolyte difficulties can be achieved by construction of a proximal graft stoma.

Infectious Complications

The risk of infection in the transplant patient has been extensively studied and reviewed (DUMMER et al. 1983; RUBIN et al. 1981). This problem is especially important in the intestinal transplant recipient because the bowel, in contrast to other viscera, is not inherently sterile. Even with conventional oral antibiotic preparations, the small bowel harbors significant numbers of bacteria and fungi (PARKER and O'LEARY 1978).

Bowel allografts can be prepared easily with antibiotics and cathartics in a living related donor. This would be more difficult in cadaver donors. A limited attempt to purge the bowel would certainly be indicated prior to harvesting. If the allograft were to be placed in continuity (with anastomoses), a further wash with antibiotic solutions would be advisable prior to implantation. If stomas are to be constructed, the donor or recipient bowel need never be opened while the peritoneal cavity or wound is open. Maturation of the stomal openings of the graft could even be deferred until wound healing had begun, thereby lowering the risk of a wound infection. Patients in need of intestinal transplants are nutritionally depleted and are therefore at a very high risk for complications associated with infection or wound healing (IRVIN 1978).

If intestinal anastomoses are to be performed at the time of the grafting, the potential for contamination of the operative field is high. BALLINGER et al. (1962) noted infections at the site of the mesenteric vascular anastomoses in autotransplanted animals undergoing immediate intestinal anastomoses. Such infections may result in massive hemorrhage or enteroarterial fistulae. However, if intestinal continuity is not established until after the vessels have healed, such complications are less likely to occur.

The effect of infection on allograft function and rejection deserves further close scrutiny. In the course of allograft rejection, HOLMES et al. (1971) detected the formation of abcesses in the crypt lumen of degenerating villi. They attributed progressive bacterial infection to the initial epithelial damage. The same authors also found that *Escherichia coli* and streptococci frequently cause infections in intestinal transplants in dogs and require antibiotic treatment (HOLMES et al. 1970). The blind jejunal pouch has also been subject to infection (KUNLIN et al. 1971). In mucosal biopsies from infected pouches, epithelial lesions of rejection appeared to be more advanced than those in the noninfected grafts at an equivalent time after transplantation. This implies a cross-reactivity between the bacterial antigens and transplantation antigens, which may be a unique problem in intestinal transplantation, but which is well recognized in immunobiology. TOLEDO-PEREYA et al. (1974) showed prolonged intestinal allograft survival when the donors were treated preoperatively with a mechanical and antibiotic bowel preparation and recipients were given parenteral antibiotics postoperatively [control mean survival time (MST) of 6 days vs antibiotic-treated group with MST of 26 days]. It appears, therefore, that any technique which lowers intraluminal bacterial counts in the intestinal grafts and maintains them at low levels during the initial post-transplant period might be beneficial, from the perspective of infections and potential immunologic problems. Once a graft is placed in continuity, its bacterial flora cannot be readily manipulated. On the other hand, if both proximal and distal stomas are accessible, antibiotic lavage of the graft can be performed at closure and at frequent intervals. With lower bacterial counts, rejection may be milder and less frequent, while conversely, fewer rejection episodes may leave the mucosal epithelium more resistant to infection.

Blind Loop Syndromes

Besides the obvious risk of infections complications in the transplant recipient, there are other complications associated with increased numbers of bacteria in the intestinal lumen. This situation is known to arise in patients who develop stagnation of small-bowel contents as a result of strictures, stenosis, fistulae, diverticula, or blind pouch formation (KING and TOSKES 1979). The bacterial flora are altered in both number and kind, which may lead to nutritional deficiencies, as bacteria compete with the host for nutrients and vitamins. Fat malabsorption, steatorrhea, loss of fat-soluble vitamins, and even direct mucosal damage may occur.

The effects of denervation dysmotility, immunosuppressive drugs, and possible narrowing at anastomosis sites may predispose the recipient of an in-continuity intestinal allograft to a bacterial overgrowth syndrome. Changes in the absorption of radiolabeled glucose by infected intestinal segments were noted by HOLMES et al. (1970). The etiology of malabsorption by an intestinal allograft would be difficult to define unless a stoma were available for inspection, biopsy, and culture.

Effects of Intestinal Exclusion

Long-term exclusion of an intestinal segment from the rest of the host's GI tract could result in altered function of the intestinal mucosa. The effects of pancreatic enzymes on brush-border proteins and the role of intestinal hormones and growth factors may be relevant to intestinal transplantation, but are poorly understood at present. However, even when an intestinal segment is isolated with two stomas, enteral feeding with elemental formulae is feasible. Once lymphatic regeneration occurs (after approximately 6 weeks), short- or medium-chain triglycerides could be employed (STANFORD and HARDY 1974). Feeding by the enteral route might permit discontinuation of intravenous alimentation and allow precise monitoring of graft function.

When to Anastomose

If stomas are created, assuming rejection is controlled and the graft has proven functional, establishment of continuity with the remainder of the host GI tract could be delayed until the vascular connections are well healed and levels of immunosuppressive drugs are lower than in the immediate post-transplant period, thus decreasing the risk of anastomotic disruptions. Re-establishment of continuity will be safest when the patient's nutritional status is improved, the graft is functional, and the initial rejection episodes are controlled.

Conclusion

We conclude that, at present, placement of an intestinal allograft in continuity at the time of transplantation does not appear to be the safest or wisest strategy that can be used. A stoma appears necessary for biopsies, studies of motility, evaluation of electrical activity, and absorption studies. Some or all of these tests are necessary to diagnose rejection and/or malabsorption. An isolated pouch can be used for many of these tests but not for determination of intraluminal infection. The immediate dangers of an acute intestinal anastomosis in immunosuppressed and malnourished recipients are numerous and include infections, vascular complications, and sepsis. Segmental intestinal transplantation with stoma(s) is technically easiest to construct in a most rapid fashion, is safest for the host, permits constant evaluation of the graft via the stoma, and therefore results in most rational management of the patient, allowing for adequate nutrition through the isolated segment. Reestablishment of continuity of the recipient's GI tract would be safest and most beneficial once graft viability is well established and the recipient's risks from another operation are decreased, primarily by improved nutrition and decreased immunosuppression.

References

Ahonen A, Nemlander A, Wiktorowitz K, von Willebrand E, Hekali R, Lalla M, Hayry P (1983) Effect of cyclosporine on wound healing. Transplant Proc 15:3092

Alican F, Hardy JD, Cayiri M, Varner JE, Moynihan PC, Turner MD, Anas P (1971) Intestinal transplantation: Laboratory experience and report of a clinical case. Am J Surg 121:150

Aszodi A, Ponsky L (1984) Effects of corticosteroid on the healing bowel anastomosis. Am Surg 50:546

Atkinson K, Britten K, Paull P, Farrell C, Concannon A, Dodds A, Biggs J (1983) Detrimental effect of intestinal disease on absorption of orally administered cyclosporine. Transplant Proc 15:2446

Ballinger WF, Christy MG, Ashby WB (1962) Auto-transplantation of the small intestine: The effect of denervation. Surgery 52:151

Cassidy S, Verdenheimer MC (1985) Complications of intestinal stomas. Probl Gen Surg 2:545

Cohen WB, Hardy MA, Quint J, State D (1969) Absorptive function in canine jejunal autografts and allografts. Surgery 65:440

Cohen Z, Nordgren SR, Mackenzie RD, Lossing AG, Stiller CR, Langer B (1983) Pharmacokinetics of cyclosporine in a canine intestinal transplantation model. Transplant Proc 15:3013

Cohen Z, Nordgren SR, Lossing AC, Cullen J, Craddock G, Langer B (1984) Morphologic studies of intestinal allograft rejection. Immunosuppression with cyclosporine. Dis Colon Rectum 27:228

Craddock GN, Nordgren SR, Reznick RK, Gilas T, Lossing AG, Cohen Z, Stiller CR, Cullen JB, Langer B (1983) Small bowel transplantation in the dog using cyclosporine. Transplantation 35:284

Deltz E, Ulrichs K, Engemann R, Schack T, Friedrichs B, Muller-Ruchholtz W, Muller-Hermelink HK, Thiede A (1983) Prevention of graft-versus-host reaction following small bowel transplantation by temporary cyclosporine treatment. Transplant Proc 15:3027

Dilez-Perez HS, McClure J, Bedetti C, Hong H, DeSantibanes E, Shaw Jr BW, Thiel DV, Iwatsuki S, Starzl TE (1984) Successful small bowel allotransplantation in dogs with cyclosporine and prednisone. Transplantation 37:126

Dummer JS, Hardy A, Poorsattar A, Ho M (1983) Early infections in kidney, heart and liver transplant recipients on cyclosporine. Transplantation 36:259

Ehrlich HP, Hunt TK (1969) The effect of cortisone and anabolic steroids on the tensile strength of healing wounds. Ann Surg 170:203

Fortner JG, Sichuk G, Litwin SD, Beattie EJ (1972) Immunological responses to an intestinal allograft with HL-A identical donor-recipient. Transplantation 14:531

Gallagher ND, Harrison DD, Skyring AP (1962) Fluid and electrolyte imbalances in patients with long-established ileostomies. Gut 3:219

Hardy MA, Quint J, Cohen WB, State D (1968) ^{14}C-D-glucose absorption in heterotopic jejunal allografts. Gastroenterology 54:1295

Hardy MA, Quint J, State D (1970) Effect of anti-lymphocyte serum and other immunosuppressive agents on canine jejunal allografts. Ann Surg 171:51

Holmes JT, Yeh SDJ, Winawer SJ, Kawano N, Fortner JG (1970) Absorption studies in canine jejunal allografts. Ann Surg 174:101

Holmes JT, Klein MS, Winawer SJ, Fortner JG (1971) Morphological studies of rejection in canine jejunal allografts. Gastroenterology 61:693

Irwin TT (1978) Effects of malnutrion and hyperalimentation on wound healing. Surg Gynecol Obstet 146:33

Jonsson K, Jiborn H, Zederfeldt B (1983) Breaking strength of small intestinal anastomoses. Am J Surg 145:800

King CE, Toskes PP (1979) Small intestine bacterial overgrowth. Gastroenterology 76:1035

Kirkman RL, Lear PA, Madara JL, Tilney NL (1984) Small intestinal transplantation in the rat: Immunology and function. Surgery 96:280

Kort WJ, Westbroek DL, MacDiken I, Lamijer LDF (1973) Orthotopic total small bowel transplantation in the rat. Eur Surg Res 5:81

Kunlin A, Gaston JP, Shiu MH, Winawer SJ, Fortner JG (1971) The isolated allograft pouch: A useful method for monitoring small bowel allografts. Surg Forum 22:237

Lee KKW, Schraut WH (1985) In vitro allograft irradiation prevents graft-versus-host disease in small bowel transplantation. J Surg Res 38:364

Lillehei RC, Idezuki J, Feemster JA, Dietzmann RH, Kelly WD, Merkel FK, Goetz FC, Lyons GW, Manax WG (1967) Transplantation of stomach, intestine and pancreas: Experimental and clinical observations. Surgery 62:721

Lossing A, Nordgren S, Cohen Z, Cullen J, Craddock G, Langer B (1983) Histologic monitoring of rejection in small intestinal transplantation. Transplant Proc 14:643

Mackenzie R, Nordgren S, Lossing A, Craddock G, Cohen Z, Stiller C, Langer B (1982) Cyclosporine A absorption in canine small intestinal transplantation. Transplant Proc 14:646

Madara JL, Kirkman RL (1985) Structure and functional evolution of jejunal allograft rejection in rats and the ameliorating effects of cyclosporine therapy. J Clin Invest 75:502

Monchick GJ, Russel PS (1971) Transplantation of small bowel in the rat: Technical and immunologic considerations. Surgery 70:693

Morowitz DA, Kirsner JB (1981) Ileostomy in ulcerative colitis: A questionnaire study of 1803 patients. Am J Surg 141:370

Nordgren S, Cohen Z, Mackenzie R, Finkelstein D, Greenberg G, Langer B (1984) Functional monitors of rejection in small intestinal transplants. Am J Surg 147:153

Olivier C, Rettori R, Olivier C, Baur O, Roux J (1969) Un cas de transplantation orthotopique de jejuno-iléon et des colons droit et transverse. Presse Med 77:1275

Parker TH, O'Leary JP (1978) Effect of preparation of the small intestine on microflora and post-operative wound infection. Surg Gynecol Obstet 146:379

Pritchard MD, Madara JL, Tapper MD, Kirkman RL (1985) Failure of cyclosporine to prevent small bowel allograft rejection in pigs. J Surg Res 38:553

Raju S, Didlake RH, Cayirli M, Turner MD, Grogan JB, Achard J (1984) Experimental small bowel transplantation utilizing cyclosporine. Transplantation 38:561

Reznick RK, Craddock GN, Langer B, Gilas T, Cullen JB (1982) Structure and function of small bowel allografts in the dog: Immunosuppression with cyclosporine A. Can J Surg 25:51

Ricour C, Revillon Y, Arnaud-Ballandier F, Ghnassia D, Weyne P, Lauffenberger A, Jos J, Fontaine JL, Gallix P, Vaiman M (1983) Successful small bowel allografts in piglets using cyclosporine A. Transplant Proc 15:3019

Rubin RH, Wolfson JS, Cosimi AB, Tolkoff-Rubin NE (1981) Infection in the renal transplant recipient. Am J Med 70:405

Ruiz JO, Uchida H, Schultz LS, Lillihei RC (1972) Problems in absorption and immunosuppression after entire intestinal allotransplantation. Am J Surg 123:297

Schiller WR, Suriyapa C, Mutchler JHW, Gohara SF, Anderson MC (1973) Motility changes associated with canine intestinal allografting. J Surg Res 15:379

Stanford WP, Hardy MA (1974) Fatty acid absorption in jejunal autograft and allograft. Surgery 75:495–502

Toledo-Pereyra LH, Raij L, Simmons RL, Najarian JS (1974) Role of endotoxin and bacteria in long-term survival of preserved small-bowel allografts. Surgery 73:474

Small-Bowel Allotransplantation in Pigs Using Cyclosporine A: Technique and Results

Y. RÉVILLON, P. GALLIX, F. ARNAUD-BATTANDIER, and C. RICOUR

Cyclosporine A (CsA) has been recently proved to be an efficient immunosuppressive drug against graft rejection. This prompted us to reconsider the possibility of intestinal graft.

Materials and Methods

From 1980 to 1983, we performed 44 allotransplantations in Large White piglets (25–53 kg). Donor and recipient were histoincompatible for only one or two haplotypes in the piglet major histocompatibility system SLA (VAIMAN et al. 1971), and lymphocyte culture was positive in all but one case.

According to the CsA immunosuppressive treatment they received, the piglets were separated into four groups (Table 1). Group 1 ($n = 4$) received neither CsA nor any other immunosuppressive therapy.

The other three groups were treated with CsA. The dose of CsA was established before treatment and not adapted to plasma levels. The recipient underwent treatment orally at a dose of 25 mg/kg per day 1–3 days before transplantation. In group 2 ($n = 10$), CsA was given intramuscularly (25 mg/kg per day for 3 days. Starting on day 4, the same dose was given orally. In group 3 ($n = 24$), CsA was given only orally at a dosage of 25 mg/kg per day, even when it was absorbed incompletely by the piglet. In group 4 ($n = 6$), CsA was started intravenously (8 mg/kg per day) for 5–10 days and then given orally.

Surgery and graft conservation were performed as described by RICOUR et al. 1981, 1983. Briefly, under general anesthesia, the graft is located and measured. The small-bowel lumen and mesenteric vessels are washed with Collins' solution at 4°C.

Table 1. Surgical procedure and results of small-bowel allotransplantation with CsA immunosuppression therapy in 44 pigs

	Group 1 $n = 4$	Group 2 $n = 10$	Group 3 A $n = 8$	Group 3 B $n = 16$	Group 4 $n = 6$
CsA	0	IM	oral	oral	IV
Transplant	stomal	stomal	stomal	continual	continual
Failure	0	3	5	10	2
Rejection	4	3	2	5	0
Survival	0	4	1	1	4

Washing of the small bowel lumen is started before clamping of the vessels of the small bowel, while washing of the mesenteric vessels is initiated just after section the vessels. The washing procedure is carried out until the lumen is clean and the mesentery discolored. The grafts are then conserved in 500 ml of the same solution in a sterile container and kept at around 4°C until the reimplantation is completed.

We always performed end-to-end orthotopic vascular anastomosis, but two different procedures were employed for the intestinal loop. In the first 22 animals (groups 1 and 2, as well as eight animals from group 3), a 2-m-long small-bowel segment was transplanted with a cutaneous enterostomy at both ends in order to have histologic control, and recipient residual bowel continuity was restablished by end-to-end anastomosis. After recovery, recipients were reoperated in order to resect the recipient small bowel and place the graft in continuity. The last operation was made particularly difficult by adhesions. In the last 22 animals (16 from group 3 and six of group 4), a 2-m-long small-bowel segment was transplanted and placed immediately in continuity with the recipient small bowel. After recovery, the animals were reoperated just for resection of the recipient small bowel.

Study Protocol

Biopsy (only on the group with enterostomy) and immunosuppressive controls were performed twice a week during the first month, once a week for the next 2 months, and once a month thereafter. Immunosuppressive controls consisted of assays of plasma CsA levels and serum complement-dependent cytotoxicity, measured as the percentage of lymphocytotoxicity, (%LCT). Acute rejection of the graft was diagnosed when the %LCT was over 50% with mucosal atrophy and lymphosis infiltration on histologic study. In case of death, an autopsy was performed and a histologic study carried out.

Results

In group 1, acute rejection (Hay et al. 1974; Thiede and Deltz 1978) with graft necrosis always occurred within 8 days. In the other groups, 16 experiments failed as a result of vascular thrombosis, and one was ended by intestinal anastomosis leakage. Two pigs died of a viral infection; one succumbed to malignant hyperthermia. Another 20 piglets survived 15–820 days. When in ten of these 20 cases acute rejection was observed, CsA was given orally. Here, the plasma CsA levels were below 200 ng/ml. In the remaining ten cases postoperative courses were uneventful from the 41st to the 280th day, with plasma CsA levels of between 250 and 1900 ng/ml. Of these pigs, eight died while they were still undergoing CsA therapy: five from progressive impairment with weight loss, one of an intraperitoneal abscess, one of bowel necrosis, and one from the general anesthesia used during biopsy. In the remaining two pigs, CsA was interrupted after 1 year. One pig died of acute rejection 50 days after CsA was stopped. The other, the only pig with a mixed negative lymphocyte culture, was sacrified 250 days after stopping CsA. At the time of sacrifice, 820 days post-transplantation, the pig was growing normally, with no gastrointestinal problems and no signs of rejection at autopsy. No hepatic or kidney alterations were observed, and no signs of graft-vs-host reaction were noted.

Discussion

Luminal and vascular washing as described by Ricour et al. (1981) enables a quick cooling down and a decrease in the germ concentration in the lumen and probably protects the mucosa against ischemia.

When immunosuppressive therapy is correct, with high CsA plasma levels, acute rejection is never observed (Nordgren et al. 1984). In our study, this was particularly true for group 4, where CsA was given intravenously. There, plasma levels were constantly high. Oral administration presents potential problems, since CsA is a liposoluble drug that requires intestinal absorption and good lymphatic transport. After transplantation, those two conditions cannot always be immediately met.

We found that frequent monitoring of CsA plasma levels and %LCT is crucial, as are histologic studies of the graft mucosa. In case of graft rejection, we advise IV immunosuppressive therapy.

Conclusion

We have shown that graft tolerance is better when CsA is given intravenously. In patients undergoing a small-bowel allograft, IV CsA as an immunosuppressive treatment and parenteral feeding as a nutritional support should be reconsidered.

Acknowledgments. The authors would like to acknowledge the skilled technical assistance of Sàmia Hamidi, Catherine Vayssettes, Sylvie Stadel, and Denis Calise.

References

Hay JM, Fagniez PL, Parc R, Kunlin A, Villiers P, Vaiman M (1974) Résultats de l'allotransplantation orthotopique de l'intestin grêle chez le porc. Ann Chir 28:1063–1067

Nordgren S, Cohen Z, Mackenzie R, Finkelstein D, Greeberg GR, Langer B (1984) Functional monitors of rejection in small intestinal transplants. Am Surg 147:152–156

Ricour C, Révillon Y, Pletync M, Laufenburger A, Jehannin B, Ghnassia D, Duval C, Ghnassia JC, Jos J, Fontaine JL, Navarro J, Schmitz J, Gallix P (1981) Conservation hypothermique et autotransplantation du grêle chez le porcelet. Gastroenterol Clin Biol 5:977–986

Ricour C, Révillon Y, Arnaud-Battandier F, Ghnassia D, Weyne P, Laufenburger A, Jos J, Fontaine J-L, Gallix P, Vaiman M (1983) Successful small bowel allografts in piglets using cyclosporine. Transplant Proc 15/4:3019–3026

Thiede A, Deltz E (1978) Morphological reaction in transplanted small intestine using immunogenetically defined rat strain combinations. Langenb. Arch Chir 346:119–124

Vaiman M, Renard C, Lafage P, Ameteau J, Nizza P (1971) Determination d'un système d'histocompatibilité chez le pore: le système S.L.A. Ann Biol Animal Biochem 11:41

Session 6: Summary

S. Nordgren

In this session, various technical aspects of small-intestinal transplantation have been highlighted. The surgical manipulation of the host and graft in order to create a synergistic effect on immunosuppressive treatment has been emphasized, as has the handling of the two ends of an intestinal allograft in a clinical situation. The arguments for and against the creation of intestinal stomas were reviewed, and it was concluded that intestinal stomas will be necessary in the early post-transplant period and most likely during the long term as well. However, the development of histologic criteria for the diagnosis of rejection is hampered by the lack of long-term survivors. Established histologic criteria are valid only during the first 2 weeks, and data from experimental animals surviving more than 2 weeks with an intestinal transplant suggests that the histologic changes observed in biopsies from intestinal allografts in or out of continuity do not show the sequence of events known to occur in acute rejection (own unpublished observations).

It was reported from Ricour and his collaborators in Paris that a program for clinical intestinal transplantation has been developed and has been approved by the hospital authorities. The surgical technique has been developed in a pig model and was presented here. Collin's solution will be used for perfusion and emphasis is put on irrigation of the intestinal lumen with antibiotics.

Session 7
Clinical Considerations

Physical and Psychological Preparedness of Short-Bowel Patients for Small-Bowel Transplantation

J. M. Müller, H. W. Keller, U. Brenner, M. Walter, and W. Holzmüller

There is no clear clinical or pathologic definition of the short-bowel syndrome. According to Irving (1983), chronic gut failure is present when the patient is unable to absorb enough nutrients from the intestinal tract to preserve health and a feeling of well-being. When the causes of short-bowel syndrome are considered, patients can be divided into three groups. The first group has an absolute decrease in absorptive surface owing to subtotal resection of the small intestine performed on account of mesenterial arterial or venous thrombosis. The remaining gut (usually the duodenum, the first few centimeters of the jejunum, and the large colon distal to the splenic flexure), is seldom in a position to effect necessary absorption. The second group of patients has a relative decrease in small-bowel surface caused by diffuse disease of the small intestine, such as Crohn's disease or radiation enteritis. The third group of patients has an absence of gut motility, which in turn leads to chronic intestinal malabsorption. Scleroderma and ideopathic pseudo-obstruction are typical symptoms in this group.

Exact figures on the incidence of short-bowel syndrome in the Federal Republic of Germany are not available. Based on American statistics, an incidence of four cases per million of the general population is to be expected.

Treatment of the Short-Bowel-Syndrome

The ideal therapy for patients displaying short-bowel syndrome, especially those in group I, would be small-bowel transplantation. However, clinical application of this solution has shown that, apart from a few rare exceptions, long-term parenteral nutrition is presently the only acceptable method of preventing these patients from starving.

Therapy immediately following extensive bowel resection requires IV nutrition and bowel rest. During the first 2 months of therapy, the main risk to the patients is from excessive fluid and electrolyte losses. Allowances for these losses have to be made in setting up infusion plans. In the transitional phase which follows, parenteral nutrition is continued during initial administration of enteral nutrition. The use of chemically defined diets, given continuously by an infusion pump, is usually indicated. However we usually reserve this technique for anorectic patients and in other patients attempt to introduce an oral diet which covers some of their total needs. The fat content of the diet has to be kept low (30–50 g) in order to reduce stool frequency and to control steatorrhea. This also helps to reduce the loss of calcium, magnesium, and zinc. If the entire colon has been preserved, the amount of oxalate and lactose in the diet must be restricted. These dietary measures are supplemented by any necessary drug therapy, e. g., antidiarrhea preparations, cimetidine, cholesteramine, or antibiotics.

It is usually clear within 1 or 2 years after surgery to what extent the patients' oral nutrition must be supplemented by parenteral nutrition. In order to decrease the length of the hospital stay, the patient is admitted into a home parenteral nutrition program as soon as extra medical or nursing assistance is no longer required. A special catheter is implanted for long-term parenteral nutrition (BROVIAC et al. 1973; KELLER et al. 1983), after which the patient is taught step-by-step the techniques necessary (MÜLLER 1982) for carrying on parenteral nutrition at home. After discharge, follow-up of metabolic parameters takes place in the clinic in close cooperation with the patient's personal physician. The absorptive capacity of the remaining bowel should be tested at 3- to 6-month intervals, particularly during the first 2 years. This allows us to change from parenteral nutrition, which has a high complication rate, to an oral nutritional program at the earliest possible stage.

Experience with Short-Bowel Patients

Between 1978 and 1985, 26 patients with short-bowel syndrome were treated in the University of Cologne's surgical department (Table 1). The reason for the occurrence of short-bowel syndrome in half of these patients was a subtotal small-intestinal resection following vascular occlusion of the small intestine. Of the 26 patients, seven died postoperatively. Of the patients who received parenteral nutrition at home, eight died between 3 and 13 months after discharge from the hospital. In six of these patients, death was due to the underlying disease. One patient who had undergone

Table 1. Outcome of 26 patients with short-bowel syndrome treated between 1978 and 1985

Cause of short-bowel syndrome	Patients (*n*)	Mortality In hospital	Mortality During HTPN	Mean survival time (months)
Basal interaction with resection:	13	5	3	
Thrombosis: mesenteric vein	7	1	1	8
Thrombosis: mesenteric artery	6	4	2	6.5
Inflammatory bowel disease with resection	3	0	1	13
Malignancy with resection radiation	4	1	3	7.3
Radiation arthritis	2	1	1	11
Multiple abdominal surgery	3	0	0	0
Pseudo-obstruction	1	0	0	0
Total	26	7	8	8.4

HTPN, home total parenteral nutrition

parenteral nutrition at home had to be admitted to the clinic after developing severe metabolic disturbances. This patient underwent several operations for peripheral vascular disease, as well as a subtotal small-intestinal resection for mesenteric thrombosis. Owing to the long hospital stay, reintegration into the family situation was very difficult; lack of support on the part of the family led to the patient's wish to commit suicide. The circumstances prevent a clear explanation for the severe metabolic disturbances which brought about this patient's death. One other patient died owing to septic shock which was brought on by catheter infection. Neither the patient's personality nor the domestic situation were adequate for taking the precautions necessary for home parenteral nutrition, which led to catheter sepsis that occurred at regular intervals. Of the 11 surviving patients, seven have returned to their former jobs, five on a full-time and two on a part-time basis. The remaining four are unable to work. However, they are all in a position to leave the house without assistance and to carry out parenteral nutrition by themselves.

In order to clarify whether these patients could be considered potential candidates for small-bowel transplantation, we examined them to see if they were in a condition to be operated on. There were no limitations in cardiopulmonary function which could be seen as increasing the risk of surgery in any of the patients (Table 2). To a large extent their nutritional status was normal (Table 3). The patients' body weight was 9% less than optimal body weight; this underweight was due to a reduction in the amount of body fat. The fat-free body mass, muscle strength measured using a handgrip dynamometer, and the protein compartment were all within normal limits. Using the nutritional index developed by our department to assess the risk of the operation, we concluded that there was no increased operative risk from the nutritional point of view.

Table 2. Cardiopulmonary function in 11 patients with short-bowel syndrome

Patients *(n)*	11	
male *(n)*	3	
female *(n)*	8	
average age (years)	39 (range, 11–59)	
average duration of HPN (months)	22.3 (range, 8–74)	
Cardiopulmonary parameters		
ECG		
normal *(n)*	10	
left anterior hemiblock *(n)*	1	
	Output	% Normal
Residual volume	3.5 L	143
Total lung capacity	6.8 L	116
Residual volume as a percentage of total lung capacity	51%	124
VC_{max}	3.4 L	102
VC_{in}	3.4 L	102
FEV_1	2.4 L	98

HPN, home parenteral nutrition; FEV_1, forced expiratory volume in 1 s; VC_{max}, vital capacity (maximum); VC_{in}, vital capacity (inspiratory)

Table 3. Nutritional status of 11 patients with short-bowel syndrome

Body weight (kg)	59.3 ± 6.7	91% of optimum	
Triceps skinfold (mm)	11.11 ± 4.01	99% of standard	
Midarm circumference (cm)	34.1 ± 3.9	98% of standard	
Dynanometry (kp)	33.5 ± 6.8	107% of standard	
Total protein (g/dl)	6.8 ± 0.6		
Albumin (g/dl)	3.7 ± 0.5		
Prealbumin (mg/dl)	23.6 ± 7.3		
Parenteral nutrition index		Mullen Index (multifactorial index of nutritional status) *(n)*	Department of Surgery, University of Cologne *(n)*
high risk			
medium risk		2	
low risk		9	11

We were able to detect abnormal metabolic changes in only three patients, all of whom showed signs of intrahepatic cholestasis. Liver biopsies showed fatty infiltration of the peripheral type and pericholangitis, which was responsible for raised transaminase and alkaline phosphatase levels in these patients. There was no clear explanation for these liver changes and in reviewing the reference material available (DUDRICK and LONG 1976; GHADIMI et al. 1971; JOHNSTON et al. 1972), the most likely cause seems to be an excessive amount of glucose in the infusion scheme. To allow the patients more freedom of movement, we infused up to 300 g glucose within 8 h overnight. This, in addition to possibly pre-existing liver disease due to surgery or illness, could be the reason for elevated liver enzyme levels. In summary, in this group of patients there were no essential objective findings which would increase the risk of any planned major surgery.

In order to find out whether these patients would be willing to undergo the risk of small-bowel transplantation we posed two simple questions. Our first question was: "Small-bowel transplantation has been successful in animal experiments and has now reached the stage of clinical testing. Would you be prepared to take part in a program for small-bowel transplantation?" Seven of the patients gave a positive response while four said no. An interesting point for us was that six of the seven patients receiving home parenteral nutrition who were working full- or part-time were prepared to take part in the program. However, only one of four patients who were unable to work showed the same willingness.

Our second question was: "Small-bowel transplantation has up to now been carried out on only a few patients with the short-bowel syndrome. None of these operations has been a total success. One would have to say that the health of patients undergoing small-bowel transplantation could deteriorate considerably if the operation were not successful. Would you still be prepared to take on the risk of transplantation?" Under the circumstances, only one patient was prepared to continue to consider the possibility of small-bowel transplantation and requested further information on the operations carried out to date.

References

Broviac JM, Cole JJ, Scribner BB (1973) A silicone rubber atrial catheter for prolonged parenteral alimentation. Surg Gynecol Obstet 136:602

Dudrick S, Long JM (1976) Applications and hazards of intravenous hyperalimentation. Ann Rev Med 28:517

Ghadimi H, Abaci F, Kumar S, Rath M (1971) Biochemical aspects of intravenous alimentation. Pediatrics 49:955

Irving M (1983) Intestinal failure and its treatment by home parenteral nutrition. In: Johnston IDA (ed) Home parenteral nutrition. MTP Press, Lancaster, p 62

Johnston JD, Albritton WL, Sunshine P (1972) Hyperammonemia accompanying parenteral nutrition in newborn infants. J Pediatr 81:154

Keller HW, Müller JM, Pichlmaier H (1983) "Peel-away-introducer": Eine neue Technik zur Implantation des Langzeit-Katheters zur ambulanten parenteralen Ernährung. Infusionstherapie 10:79

Müller JM (1982) Die parenterale Ernährung zu Hause: Ein Handbuch für Patienten. Travenol, Munich

Procurement of Intestinal Allografts from Living Related and from Cadaver Donors

W. H. SCHRAUT and K. K. W. LEE

Introduction

Small-bowel transplantation has been shown to be technically feasible (LILLEHEI et al. 1959; MONCHIK and RUSSEL 1971; CRADDOCK et al. 1981), and it may become a clinical reality with the advent of effective immunosuppressive agents such as cyclosporine A (CRADDOCK et al. 1981; LEE and SCHRAUT 1986). However, safe and efficient strategies for procuring the small intestine either alone (from a living related donor) or together with other organ grafts (from a cadaver donor) need to be devised. Furthermore, effective methods of preserving the small intestine during the interval between harvesting and implantation are required. These will involve cold storage with or without vascular or luminal perfusion.

We studied and evaluated various aspects of the procurement of small-bowel allografts from living related and from cadaver donors in combination with the harvesting of other abdominal organs. This involved mock harvesting of the small bowel during autopsy and at the time of harvesting of kidney, liver, and pancreas grafts intended for clinical use. It was our aim to develop strategies that will allow the simultaneous and safe harvesting of these other organs in conjunction with a small-bowel graft.

Small-Bowel Allograft from a Living Related Donor

Obviously, for small-bowel transplantation, a living related donor with matching blood type and histocompatibility is ideal. The availability of such a donor allows scheduling of simultaneous operative procedures for harvesting and for implantation, so that prolonged graft ischemia and the need for organ preservation are avoided. However, the risk to the donor must be realized: The donor loses 150–200 cm of functioning small bowel, a loss which, in theory, should not lead to nutritional compromise but may do so in practice. Which segment of the small intestine (jejunum or ileum) is more suitable for harvesting and transplantation is an unresolved issue. There is evidence (LOSSING et al. 1982) that rejection is less rapid for the jejunum than for the ileum, possibly because the jejunum contains fewer immunogenic leukocytes.

The technical aspects of the donor operation, however, may be of major importance in the choice of the intestinal segment. If a segment of mid- or upper jejunum is to be removed, it is highly improbable that a graft of such length can be based on a major jejunal vascular pedicle alone. Therefore, a segment of the mesenteric artery and vein must be removed for a safe vascular anastomosis between graft and recipient (Fig. 1). In this situation, end-to-end reconstructive anastomoses of the mesenteric vessels in the donor become necessary; of these, the venous anastomosis involves a particular risk of thrombosis, which leads to loss of the donor's entire distal small bowel and cecum. Preliminary mesenteric angiography is a sine qua non for the living related donor of a small-bowel allograft. In donors with a well-developed arcade between the right colic and ileocecal arteries, the midileum can be harvested based on the mesenteric vessels, without the need for reconstructive vascular anastomoses. The

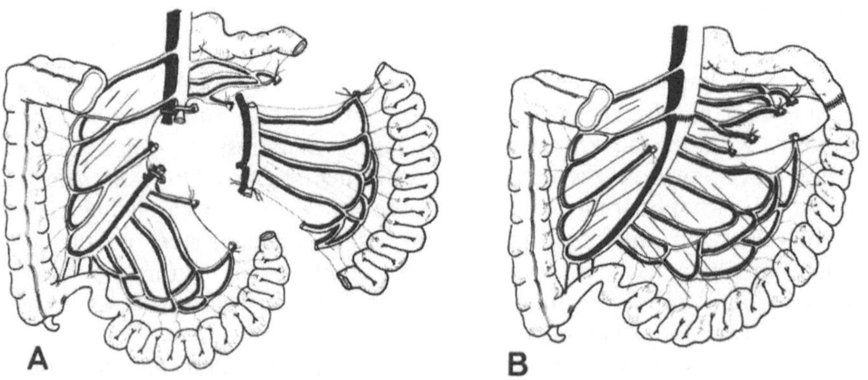

Fig. 1A, B. Harvesting of a segment of jejunum from a living related donor. For a well-vascularized jejunal allograft, it is necessary to remove a section of the superior mesenteric artery and vein with the allograft **(A).** This requires end-to-end vascular anastomoses between the proximal and distal stumps of the mesenteric vessels **(B)**

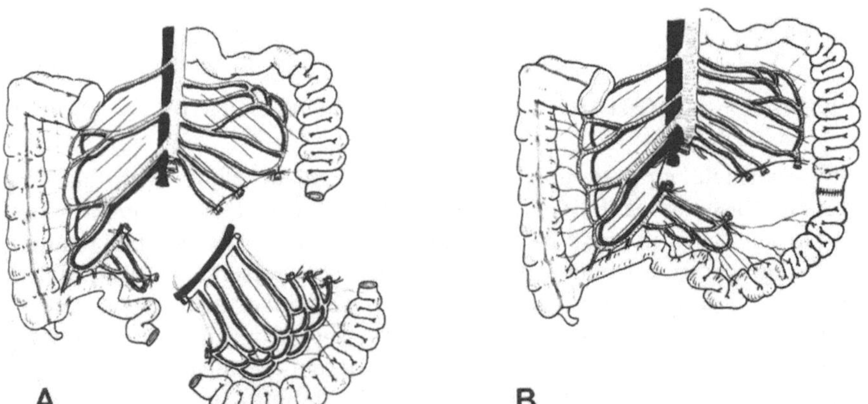

Fig. 2A, B. Harvesting of a segment of ileum from a living related donor. The terminal ileum, approximately 30 cm long, is left with the donor **(A).** This is possible because a sufficient vascular arcade and sufficient connections exist between the right colonic vessels and the terminal ileum. Therefore, the ileocecal artery and vein, which otherwise provide the major blood supply to the cecum and terminal ileum, can be ligated without jeopardizing ileocecal viability. A safe anastomosis can be constructed **(B)**

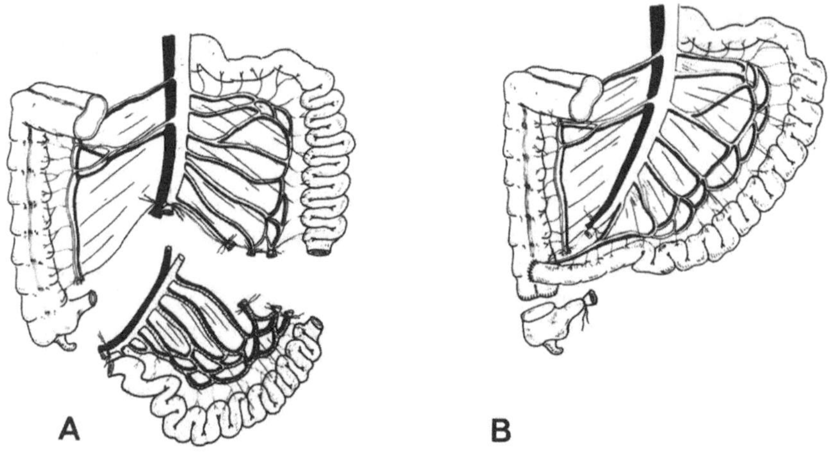

Fig. 3 A, B. Harvesting of the ileum, including the terminal ileum, from a living related donor. The distal ileocecal artery is retained with the small-bowel graft **(A)**; therefore, vascular anastomoses are unnecessary in the donor. If the blood supply is insufficient, the cecum is removed with the graft. Intestinal continuity is re-established by an ileo-ascending-intestinal anastomosis **(B)**

blood supply to the distal ileal stump is sufficient in such a case to allow a safe intestinal anastomosis (Fig. 2). All of these considerations, however, can be disregarded if one rejects the (disputed) importance of preserving the donor's ileocecal region and valve and uses the distal ileum as a graft. In this situation, the distal small bowel can be removed with or without removal of the cecum, and the donor's gastrointestinal continuity can be re-established by an ileo-ascending-intestinal anastomosis (Fig. 3). Vascular anastomoses in the donor are then unnecessary.

The actual steps of the donor operation, which, of course, would be preceded by adequate bowel preparation, involve dissection of the appropriate vessels, administration of heparin, removal of the bowel graft followed by immediate flushing of the vasculature with a cold (4° C) crystalloid solution such as Ringer's or Collins' solution, closure of the intestinal lumen at the site of resection with an intestinal stapling device, removal of the bowel graft, and subsequent irrigation of the gut lumen with a cold electrolyte solution containing 0.05% neomycin. The allograft can then be implanted immediately into the recipient, who has been prepared in the meantime.

Harvesting of the Small-Bowel Graft from a Cadaver Donor

According to Starzl et al. (1984), "A uniform procedure should be developed which is flexible enough to allow the excision of various organ combinations without jeopardy to any of the individual grafts." In the procurement of human cadaver organ grafts, the intestine will always be the last organ to be harvested because its lumen is not sterile. The kidneys, followed by the liver or pancreas and heart, must be removed by the procurement team before the intestinal tract is transected.

Concerning the appropriate donor, the same requirements exist for small-intestinal grafts as those demanded by other organ grafts. In an unstable cadaver donor who requires vasopressor support, kidney removal may be all that is possible. Just as cardiovascular instability with splanchnic vasoconstriction and hypoperfusion leads to impairment of the liver and prevents its use for transplantation, it also causes intestinal ischemia, rendering that organ useless. Furthermore, the donor of a small-bowel allograft should be geographically close to the prospective recipient of the allograft (preferably in the same hospital). At present, research on preservation and transport of small-bowel allografts is relatively new, and unresolved issues remain. These potential problems of small-bowel transplantation, however, should not complicate initial attempts at its clinical application, which may be attempted before effective preservation techniques become available.

If transplantation in an adult is anticipated, an adult donor would seem appropriate. However, it is likely that the recipient, owing to the nature of his disease, has a contracted or obliterated peritoneal cavity which will not accommodate a suitable length of small intestine from an adult donor. Technical difficulties with placement and fitting will be lessened if the intestinal graft is obtained from a pediatric donor, i.e., if a "smaller" small bowel is used. Consideration might also be given to peoperative enlargement of the recipient's peritoneal cavity by the pneumoperitoneum technique, although one must realize the limitations of its use should the peritoneal cavity be obliterated by adhesions.

Given an appropriate donor in an appropriate location, the most important objective in harvesting is the avoidance of ischemia. Every preservation technique begins with the intraoperative infusion of cold fluids into the graft. Immediate cooling of an organ graft by intravascular infusion of a chilled electrolyte solution (Ringer's or Collins' solution) at the time of circulatory arrest was introduced into the laboratory many years ago (BIGELOW et al. 1950) and was promptly applied clinically to the preservation of kidneys and all other organs. Core cooling extends the duration of organ viability many-fold and allows the subsequent unhurried application, if desired, of other, more sophisticated preservation measures. The effectiveness of immediate internal cooling by in situ infusion of a cold (4°C) electrolyte solution was demonstrated by LILLEHEI et al. (1959) for small-bowel grafts.

Harvesting of the Small-Bowel Graft Together with the Kidneys

This procedure begins with a midline incision made from the xiphoid or suprasternal notch to the symphysis pubis. All multiple-organ removals can be considered as modifications of the harvesting techniques for cadaver kidneys, which have been described by MERKEL et al. (1972) and by many other groups. In this technique, the small and large intestines are mobilized completely from the retroperitoneum, and both ureters and kidneys are identified. For simple kidney procurement, the portal structures and the superior mesenteric artery are ligated and divided. This, of course, is not possible if harvesting of the small intestine is anticipated. In this situation, the mesenteric vessels have to be dissected and, in particular, the junction between the superior mesenteric vein and splenic vein has to be identified. This involves ligation and division of the colonic vessels, the inferior gastroduodenal arcade, and two to four of the uppermost jejunal and duodenal vessels. In this way, the vascular (mesenteric) pedicle becomes long enough for easy vascular anastomoses and for exteriorization of the graft by enterostomas (Fig. 4). In the course of the dissection, the entire length of the intra-abdominal aorta is exposed; this requires mobilization of the spleen and of the tail of the pancreas (Fig. 5). In turn, this allows aortic cross-clamping either above or below the celiac axis. When the retroperitoneal dissection has been completed, the

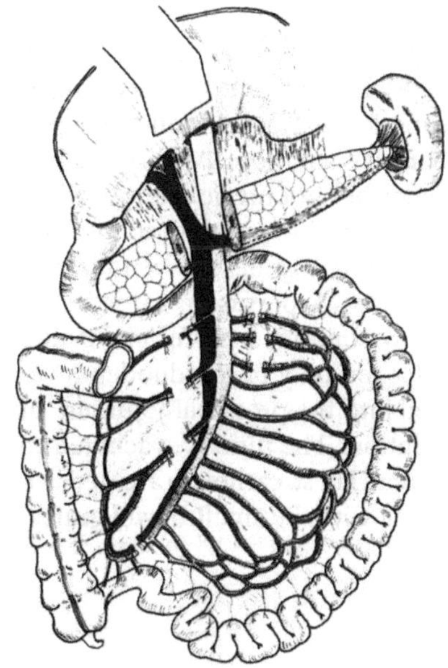

Fig. 4. Harvesting of the intestinal allograft from a cadaver donor. The vascular pedicle for the entire small-bowel graft is prepared by dissection of the superior mesenteric artery from its origin to the first and second jejunal branches. The superior mesenteric vein, splenic vein, and portal vein are also dissected. For a sufficiently long mesenteric pedicle, several jejunal vessels, the pancreatoduodenal vessels, and the short branches to the fourth portion of the duodenum are ligated and divided

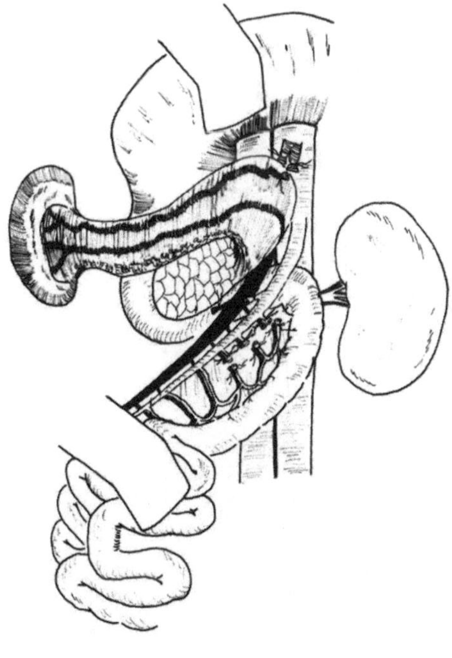

Fig. 5. Harvesting of the intestinal allograft from a cadaveric donor. The retroperitoneal structures are dissected free, and the superior mesenteric artery is exposed at its origin from the aorta. Complete retroperitoneal dissection requires mobilization of the spleen and the tail of the pancreas, with reflection of these organs and of the small bowel toward the patient's right side

infrarenal aorta an vena cava are encircled, ligated, and divided. This is followed by mobilization of both vessels in a superior direction, with ligation and division of the inferior mesenteric artery and of two or three sets of lumbar branches. Heparin (3 mg/kg) and an α-blocking agent are administered. An infusion catheter is then introduced into the aorta, and a drainage catheter is inserted into the distal end of the inferior vena cava and into the portal vein (Fig. 6). Cooling is begun, and when the kidneys and ureters have been mobilized completely, the aorta is cross-clamped above the superior mesenteric artery. For ready access to the superior mesenteric artery, it is advisable to ligate or cross-clamp the celiac axis und place the aortic occlusion clamp superiorly. Then, in situ organ perfusion and cooling are begun with either Collins' or Ringer's solution. After the infusion of 2–3 liters, the kidneys are removed, and the superior mesenteric artery is divided at its root, preferably with a small cuff of aorta. The superior mesenteric vein or, if possible, the portal vein is divided, thereby providing a generous venous pedicle for a portocaval or portoportal venous anastomosis. A perfusion catheter (soft-tipped) is placed into the mesenteric artery to allow continued perfusion, if desired. At this point, the small-bowel graft remains attached only to the duodenum and cecum. Next, a larger-bore infusion catheter is tied into the proximal jejunum, and the intestinal lumen is rinsed with cold Ringer's solution. The fluid is evacuated through a similar large-bore catheter in the terminal ileum. These catheters are tied in securely so that they can be removed from the donor along with the small-bowel graft (Fig. 7). The graft is then placed on ice and is either

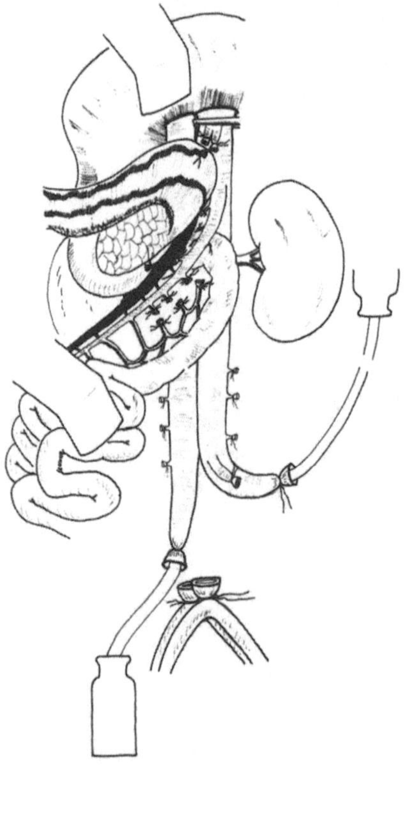

Fig. 6. The retroperitoneal dissection is complete. The aorta and inferior vena cava have been ligated at their bifurcation. Catheters have been introduced into the distal aorta (for infusion) and the inferior vena cava (for drainage). The aorta and inferior vena cava are mobilized in a superior direction, which requires ligation and division of several pairs of lumbar vessels. Following cross-clamping of the aorta, core cooling of the kidneys and small bowel is begun

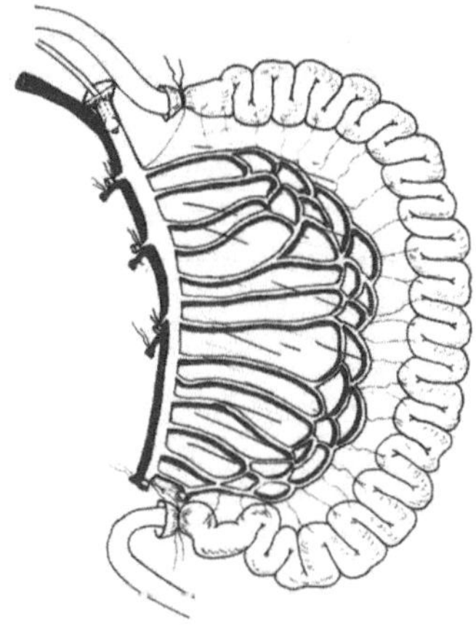

Fig. 7. The small-bowel allograft has been removed from the donor's abdomen. A soft-tipped catheter is placed into the superior mesenteric artery to allow infusion of cold solutions, if desired. Large-bore catheters have been tied into the jejunal and ileal stumps for flushing and further cooling of the bowel graft

simply stored (in hypothermia) or perfused intravascularly or intraluminally until it is implanted.

Harvesting of the Small-Bowel Graft Together with Kidneys and Liver
The donor's abdomen and chest are opened through a midline incision. A complete retroperitoneal dissection of the large vessels, kidneys, and ureters is undertaken as outlined earlier. The removal of the liver requires dissection of the celiac axis, the portal structures, and the splenic and superior mesenteric veins and arteries. Again, the mesenteric root is mobilized and freed from the duodenum, pancreas, and upper jejunum. Dividing the neck of the pancreas greatly facilitates the dissection of the portal structures. Following this extensive retroperitoneal dissection, the liver is mobilized from the diaphragm. Catheters are placed in the infrarenal aorta and cava, and heparin and an α-blocker are administered. An infusion catheter is inserted in the splenic vein to allow precooling of the liver. Because the portal venous flow still includes inflow through the mesenteric vessels, the degree of precooling of the liver that occurs with liver harvesting alone cannot be achieved. It may become necessary either to shorten the precooling phase or to infuse cold crystalloid solution into the infrarenal aorta, thereby allowing backflow into the mesenteric circulation. When the precooling phase has been completed, the aorta and inferior vena cava are mobilized, and core cooling is begun with aortic cross-clamping and immediate infusion of 2–3 liters of cold crystalloid solution. During this cooling period, it becomes necessary to drain the vena cava and the portal system (right atrial vent) to prevent venous engorgement. The kidneys and liver are then removed according to established techniques. The superior mesenteric artery is divided, preferably with an aortic cuff, and a catheter is placed for perfusion. With the removal of the kidneys and liver, the small bowel is the last organ remaining in the abdomen and remains attached at the duodenum and cecum. Its harvesting is completed as outlined previously.

Harvesting of the Small-Bowel Graft Together with Kidneys and Pancreas
This procedure parallels the previously described approaches in the initial steps, amounting to a complete retroperitoneal dissection of both the vena cava and the intra-abdominal aorta with its branches. The superior mesenteric artery and vein are

encircled where they emerge beneath the pancreas. Harvesting of the pancreas requires division of the superior mesenteric vein as it joins the splenic vein. This leaves a short vascular pedicle which is lengthened by ligation and division of several (one to four) jejunal vascular arcades. Although the proximal jejunum is lost, the remaining small-bowel graft is sufficiently long (> 200 cm). In the removal of kidneys, pancreas, and small bowel, the previously outlined steps of precooling, organ cooling, organ removal, and organ storage are followed.

Summary

The procurement of a segment of ileum rather than jejunum from an available living related donor promises to be the safest procedure for the donor. A healthy, nutritionally uncompromised adult should be able to donate 150 or possibly 200 cm of small bowel without compromise of the intestinal absorptive capacity and thus nutritional balance.

Techniques are available which permit removal of several abdominal organs, kidney, liver or pancreas, and the small intestine, from the same cadaver donor without jeopardy to any of the individual grafts. If is inevitable that the small intestine, because of its bacteria content, will be the last organ to be removed from the donor. Thus, the carefully timed and controlled infusion of cold solutions into the aorta and mesenteric artery is of major importance. For the time of ischemia to be kept as short as possible, the strategies and techniques to be used must be practiced. This is possible, in our experience, in conjunction with clinical organ harvest and does not interfere with the viability of kidneys, liver, or pancreas.

References

Bigelow WG, Lindsay WK, Harrison RC, Gordon RA, Greenwood WF (1950) Oxygen transport and utilization in dogs at low body temperatures. Am J Physiol 160:125–137

Craddock GN, Reznick RK, Langer B, Wolman WG, Cullen JB (1981) Structure and function of small bowel allografts treated with cyclosporin A. Surg Forum 32:350–352

Lee KKW, Schraut WH (1986) Structure and function of orthotopic small-bowel allografts in rats treated with cyclosporin A. Am J Surg (to be published)

Lillehei RC, Goott B, Miller FA (1959) The physiological response of the small bowel of the dog to ischemia including prolonged in vitro preservation of the bowel with successful replacement and survival. Ann Surg 150:543–560

Lossing A, Nordgren S, Cohen Z, Cullen J, Craddock G, Langer B (1982) Histologic monitoring of rejection in small intestinal transplantation. Transplant Proc 14:643–645

Merkel FK, Jonasson O, Bergan JJ (1972) Procurement of cadaver donor organs; evisceration technique. Transplant Proc 4:585–589

Monchik GJ, Russel PS (1971) Transplantation of the small bowel in the rat: Technical and immunological considerations. Surgery 70:693–702

Starzl TE, Hakala TR, Shar BW Jr, Hardesty RL, Rosenthal TJ, Griffith BP, Iwatsuke S, Bahnson HT (1984) A flexible procedure for multiple cadaveric organ procurement. Surg Gynecol Obstet 158:223–230

Session 7: Summary

M. A. Hardy

This section addressed the questions of (a) who should be considered as a potential recipient of an intestinal transplant, (b) the characteristics of potential donors, and (c) technical considerations in the removal and preservation of an intestinal allograft.

Of the patients who could possibly benefit from a successful small-bowel transplant, only a small number should be considered in the initial trials to be held in the future. In describing the ideal recipient of the initial intestinal transplant, Muller, as well as most of the clinicians participating in this workshop, concluded that this should be a 20- to 30-year-old individual who has suffered a superior mesenteric vein occlusion and whose only previous abdominal operation was removal of the gangrenous small intestine. Elderly patients who have superior mesenteric artery occlusion stemming from atherosclerosis, patients with Crohn's disease or radiation enteritis, and those who have had multiple previous abdominal operations will be unacceptable candidates early on.

The group from Cologne emphasized the use of objective criteria for determining the suitability of an intestinal transplant recipient. The importance of TPN as a means of maintaining potential recipients in acceptable physical condition was stressed. The preceding report also highlights the need for the psychologic evaluation of potential intestinal allograft recipients. On the basis of previous experience with other organ allograft recipients, stability, reliability, and family support have been found to be paramount in importance when considering successful outcomes. The use of objective psychologic testing and, in particular, careful psychiatric evaluations of potential recipients of intestinal allografts cannot be sufficiently emphasized and will be vital to the success of the inital trials of intestinal transplantation.

The second area considered in this section concerns our ability to select a suitable donor and how the method of graft excision and preservation will affect its function. The considerations of who should be the donor, how the graft should be removed and preserved, and which portion of the intestine should be transplanted need to be carefully examined in the initial clinical trials. Members of this workshop agreed that, in the initial trials, intestinal allografts should be procured primarily from heart-beating cadavers who have been hospitalized for a relatively short time, who have had no episodes of hypotension, and who are primarily renal organ donors. This approach will optimize the state of the intestinal allograft to be transplanted, particularly in relation to the adequacy of arterial and venous patches to be used in future anastomoses. Practice in small-intestine retrieval, perfusion, and preservation should be initiated by the interested groups as early as possible in order to determine and standardize the best methods of retrieval and perfusion. In their study of small-intestine isografts in rats, Schraut and Lee emphasized that biopsy of the intestine immediately following preservation is not helpful and that in vivo follow-up examination is necessary to determine the success of preservation methods. In the discussion of this interesting presentation, it was unanimously agreed that, in the initial clinical trials, no long-term preservation of intestinal allografts should be necessary and should be avoided. Immediate transplantation, following retrieval, would maximize the preservation of mucosal integrity, prevent submucosal fibrosis, and therefore permit maximal recovery of absorptive function at the earliest time. In the course of the discussion on donor preparation and evaluation, it was reiterated that preservation procedures of the intestine need to consider intraluminal irrigation and the use of antibiotics to decrease the bacterial intestinal flora, perhaps even to eliminate it.

In conclusion, the session on clinical considerations of the potential recipient and donor evaluation thoroughly explored important variables which undoubtedly will be the major determining factors of success in initial clinicals trials of intestinal transplantation.

Session 8

Nutritional Support Prior to and During Intestinal Transplantation

Experience in Home Parenteral Nutrition and Indications for Small-Bowel Transplantation

S. L. Wolman, K. N. Jeejeebhoy, S. Stewart, and P. D. Greig

Introduction

The advent of improved surgical techniques and recent advances in immunosuppressive therapy have prompted a re-examination of small-bowel transplantation. The expanding scope of renal, cardiac, and lung transplantation indicates that small-bowel transplantation will likely find its niche in clinical medicine. As with renal dialysis, parenteral nutrition can maintain life in the presence of organ failure, but this technique is not without its problems.

An examination of the indications and results of home parenteral nutrition (HTPN) is an appropriate method by which recommendations for further alternative therapy can be made. Since HTPN began in 1970, its effectiveness in the treatment of severe organ failure has been shown. Subsequently, its indications have been widened, and at present patients who receive HTPN fall into two quite separate groups. The first group consists of patients who will have permanent HTPN because of short bowel or bowel with inadequate function due to a disease which causes either malabsorption or obstruction or both. The obstruction may be physical or due to a motility disorder. The second group of HTPN patients are those who are primarily on parenteral nutrition as a means of palliation. These may be patients with Crohn's disease who have a highly active form of the disease and cannot maintain their nutritional status. Improving nutritional status, whether by means of parenteral or enteral nutritional support, is becoming acknowledged as an effective form of therapy in these patients (Lochs et al. 1983). Other patients with Crohn's disease may have bowel obstruction, and if the surrounding inflammation is allowed to subside, the obstruction may subside as well. Patients with gastric outlet obstruction due to peptic ulcer disease or postoperative complications may follow a similar course. Another group of increasing numbers includes patients with cancer and abdominal metastases which cause obstruction, but which do not show signs of extensive spread and imminent death. It seems reasonable to provide these patients with parenteral nutrition and allow them to return home to their families for the duration of their illness. This group of patients is not expected to remain on HTPN on a permanent basis, and I refer to them as the palliative HTPN group. These patients would not be candidates for small-bowel transplantation. The remainder of this examination of HTPN will exclude these patients unless specifically mentioned. In our program, this palliative group comprises only 15% of all patients.

Toronto General Hospital's HTPN program is the prime provider of HTPN for the Province of Ontario, which has a population of 8.8 million (1983). Since the inception of the program in 1970, 111 patients have been parenterally supported, 64 of whom are female and 47 male. The mean age is 44, ranging from 16 to 76 years. So far, the hospital has provided 98 665 patient days of support, equivalent to 270 patient years.

Description of Patients on Parenteral Nutrition

In examining the possible candidates for small-bowel transplantation, a review of the diagnoses which precipitated parenteral nutrition is in order (Table 1). Fifty-seven percent of patients had short bowel as a result of resection for bowel infarction, Crohn's disease, volvulus, or Gardener's syndrome. Nineteen percent had bowel obstruction which was not thought to be reversible. This excludes those patients with Crohn's disease, where reversal might be possible. The breakdown of obstruction by diagnosis is seen in Table 1. Another 10% of patients had inadequate bowel function due to celiac disease, radiation enteritis, or microulcerative jejunitis. The remainder of the diagnoses include to patients in the palliative HTPN group, who would not be candidates for small-bowel transplantation. An examination of the time period for parenteral nutrition reveals that the majority (94) of these patients have been receiving this type of nutrition for 0–5 years, while only small numbers have accrued in the 5–10- and 10–15-year time periods (11 and 4 respectively). This is due in part to patient attrition; however, the main reason is increased awareness of this program in

Table 1. Diagnoses

	Diagnosis	Cases *(n)*
Short-bowel syndrome:	Bowel infarction	26
	Secondary Crohn's disease	27
	Volvulus	8
	Gardener's syndrome	2
Bowel obstruction:	Crohn's disease[a]	8
	Pseudo-obstruction	12
	Radiation enteritis	2
	Scleroderma	5
	Panniculitis	2
Inadequate function:	Celiac disease	2
	Radiation enteritis	7
	Microulcerative jejunitis	1
Cancer:[a]	Lymphoma	1
	Gastric cancer	1
	Pancreatic cancer	1
	Ureter cancer	1
Postgastric surgery:	Dumping syndrome	3
	Outlet obstruction	1
Other:[a]	Ulcerative colitis	1

[a] Diagnoses of patients in the palliative HTPN group.

Ontario and increased emphasis on treatment of patients who could not survive before the advent of HTPN. Of course, as our use increases and our expertise becomes greater, we have become more willing to place patients from the palliative group on HTPN.

An examination of the patients with each diagnoses (Table 2) reveals that the patients with bowel infarction have a mean age of 49 and are older than any other segment of the population studied. This just failed to reach statistical significance. It is also noted that this group spent the lowest mean time on parenteral nutrition. Bowel infarction patients have the greatest number of admission days to the hospital and a significantly lower percentage of outpatient days. Of the 111 patients, 31 have died, with figures almost the same for both males and females (16 males, 15 females). When the deaths were examined with respect to diagnosis, it was found that the patients with bowel infarction had a significantly higher mortality (Table 3). An examination was made of the immediate causes of death, which included sepsis in 15 cases, hepatic failure in four, renal failure in four, cancer in four, and myocardial infarction in two cases. There was one suicide and one refusal to continue parenteral nutrition, as well as one death by pneumonia and one from pulmonary fibrosis. In two cases, the immediate cause of death was unknown.

Table 2. Diagnosis and HTPN Administration

Diagnosis	Mean age	Mean time on HTPN (days)	Length of in-patient treatment (days)	Length of out-patient treatment (%)
Bowel infarction	49	1008	193	81*
Crohn's disease	39	1078	97	91
Volvulus	40	1483	129	91
Pseudo-obstruction	38	1363	45	97
Crohn's obstruction[a]	23	373	10	97

* $P < 0.05$
[a] Palliative HTPN.

Table 3. Mortality in patients on HTPN

	Deaths *(n)*	Diagnosis of primary disease
Bowel infarction	14	26*
Volvulus	3	8
Crohn's disease	3	27
Cancer	3	5
Scleroderma	2	5
Pseudo-obstruction	1	12
Radiation enteritis	2	7
Celiac disease	1	2
Gastric problems	1	4
Gardener's syndrome	1	2

* $P < 0.001$

Since sepsis was listed as a cause of death and it is well known that catheter sepsis is one of the major complications of parenteral nutrition, catheter sepsis rates were examined. Over the period of examination, 192 catheters were used with a mean duration of 1.4 years. Forty-four catheters were removed after sepsis was observed, and 89 catheters were implicated in septic episodes, but were treated medically and not removed. No relationship was found between the number of line removals or the number of infectious episodes and the subsequent outcome of the patients. It was concluded that patients with bowel infarction died of multiorgan failure; sepsis played a role in most cases. It was noted that 11 patients had recurrent abdominal sepsis, and seven of these patients subsequently died ($P < 0.05$). The occurrence of abdominal sepsis was distributed throughout the group of patients with bowel infarction, volvulus, and Crohn's disease. When the survivors are separated from the nonsurvivors and the length of time on parenteral nutrition is examined, it is still evident that the patients who died survived more than 1.5 years on the average (Table 4). Patients with bowel infarction were at home 73% of the time, while patients with volvulus and Crohn's disease who eventually died were at home only 46% and 32% of the time respectively. This indicates that patients with bowel infarction have a similar degree of chronic illness, whether or not they are destined to survive. Among the patients who did not survive, those with volvulus and Crohn's disease have a far greater chronic morbidity.

Table 4. Survivors and nonsurvivors among 111 patients on HTPN

Diagnosis	Survivors				Nonsurvivors			
		Age	Length of suvival	Treatment as out-patient		Age	Length of suvival	Days of treatment as out-patient
	(*n*)	(years)	(days)	(%)	(*n*)	(years)	(days)	(%)
Bowel infarction	12	45	1523	80	14	53	718	73
Volvulus	5	43	2010	94	3	34	603	46
Crohn's disease	24	39	1094	91	3	46	866	32
Cancer	0	0	0	0	3	53	483	0
Pseudo-obstruction	11	35	1484	97	0	0	0	0

Complications of Parenteral Nutrition

Examining the complications of parenteral nutrition should reveal the causes of increased morbidity and mortality in these patients. Jaundice was observed in 20 of the patients, and of these, 12 patients died, ($P < 0.01$). It has been observed in our institution, and in others, that patients on parenteral nutrition develop hepatic lesions characterized by steatosis and cholestasis. It has been suggested that these abnormalities are due to excessive calories or excessive amounts of carbohydrate calories (Meguid et al. 1982; Buzby et al. 1981; Robin et al. 1981; Carpentier et al. 1981; Allardyce et al. 1978), excessive tryptophan metabolites (Grant et al. 1977), amino acid excess or imbalance (PREISIG and RENNERT 1977; BLITZER et al. 1980; COOK and HUTT 1967), portal endotoxemia (CAPRION et al. 1983), lithocholate toxicity (FOUIN-FORTUNET et al. 1982), carnitine deficiency (PENN et al. 1980, 1981), or essential fatty acid deficiency (RICHARDSON and SGOUTAS 1975). These problems are potentially amenable to therapy. Some of these patients may have acquired hepatitis B surface antigen or non-A, non-B hepatitis during resuscitation. These two problems are not amenable to therapy. There are patients in whom non of these mechanisms seems to be involved. It is postulated that the absence of the bowel and the influence of gut hormones leads to cholestasis and secondary liver disease. If this is in fact the case, small-bowel transplantation could reverse the abnormalities and prevent further hepatic deteriorition, which is associated with increased mortality.

Another major complication of parenteral nutrition is metabolic bone disease. Our observations of the presence of osteomalacia have been presented in a previous publication (SHIKE et al. 1980). It has also been suggested that phosphate deficiency or hypophosphatemia (KLEIN et al. 1980; HAUSSLER and MCCAIN 1977), excessive phosphate (KLEIN et al. 1980; PARFITT et al. 1979), copper deficiency (SOLOMONS 1981), steroids, and heparin (BAYLINK 1983) can contribute to osteomalacia. Certainly all of these factors are potentially reversible. On the other hand, it may be true that these patients experience increased sensitivity to vitamin D (SHIKE et al. 1980) or vitamin D deficiency (KLEIN et al. 1981). There may also be an increase in calciuria caused by sulfate (COLE and ZLOTKIN 1983) in the solutions used or the possibility that these bone lesions are due to aluminum toxicity (OTT et al. 1983). There is also concern about the protein load and its role in producing hypercalciuria (MARGEN et al. 1974; BENGOA et al. 1983; WOOD et al. 1984). At present, no single pathogenesis is evident, and if there are multiple factors playing a role in the generation of metabolic bone disease in parenteral nutrition, there is presently no specific management available that has been universally effective. While mortality in these patients is not increased, there is certainly increased morbidity owing to excessive bone pain and fractures. Successful small-bowel transplantation could possibly reverse this process and ameliorate this problem.

We also observed 14 episodes of pancreatitis, of which six were inpatients who eventually died. However, the association of this disease with mortality was not significant. For the most part, pancreatitis was resolved and was not a major factor in morbidity. We believe that this can be avoided by carefully monitoring serum calcium levels (IZSAK et al. 1980). Superior vena cava obstruction, a severe complication of parenteral nutrition, is significantly associated with mortality and can be avoided by carefully monitoring catheter placement and by keeping the osmolality of the solutions to a minimum.

Many patients on HTPN experience depression. It is difficult to determine whether this depression is a result of their illness or whether it is primarily associated with their treatment. Nevertheless, a significantly higher number of patients died who had experienced depression. It could also be argued that these patients were more severely ill, thus giving them more reason for depression. On the other hand, the patients' despondency may have caused them to be less fastidious in their care of the catheter systems and in maintenance of their general health and may have directly or indirectly contributed to their ultimate death. In the patient who refused parenteral nutrition and the patient who committed suicide, death was quite clearly the result of major psychiatric difficulties. It is well accepted that renal transplantation patients have a more satisfactory quality of life than those on dialysis regimens. Successful small-bowel transplantation could produce similar effects and result in less depression and a better quality of life for many patients with gastrointestinal tract failure.

Indications and Contraindications for Small-Bowel Transplantation

From this examination of the results of HTPN some proposals for the indications for small-bowel transplantation can be made. At present, with the success of HTPN I do not believe there is any absolute indication for small-bowel transplantation, although there are relative indications. Among these, severe liver disease and severe depression must appear at the top of the list, since they ultimately result in increased morbidity and mortality. Severe metabolic bone disease, although not associated with increased mortality, certainly greatly increases morbidity and is a major factor affecting the quality of life. Another relative indication for small-bowel transplantation is the patient who lacks organ function, has been on HTPN and as a result of thrombosis has exhausted all venous access. Considering the innovative surgical approaches available, I think that this group of patients may not be a very large. In these patients, a Goretex constructed arteriovenous fistula should be considered as another alternative. Another potentially serious problem occurs in the patient who has excessive jejunostomal outputs which are difficult to control and result in dehydration and chronic renal disease and/or pancreatitis. We have several patients with this problem; many medical regimens carried out to alleviate it have met with only limited success. The final relative indication is solution-patient incompatability. In our institution, this has not proven to be a major factor, although some patients complain of excessive nausea and headaches while their solution is being infused. However, only one patient describes this as nearly intolerable. In this case, intolerance was primarily associated with lipid-containing infusions; the patient is presently on an all-dextrose system and is using corn oil baths to provide essential fatty acids.

The consideration of small-bowel transplantation must also include contraindications. In our patients, it has been observed that patients with bowel infarction as a cause of short-bowel syndrome have an increased mortality. However, often, these patients often have severe generalized vascular disease. These patients do well on HTPN but succumb to vascular disease at sites other than the bowel. I think severe vascular disease should be a contraindication for small-bowel transplantation. Patients with bowel infarction or volvulus are not always promptly diagnosed, and this results in abdominal sepsis, which requires adequate surgical drainage, antibiotic administration, and many months of treatment in the hospital. Despite very aggressive therapy, 11 patients have had recurrent abdominal sepsis, and of these, seven haven subsequently died. This was a significant factor associated with mortality. Continuing abdominal sepsis should be an absolute contraindication for small-bowel transplantation. Of course, cases of malignancy, as I mentioned earlier, fall under the palliative HTPN group, thus precluding small-bowel transplantation. At the moment, I do not know if age should be a relative contraindication for small-bowel transplantation. Usually, procedure that are not yet routine are attempted on patients who are in the best possible physical condition, and only after further experience can such procedures be applied in the patient population that may be more at risk, such as the elderly.

Also of interest are those diseases which result in organ failure where the cause is not actually known. Crohn's disease and pseudo-obstruction fall into this category. While I cannot consider these as relative contraindications to small-bowel transplantation at present, it is possible that transplanted bowel could acquire Crohn's disease or abnormal motility from circulating factors within the host. This would certainly change our understanding of these diseases and the role of small-bowel transplantation in their treatment.

In conclusion, indications can be made for small-bowel transplantation based on the shortcomings of HTPN. It is hoped that in the future, small-bowel transplantation will play a role in alleviating the morbidity and mortality of patients with loss of gastrointestinal tract function and provide for better quality of life.

References

Allardyce DB, Salvian AJ, Quenville NF (1978) Cholestatic jaundice during total parenteral nutrition. Can J Surg 21:332–339

Baylink DJ (1983) Glucocorticoid-induced osteoporosis. N Engl J Med 309:306–308

Bengoa JM, Sitrin MD, Wood RJ, Rosenberg IH (1983) Amino acid-induced hypercalciuria in patients on total parenteral nutrition. Am J Clin Nutr 38:264–269

Blitzer BL, Ratoosh SL (1980) (abstr) Na^+ dependent amino acid uptake inhibits hepatic taurocholate uptake: a possible mechanism of amino acid induced cholestasis. Gastroenterology 79:1005

Buzby GP, Mullen JL, Stein TP et al. (1981) Manipulation of TPN caloric substrate and fatty infiltration of the liver. J Surg Res 31:46–54

Caprion JP, Herve MA, Gineston JL et al. (1983) Metronidazole in prevention of cholestasis associated with total parenteral nutrition. Lancet 1:446–447

Carpentier YA, Van Brandt M (1981) Effect of total parenteral nutrition on liver function. Acta Chir Belg 2–3:141–144

Cook GC, Hutt MSR (1967) The liver after kwashiorkor. Br Med J 3:454–457

Cole DEC, Zlotkin SH (1983) Increased sulfate as an etiological factor in the hypercalciuria associated with total parenteral nutrition. Am J Clin Nutr 37:108–113

Fouin-Fortunet H, Quernec L, Erlinger S et al. (1982) Hepatic alterations during total parenteral nutrition in patients with inflammatory bowel disease: a possible consequence of lithocholate toxicity. Gastroenterology 82:939–937

Grant JP, Cox CE, Kleinman LM et al (1977) Serum hepatic enzyme and bilirubin elevations during parenteral nutrition. Surg Gynecol Obstet 145:573

Haussler MR, McCain TA (1977) Basic and clinical concepts related to vitamin D metabolism and action. N Engl J Med 297:1041–1048

Izsak EM, Shike M, Roulet M, Jeejeebhoy KN (1980) Pancreatitis in association with hypercalcemia in patients receiving total parenteral nutrition. Gastroenterology 79:555–558

Klein GL, Ament ME, Bleustone R et al (1980) Bone disease associated with total parenteral nutrition. Lancet 2:1041–1044

Klein GL, Horst RL, Norman AW, Ament ME, Slatopolsky E, Coburn JW (1981) Reduced serum levels of 1,25-dihydroxyvitamin D during long-term total parenteral nutrition. Ann Intern Med 94:638–643

Lochs H, Meryn S, Marosi L, Ferenci P, Hortnagl H (1983) Has total bowel rest a beneficial effect in the treatment of Crohn's disease? Clin Nutr 2:61–64

Margen S, Chu JY, Kaufmann A, Galloway DH (1974) Studies in calcium metabolism. I. The calciuretic effect of dietary protein. Am J Clin Nutr 27:584

Meguid MM, Schimmel E, Johnson WC et al (1982) Reduced metabolic complications in total parenteral nutrition: pilot study using fat to replace one-third of glucose calories. JPEN 6:304–307

Ott SM, Maloney NA, Klein GL, Alfrey AC, Ament ME, Coburn JW, Sherrard DJ (1983) Aluminum is associated with low bone formation in patients receiving chronic parenteral nutrition. Ann Intern Med 98:910–914

Parfitt AM, Oliver I, Vallanueva AR (1979) Bone histology in metabolic bone disease: the diagnostic value of bone biopsy. Orthop Clin North Am 10:329–345

Penn D, Schmidt-Sommerfeld E, Wolf H (1980) Carnitine deficiency in human premature infants receiving total parenteral nutrition. Early Hum Dev 4:23–24

Penn D, Schmidt-Sommerfeld E, Pascer F (1981) Decreased tissue carnitine concentrations in newborn infants receiving total parenteral nutrition. J Pediatr 98:976–978

Preisig R, Rennert O (1977) (abstr) Biliary transport and cholestatic effects of amino acids. Gastroenterology 73:1240

Richardson TR, Sgoutas D (1975) Essential fatty acid deficiency in four adult patients during total parenteral nutrition. Am J Clin Nutr 29:258–263

Robin AP, Carpentier YA, Askanazi J et al. (1981) Metabolic consequences of hypercaloric glucose infusions. Acta Chir Belg 2–3:133–140

Shike M, Harrison JE, Sturtride WC et al. (1980) Metabolic bone disease in patients receiving long-term total parenteral nutrition. Ann Intern Med 92:343–350

Solomons NW (1981) On the assessment of trace mineral nutriture in patients on total parenteral nutrition. Nutr Supp Serv 1:13–16

Wood RJ, Sitrin MD, Rosenberg IH (1984) Calciuria in total parenteral nutrition: effects of amino acids and glucose in rats. Am J Clin Nutr 40:101–106

Enteral and Parenteral Feeding of Patients with Short-Bowel Syndrome

B. LÜNSTEDT

Introduction

Short-bowel syndrome is a clinical entity that may occur in patients with extensive loss of intestinal mass, resulting in the breakdown of nutrient and electrolyte balance. These patients require intensive nutritional care and a special and individualized nutritional support program to stabilize their condition and prevent major complications. The largest group of patients with the short-bowel syndrome includes survivors of intestinal infarction, often elderly patients, but also neonates with congenital malformations. Crohn's disease and strangulation obstruction due to volvulus are other possible reasons for massive bowel resection.

Several factors may determine the severity and prognosis of patients with short-gut syndrome. Residual small intestine amounting to less than 25% of the normal length makes adequate nutritional supply very difficult. Loss of the ileum or the ileocecal valve enhances these problems by allowing no resoption of fat and increasing the diarrhea rate. A combination of small-bowel resection and total or partial colectomy may also increase the rate of complications. The clinical problems often start in the early postoperative phase with massive diarrhea, loss of electrolytes, and gastric hypersecretion. Since fat absorption is impaired in these patients, fat-soluble vitamin deficiencies (vitamins A, D, E, and K) will occur. Bile salt malabsorption and stone formation in the gallbladder and nephrolithiasis are other possible complications of short-bowel syndrome.

The patient's ability to tolerate the loss of a major portion of the intestine depends on the adaptive response of the remaining bowel. This adaptive phase may take weeks or months, and in the interim, adequate nutrition must be provided to prevent nutritional deficits.

Nutritional Management

Total parenteral nutrition (TPN) will be necessary initially to allow restoration of protein, energy, and mineral metabolism. Oral or enteral feeding should also be available to the patient during this phase of adaptation, as the principal stimulus for intestinal hyperplasia seems to be luminal nutrition (FELDMAN et al. 1976; LEVINE et al. 1976). Hormones, endogenous secretions, and neurovascular factors require luminal nutrients to initiate their effects. Most patients with short-bowel syndrome

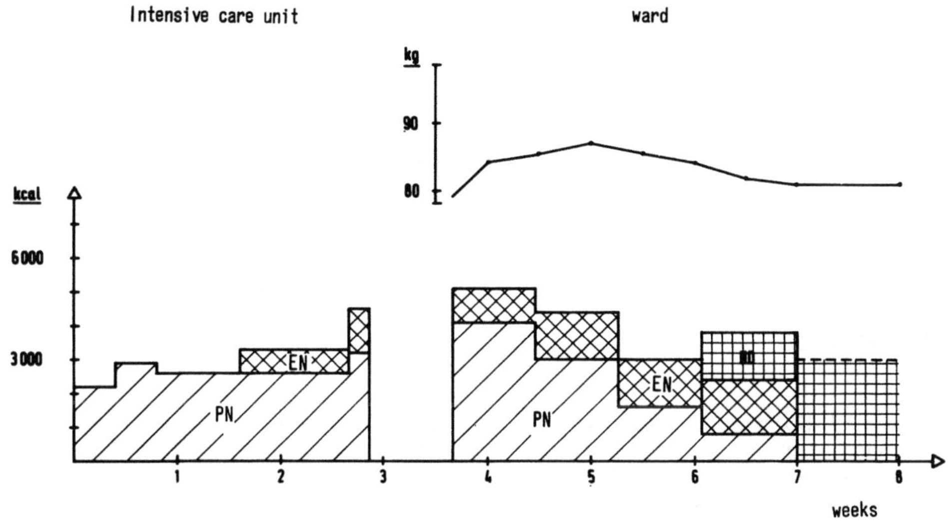

Fig. 1. Nutritional management after massive bowel resection. *PN,* parenteral nutrition; *EN,* enteral nutrition; *ND,* normal diet

will be able to achieve long-term homeostasis with oral diets, but need partial parenteral support during the adaptive phase. However, individual reactions are so variable that it is very difficult to project which patients will succeed and which will fail. Diet therapy must be individually tailored for successful long-term therapy. The optimal success we can achieve in patients with massive short-bowel resection is demonstrated in Fig. 1.

In most patients, as oral intake increases and absorption improves, parenteral nutrition is decreased and may be discontinued after some weeks. During TPN therapy, we correct essential fatty acid and trace element deficiencies which may develop in patients with massive diarrhea. Patients with acutely developed short-bowel syndrome receive normal amounts of calories per kg body weight per day (400–500 g carbohydrates, 100–120 g amino acids, and 100 g fat emulsion).

Enteral tube feeding should be started as soon as possible unless it is contraindicated because of intestinal obstruction, nausea, or increasing diarrhea. Continuous enteral tube feeding using an oligopeptide diet is administered by a volumetric pump. Initially, small volumes (25–50 ml/h) of this diet diluted to isotonicity should be used. In this phase, attention must be paid to serum electrolytes and to intake and output. Pharmacologic control of diarrhea is often not very successful, but loperamide and other drugs can be helpful. Continuous enteral tube feeding should be aimed at providing enough calories and protein to maintain body weight and nitrogen balance. Oral intake should be allowed, if possible. However, some patients with short-bowel syndrome never achieve homeostasis without chronic TPN. With the development of new techniques allowing chronic access to the central venous system, home TPN has become a reality and facilitates discharge from the hospital. This procedure should be reserved for specialized centers only. The long-term management of patients with short-bowel syndrome should be directed toward minimizing and preventing complications such as vitamin and mineral malabsorption.

Conclusion

The advent of total parenteral and special enteral nutrition has considerably improved the ability to correct and prevent malnutrition in these patients. However, these patients often become both psychologically and medically tied to TPN therapy, and the quality of their life is extremely bad. The possibility of short-bowel transplantation in the future seems to be the only means of increasing quality of life for these patients.

References

Feldman EJ, Dowling RH, McNaughton J (1976) Effect of oral versus intravenous nutrition on intestinal adaptation after small bowel resection in the dog. Gastroenterology 70:712–719

Levine GM, Deven JJ, Yezdimio E (1976) Small bowel resection: Oral intake is the stimulus for hyperplasia. Am J Dig Dis 21:542–546

Methods of Perioperative Nutritional Support and Their Possible Application in Small-Bowel Transplantation

K. H. VESTWEBER, B. VIELL, and H. TROIDL

Parenteral nutrition in the perioperative period, as well as long-term parenteral support, are often used in surgical units, and medical staff is usually well trained in its administration. Enteral nutrition is not as attractive for research, and for a long time was not highly regarded even though it is a physiologic means of nutrition. This report deals with the question of the possible uses of enteral support in surgical patients.

Methods of Application

Oral alimentation, which is preferable, is often not possible during the postoperative period for various reasons. Nasoenteral feeding tubes can be used to give alimentation. However, wide or stiff tubes should not be used as they bring about corrosive and infectious side effects in the nasopharynx and esophagus (PADILLA et al. 1979; TOROSIAN and ROMBEAU 1980). Flexible and fine-bore tubes can be placed during surgery (HULTEN et al. 1980; PADILLA et al. 1979). Postoperatively, exact placement is possible with endoscopic assistance (ATKINSON et al. 1979; KAUTZ et al. 1981; MEISSNER and WEISSENHOFER 1978). Favorable results have been reported using combination tubes, which decompress the esophagus and stomach and feed into the jejunum (LORRAIN and PAGE 1965; MOSS 1963, 1966; MOSS and FREIDMAN 1977). The disadvantage of this tube is its large size.

The use of this type of nutrition is limited, as many patients do not tolerate nasoenteral tubes (BAUER et al. 1984).

The use of transcutaneous tubes is a possible alternative to the administration of nutrition via nasoenteral tubes. Pharyngostomies (LYONS 1974; SHUMRICK 1967), esophagostomies (FITH-HUGH and SLY 1967; GRAHAM and ROYSER 1967; HARTWELL 1975), gastrostomies (KADER 1896; STAMM 1894; WITZEL 1891), and duodenostomies (ALEXANDER-WILLIAMS et al. 1967) have been reported to provide possible routes for enteral substitution. Our preference is the fine needle-catheter jejunostomy (FNCJ) (DELANY et al. 1973, 1977; MCDONALD 1954; PAGE et al. 1976, 1979) in TROIDL's modification (TROIDL et al. 1983, 1984) if the patient needs an operation for any reason. In a prospective trial of about 150 patients who underwent FNCJ, there were no major complications connected with the FNCJ tube used postoperatively. Minor problems, with partial damage of the catheter material, occurred in about 24 patients (16%), especially during long-term nutrition. Infections at the catheter insertion site could be found in about five patients (3%). No fistulas, and no peritonitis were detected.

When patients do not require an abdominal operative procedure, we prefer the percutaneous endoscopic gastronomy (PEG) (Gauderer and Ponsky 1981; Hashiba et al. 1984; Larson et al. 1983; Ponsky and Gauderer 1981; Ponsky et al. 1983) in our own modification (Vestweber et al. 1984a, b, 1985a). Underlight sedation, endoscopy is performed. After transillumination of the abdominal wall, the area for direct puncture of the stomach in the left upper abdomen is determined. Under local anesthesia, a split cannula with a Foley catheter is inserted into the stomach under continuous direct endoscopy. The balloon is inflated after withdrawal of the cannula, and the catheter is fixed outside to the skin of the abdominal wall. The procedure is illustrated schematically in Fig. 1.

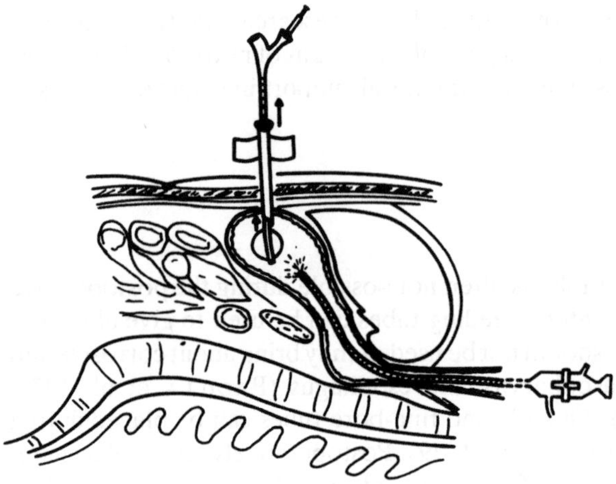

Fig. 1. Percutaneous endoscopic gastrostomy (DMW, Zbl). The inflated stomach is punctured with a split cannula under direct endoscopy. The balloon catheter can be pushed through the cannula, and the split cannula is withdrawn and broken off. The balloon is inflated, and with slight traction it holds stomach and abdominal wall in contact

Intestinal Absorption in the Perioperative Period

Substrate absorption in the small bowel is treated in many recent reports. Of great interest is the uptake of amino acids and oligopeptides, since there are several amino acid peptide diets available which can easily be fed through fine-bore tubes. Data concerning small-bowel absorption of these substances are usually derived from experiments done with healthy volunteers (Adibi and Morse 1977; Matthews and Adibi 1976). We attempted to observe events in the immediate postoperative period. We used an FNCJ first in an experimental rat model (Viell et al. 1984), and then in patients who also had a cecal fistula for decompression (Vestweber et al. 1985b). Test substances were administered in the orally preoperative period and were given via FNCJ postoperatively to test absorption. In the rats, we used tryptophan, and in humans, we used the isotope [^{15}N]leucine and the dipeptide glycyltyrosine. In the rats, a small but significant reduction in postoperative absorptive capability immediately and 1 day after operation could be observed. In humans who had received [^{15}N]leucine, a small but insignificant decrease in absorption could be observed. Figure 2 shows the bioavailability curve of [^{15}N]leucine as found in venous blood

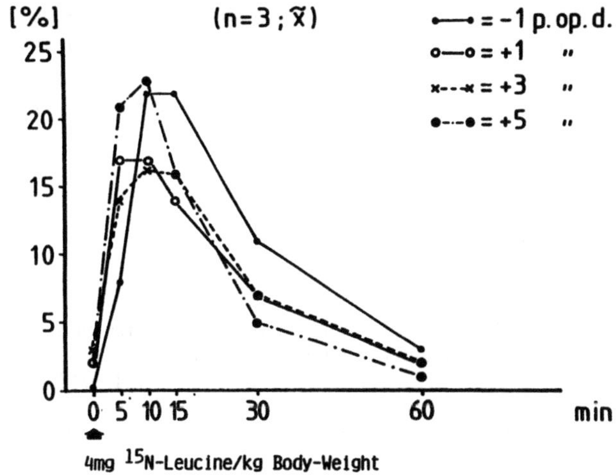

Fig. 2. Detection of ^{15}N-leucine in venous bloods samples after enteral administration (1 day preoperatively and on postoperative days 1, 3, and 5). There is a slight decrease on days 1 and 3 postoperatively, compared with 1 day preoperative and the fifth postoperative day

samples. Dipeptide absorption seems to have been unaffected (VESTWEBER et al. 1985b; VIELL et al. 1985). These results are confirmed by the analysis of cecal-fistulae secretion, wherein only a very small amount of marker substances could be detected.

Controlled Trial: Immediate Postoperative Enteral versus Parenteral Support

Clinical applicability of early postoperative feeding was tested in a controlled, randomized trial against the routine postoperative procedure of parenteral nutrition (VESTWEBER et al. 1985b). After major abdominal operations consisting of esophagectomies, gastrectomies, and pancreatic and liver surgery (n = 36), enteral nutrition with an amino acid oligopeptide diet was started on the first postoperative day. Increasing amounts of enteral support were administered, and a full amount (2800 Kcal/day) was reached on the fourth postoperative day. Parenteral nutrition was given to augment enteral administration during the first 3 postoperative days. The parenteral group received a full diet of 2800 Kcal/day and 100 g amino acids beginning at the first postoperative day. The results showed that there were no differences in clinical effectiveness; nutritional parameters were the same, as were all laboratory data. Gastrointestinal side effects such as epigastric fullness, distension of the abdomen, and diarrhea were more common in the enteral group. The costs of enteral nutrition were lower (about half the price of parenteral nutrition).

Summary

Immediate postoperative enteral nutrition with amino acid oligopeptide diets is possible and effective. Absorption of amino acids and oligopeptides shows no clinically relevant disturbances in the immediately postoperative period. Despite the intestinal side effects of enteral support, points in favor of enteral nutrition include increased hormone response, more rapid intestinal adaptation, low price, and the ease and economy of this form of long-term nutrition.

References

Adibi SA, Morse EL (1977) The number of glycine residues which limits intact absorption of glycine oligopeptides in human jejunum. J Clin Invest 60:1008

Alexander-Williams J, McLeisha AR, Guirguis AH (1967) The technique and indications for balloon catheter duodenostomy. Proc R Soc Med 69:847

Atkinson M, Walford S, Allisson SP (1979) Endoscopic insertion of fine-bore feeding tubes. Lancet 2:829

Bauer E, Gräber R, Brodtke R, Lünstedt B, Seifert J (1984) Ernährungsphysiologische, immunologische und klinische Parameter bei prospektiv randomisierten Patienten unter enteraler oder parenteraler Ernährungstherapie nach Dickdarmoperationen. Infusionsther Klin Ernähr Forsch Prax 11:165

Delany HM, Carnevale NL, Garvey JW (1973) Jejunostomy by a needle catheter technique. Surgery 73:786

Delany JM, Carnevale NJ, Garvey JW, Moss CM (1977) Postoperative nutritional support using needle catheter feeding jejunostomy. Ann Surg 186:165

Fith-Hugh GS, Sly DE (1967) Elective cervical oesophagostomy. Ann Otol Rhinol Laryngol 76:804

Gauderer MWL, Ponsky JL (1981) A simplified technique for constructing a tube feeding gastrostomy. Surg Gynecol Obstet 152:83

Graham WP, Royser HP (1967) Simplified cervical oesophagostomy for long-term extraoral feeding. Surg Gynecol Obstet 125:127

Hartwell SW Jr (1975) Surgical treatment of cervical oesophagostomy. Surg Clin North Am 55:1103

Hashiba K, Fabbri CE, Cappellnes CA, Branco PD, Birolini D, Oliveira MR (1984) Endoscopic percutaneous gastrostomy without laparotomy. Endoscopy 16:219

Hulten L, Andersson H, Bosaeus J, Fasth S, Hellberg R, Isaksson B, Magnusson O, Warnold J (1980) Enteral alimentation in the early postoperative course. J Parenter Enter Nutr 4;5:455

Kader B (1896) Zur Technik der Gastrostomie. Zentralbl Chir 23:685

Kautz G, Kohaus H, Langhans P (1981) Endoscopic insertion of feeding tubes: a new method for the management of upper digestive tract stenosis. Endoscopy 13:121

Larson DE, Fleming CR, Ott BJ, Schroeder KW (1983) Percutaneous endoscopic gastrostomy. Simplified access for enteral nutrition. Mayo Clin Proc 58: 103

Lorrain J, Page A (1965) Positive nitrogen balance and the prevention of ileus in the immediate postoperative period. Can Med Assoc J 93:546

Lyons JH (1974) Cervical pharyngostomy: a safe alternative for gastrointestinal decompression. Am J Surg 127:387

Matthews DM, Adibi SA (1976) Peptide absorption. Gastroenterology 71:151

McDonald HA (1954) Intrajejunal drip in gastric surgery. Lancet 2:1007

Meissner K, Weissenhofer W (1978) The effective placement of Miller-Abbott-Tubes under endoscopic guidance. Technical improvements. Endoscopy 10:13

Moss G (1963) Nitrogen equilibrium in the early postoperative period. Surg Forum 14:67

Moss G (1966) Postoperative decompression and feeding. Surg Gynecol Obstet 122:550

Moss G, Freidman AC (1977) Abdominal decompression: increase efficiency by esophageal aspiration utilizing a new nasogastric tube. Am J Surg 133:225

Page CP, Ryan JA, Haff RC (1976) Continual catheter administration of an elemental diet. Surg Gynecol Obstet 142:184

Page CP, Carlton PK, Andrassy RJ (1979) Safe, cost-effective postoperative nutrition; defined formula dient via needle-catheter jejunostomy. Am Surg 138:939

Padilla GV, Grant M, Wong H (1979) Subjective distresses of nasogastric tube feeding. J Parenter Enter Nutr 3:53
Ponsky JL, Gauderer MWL (1981) Percutaneous endoscopic gastrostomy: a nonoperative technique for feeding gastrostomy. Gastrointest Endost 27:9
Ponsky JL, Gauderer MWL, Stellato TA (1983) Percutaneous endoscopic gastrostomy: Review of 150 cases. Arch Surg 118:913
Shumrick DA (1967) Pyriforsinusotomy: a useful technique for temporary or permanent tube feeding. Arch Surg 94:277
Stamm M (1894) Gastrostomy by a new method. Med News 65:324
Torosian M, Rombeau JL (1980) Feeding by tube enterostomy. Surg Gynecol Obstet 150:918
Troidl H, Vestweber KH, Brotke R, Riedel A, Werner HH, Hioki K (1983) Unmittelbare postoperative enterale Ernährung mit der Elementardiät (Survimed®) mittels neuer Applikationsform einer sogenannten Feinnadel-Katheter-Jejunostomie (FNKJ). Chirurg 54:805
Troidl H, Vestweber KH, Sommer H, Tepner S (1984) Moderne Techniken der Sonderernährung. Leber Magen Darm 14:58
Vestweber KH, Troidl H, Sommer H (1984a) Perkutane endoskopische Gastrostomie. Eine einfache Technik zur enteralen Ernährung. Dtsch Med Wochenschr 109:1203
Vestweber KH, Viell B, Sommer H, Troidl H (1984b) Eine neue Technik zur enteralen Ernährung: perkutane endoskopische Gastrostomie. Langenbecks Arch Chir 364:495
Vestweber KH, Troidl H, Sommer H, Viell B, Mennigen R, Bönninghoff N, Eypasch E, Krause B (1985a) die endoskopische perkutane Gastrostomie – eine einfache Technik zur Langzeiternährung. Zbl Chir 110:913
Vestweber KH, Viell B, Troidl H, Krause B (1985b) Indikation und Ergebnisse der perioperativen enteralen Ernährung mit Formuladiäten. Z Gastroenterologie 23:82
Viell B, Vestweber KH, Korn F (1984) Die postoperative Resorptionsleistung des Rattendarmes bei Ernährung über eine Feinnadel-Katheter-Jejunostomie. Infusionsther 11:68
Viell B, Vestweber KH, Korn F, Plett G, Troidl H, Lange H, Budzikiewicz H (1986) Postoperative absorption capability of the jejunum. Gastroenterology (to be published)
Witzel O (1891) Zur Technik der Magenfistelanlegung. Zentralbl Chir 18:601

Session 8: Summary

S. L. Wolman

This session deals with nutritional support by either the parenteral or the enteral routes and its relationship to small-bowel transplantation. The first presentation, made by myself, is a review of 111 patients who were placed on home total parenteral nutrition (HTPN). This paper looks at the various causes of the loss of small-bowel function which ultimately requires HTPN, as well as the causes of morbidity and mortality in these groups of patients. At the present time, since small-bowel transplantation is not yet a routine procedure, indications must be defined so that the patients selected are those most likely to benefit from small-bowel transplantation and for whom HTPNhas some major shortcoming. Thus, some relative indications for small-bowel transplantation can be arrived at by distinguishing the portion the HTPN population that can be recognized as doing particularly poorly compared with the rest of the group. In reviewing the situation, it is seen that most of these patients have had a mean time on parenteral nutrition of approximately 3½ years, as compared with 2¾ years for those patients who require HTPN because of bowel infarction. As this is an ongoing parenteral nutrition program, it is also noted that, while those patients with bowel infarction have thus far had significantly more deaths, this current assessment does not necessarily reveal that those patients in the other disease groups will likely live longer than 3½ years on HTPN. It is also important to note that the patients with bowel infarction have spent 81% of their time out of the hospital, compared with those with other diagnoses, who spent 91%–97% of their time outside and that those patients with bowel infarction who died before this study was initiated still spent 73% of their time as outpatients, compared 80% for the HTPN group as a whole. In short, patients with bowel infarction have a shorter prognosis and less out-of-hospital time. Unfortunately, they also tend to have generalized vascular disease and are older and thus are not as good surgical candidates.

An examination of the patients indicates that severe liver disease and severe depression seem to be associated with increased morbidity and mortality. Severe metaboic bone disease is also related to increased morbidity. These may be the main relative indications for small-bowel transplantation. Other less common indications may be lack of vascular access and uncontrolled excessive jejunostomy outputs.

The second presentation concerning the enteral and parenteral feeding of patients with short-bowel syndrome by B. Lunstedt addresses the patient who has recently acquired short-bowel syndrome and delineates the objectives of parenteral nutrition at this early stage, as well as advocating the early institution of enteral feeding unless it is contraindicated by intestinal obstruction, nausea, or increasing diarrhea. He goes on from that point to discuss the various outcomes, which include both patients who are dependent on parenteral nutrition and those who subsequently adapt and can return to an oral diet.

The third paper presented by K. H. VESTWEBER, H. TROIDL, and B. VIELL outlines methods of perioperative nutritional support and their possible application in small-bowel transplantation. This paper discusses in more detail the use of the various types of nasogastric and jejunostomy feeding tubes that are available. Their experience with the fine-needle catheter jejunostomy reveals that 150 patients have been fed successfully with no major complications. Minor problems occurred in another 16%. The authors also discuss percutaneous endoscopic gastrostomy for those patients who do not require abdominal procedures.

The second part of their paper examines amino acid absorption in the early postoperative stage. Tryptophan absorption was assessed in rats, and [^{15}N]leucine and glycyltyrosine were administered in humans. These revealed that there are small and significant reductions in absorption in the rats immediately and up to 1 day postoperatively. Humans who received [^{15}N]leucine showed insignificant decreases in absorption.

A controlled trial of immediate postoperative enteral versus parenteral support, both given at the rate of 2800 Kcal/day revealed that there were no differences in clinical effectiveness. The enteral route produced some gastrointestinal side effects, but was less costly.

Session 9

Immunological and Clinical Monitoring After Transplantation

Monitoring of Small-Bowel Grafts by Mucosal Suction Biopsies

U. G. STAUFFER

In a series of papers, we previously described our experimental work on small-intestinal transplantation in minipigs of the Göttingen strain (STAUFFER 1975, 1983; STAUFFER et al. 1975, 1978a, b). One of the goals of our studies was to establish a safe control system for early recognition of vascular complications and rejection crisis in the graft. This is one of the prerequisites for the clinical application of small-intestinal transplantations in man. In this paper, we shall summarize our work on the monitoring of small-bowel grafts by sequential mucosal suction biopsies.

Materials and Methods

Surgical Procedure

A total of 142 minipigs were divided into four groups:

Group 1 consisted of four animals. A 30-cm-long jejunal segment was isolated from the intestinal continuity, an intestinal biopsy was taken, and both intestinal ends were sewn to the abdominal wall as separate enterostomies. Intestinal continuity was restored by a one-layer, end-to-end anastomosis. Several intestinal biopsies were taken at 1- to 2-day intervals. This group allowed for recognition of unspecific histologic changes at the ostia and served as controls.

Group 2 consisted of six animals. In a 100-cm-long jejunal segment, complete ischemia was produced for a period of 1–2 h. The corresponding branch of the superior mesenteric artery was proximally clamped, cannulated distally, and continuously perfused with a perfusion solution cooled down to 4°C. The jejunal loop was prolapsed outside the abdominal cavity and packed in ice. After the termination of perfusion, the arteriotomy was closed with 7/0 silk sutures. The rest of the procedure was identical to that for group 1. Several intestinal biopsies were taken before, during, and after ischemia and later on at 1- to 2-day intervals for several weeks. This group helped to determine hypoxic injuries to the intestine.

Group 3 was the first transplantation group and consisted of 72 animals. Donor and recipient were operated on simultaneously. In the donors, the abdomen was opened with a long midline incision, and the intestines were completely eventrated. In the distal part of the small intestine, a suitable 30- to 120-cm-long intestinal graft was isolated and packed in sterile ice. A cannula was inserted into the artery and a perfusion with 4°C Ringer's lactate solution was started. The recipient animals were nephrectomized on the right side, and graft vessels were anastomosed end to end to the renal vessels. Both ends of the graft were implanted into the abdominal wall as separate enterostomies. Just before establishment of circulation and 30–60 min afterward, intestinal biopsies were taken. Postoperatively, the enterostomies were examined daily, type and quantity of secretion were recorded, and two to three suction biopsies were taken from both ostia for histologic examination at 2- to 2-day intervals. In this group, the spontaneous development of the grafts and the animals was observed. No attempt was made to save the recipients by explantation of a damaged graft.

Group 4 consisted of 60 animals. In this group, the monitoring system established for groups 1–3 was tested as to its practical value. We projected that it the control system were correct, the recipient could be explanted in time and would be able to survive. The surgical procedure was identical to the one described for group 3. However, timely explantation enabling the survival of the recipient was attempted according to criteria based on observations that had been made in groups 1–3.

Histologic Studies

Qualitative Histological Assessment

About 1100 biopsies were taken. They were fixed in 4% buffered formalin, dehydrated, visualized with a magnifying glass or microscope and embedded in paraffin, and series of sections were made. About 40000 sections were then stained with hematoxylin and analyzed by routine histologic examinations.

Quantitative Morphometric Analysis

At least five strictly perpendicular sections per biopsy were submitted to quantitative morphometric analysis (Dunnhill and Whitehead 1972). This technique relies on a method described by Chalkley et al. in 1949 for determining an index for deriving the ratio of the surface to volume for three-dimensional structures *(S/V)* by analyzing two-dimensional sections. A template of 15 lines of equal length *(l)* connecting the vertices of a regular hexagonal point network is superimposed onto the histologic sections using the lamina muscularis mucosae as a baseline (see Fig. 1). We used the template designed by Weibel (1963). A cut *(c)* is counted where a line crosses the epithelium covering the mucosal surface, and a hit *(h)* is counted where the end of a line l falls over the mucosal tissue between the covering epithelium and the lamina muscularis mucosae. The number of c is proportional to the surface; the number of h is proportional to the volume. According to Chalkley, S/V is equal to $4c/lh$.

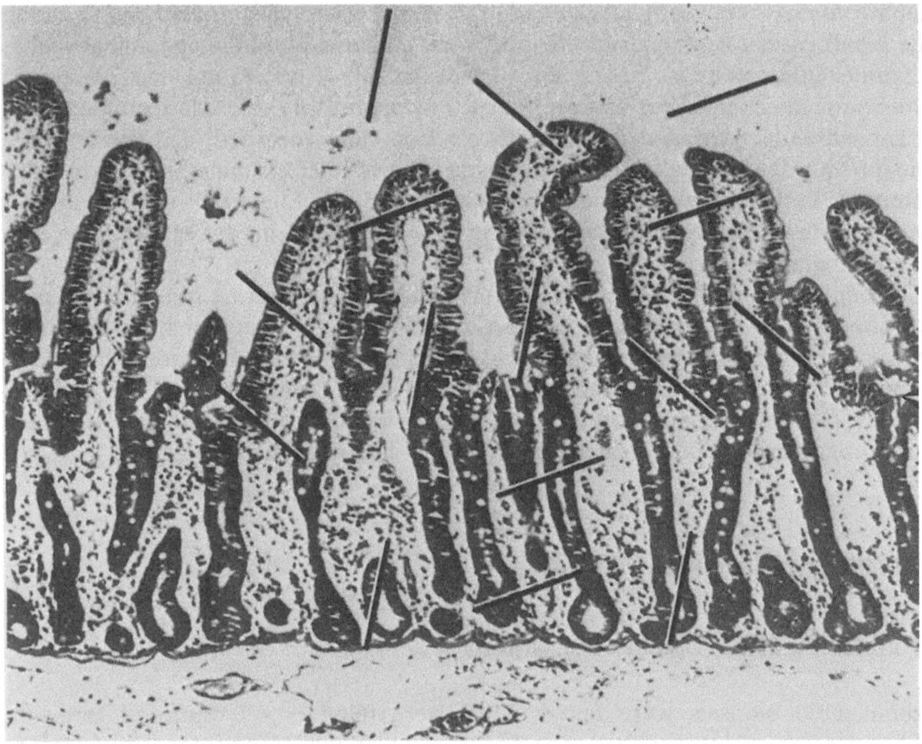

Fig. 1. A template of 15 lines of equal length *l* is superimposed over a section of a normal biopsy. Cuts are countered where the lines cross the surface epithelium, hits are counted where the lines cross the surface epithelium, hits are counted where the end points of the lines lie over the mucosa

Results

Group 1

The animals survived for many months, and the enterostomies remained patent until the animals were sacrificed. Mucosal suction biopsies taken from a depth of 3–4 cm were normal beginning from the 2nd or 3rd day. Nearer to the stoma, unspecific inflammatory changes were noticed. We concluded from group 1 that the biopsies have to be taken at a depth of at least 3–4 cm from the enterostomy opening.

Group 2

Immediately after reestablishment of circulation, marked intestinal hyperperistalsis and mucus production occurred. This lasted for the first 12–24 h during which period the enterostomies were edematous. By the 3rd day, they were again pink and inconspicuous. Even serious ischemic changes with histologically complete loss of the mucosal epithelial cells in the area of the villi were completely reversible. It could be concluded from group 2 that the reparative process was already fully established 24 h after ischemia. By the 4th postoperative day, the biopsies were again nearly normal.

Group 3

All 36 recipients survived the operation. However, six animals with an intact transplant died within the 1st postoperative week owing to hemorrhagic shock, pneumonia, mechanical ileus, or while under anesthesia during biopsy. The complications of the grafts in the remaining 30 transplantations are listed in Table 1. All 13 cases with complications at the vascular pedicle – due to either insufficiency of arterial circulation or venous thrombosis with hemorrhagic infarction of the transplants – occurred during the first 5 days. Both complications could be recognized early on by simple inspection of the enterostomies. Histologic examination could only confirm the diagnosis, but did not allow for recognition of the complications at an earlier stage. The 14 grafts with the vascular pedicle intact survived for an average of 10–18 days. Macroscopically, the initial rejection process could be recognized by edematous stomata. Within 24–72 h, these stomata became dark bluish-red and finally black. At the same time, intestinal secretion stopped, and no more biopsies could be obtained.

Table 1. Graft complications in 30 homologous small-intestinal transplants

Complication	Cases *(n)*
Deficient arterial blood supply	5
Hemorrhagic infarction	8
Rejection	14
Infection	2
Intussusception of the transplant	1

Qualitative Histologic Studies

Qualitative histologic assessment disclosed that the first microscopic changes in the biopsies suggesting the first stages of rejection could be detected 24–36 h before the first macroscopic changes were visible at the ostia. The grafts were rejected in the classical manner, usually within 2–4 days. The early loss of epithelium, especially at the tips of the villi, preceded total necrosis. Once the epithelium had been destroyed, leukocytes appeared regularly in addition to round cells as a sign of a superadded infection. In the whole series, there was no histologic evidene of graft-vs-host reaction.

Table 2. Mean values for *c*, *h*, and *c/lh* in normal small-intestinal biopsies of 27 young minipigs. (From Dunnhill and Whitehead 1972)

$\bar{c}$	11.835 ± 0.99
$\bar{h}$	20.191 ± 2.46
$\bar{c}/l\bar{h}$	0.428 ± 0.07

Quantitative Morphometric Analysis

Table 2 summarizes the mean values of *c, h,* and *c/lh* with standard deviations for 27 normal intestinal biopsies from young minipigs. Figure 2 illustrates the changes in *S/V (c/lh)* in sequential biopsies of one of our transplants in group 3. After transplantation, *c/lh* decreases 1–2 days, owing to postoperative edema. The functional surface decreases, which leads to a reduction in the number of cuts *c*. The volume of the mucosa, however, remains more or less constant during that time. As the edema disappears, the curve goes up again, a result of the reconstruction phase. Here, the villi lengthen and become thinner, which causes the number of cuts *c* to increase more rapidly than the number of hits *h*. As the rejection process begins, *c/lh* decreases again. This shows that the surface (especially the epithelial cells) is more sensitive to the rejection process than the total volume of the mucosa. Later on, the curve is again flatter. This means that, in a later stage of the rejection process with marked atrophy of the mucosa, volume and surface decrease at a similar rate. At this stage, the absolute number of *c* and *h* permits some evaluation of the actual state of the mucosa.

Quantitative morphometric analysis enabled us, to recognize a beginning rejection crisis 3–4 days before macroscopic changes at the ostia were seen and 24–36 h before the first and still inconclusive histologic changes could be found at normal histologic assessment of the biopsies.

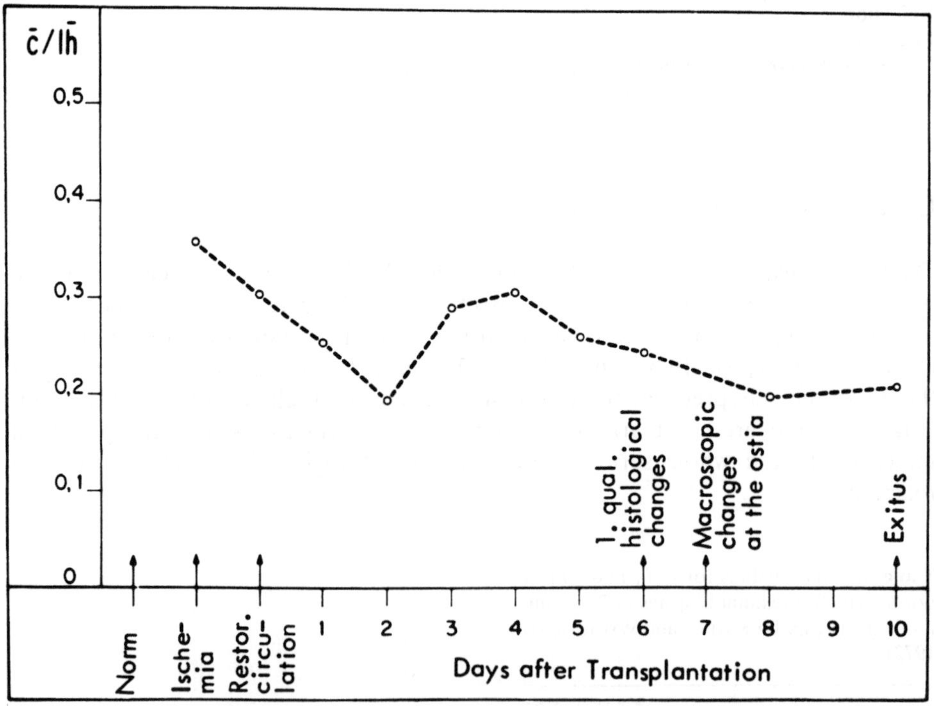

Fig. 2. Quantitative morphometric analysis of sequential mucosal biopsies. The changes in the ratio of surface to volume *(c/lh)* in sequential biopsies of one of our transplants is demonstrated. (From Dunnhill and Whitehead 1972)

Group 4

Table 3 shows graft complications in 23 primarily successful small-intestinal transplantations. Hemorrhagic infarction occurred in six cases, deficient arterial circulation was found in six cases, and in 11 animals, rejection occurred. All six cases of hemorrhagic infarction occurred within 48 h after transplantation. Five of the grafts were subjected to emergency explantation several hours after diagnosis, and all five animals survived. In one animal, the hemorrhagic infarction was unfortunately recognized too late, and the animal died before explantation could be attempted. In this case, the enterostomata were not inspected until the 3rd day, as its postoperative condition was too poor for it to sustain anesthesia. In pigs, general anesthesia must be administered while dressings are changed, ostia inspected, and biopsies performed. (In humans, this entire procedure is painless, thus precluding the use of anesthesia.) The six cases of deficient arterial circulation all occurred between day 2 and 5. In the 11 animals whose vascular pedicle remained intact, rejection crisis started between days 4 and 18. All 11 grafts were explanted within 36 h after diagnosis of a severe irreversible rejection crisis, defined as three falling points upon quantitative morphometric analysis of the biopsies (see also Fig. 2). Of these 11 animals, ten survived for weeks or months. One animal was found dead in its cage 2 h after explantation; the autopsy showed massive aspiration into the lungs. The results for group 4 confirm the validity fo the monitoring systems that were used in groups 1–3.

Table 3. Graft complications in primarily successful small-intestinal transplantations

Complication	Cases *(n)*
Hemorrhagic infarction	6
Deficient arterial circulation	6
Rejection	11
Total	23

Discussion

Quantative morphometric analysis was used in small intestinal transplantations for the first time in this series. This method enabled us to recognize rejection crisis 3–4 days before macroscopic changes at the ostia could be observed and 24–36 h before initial and inconclusive histologic changes could be detected upon normal histologic assessment of the biopsies. We concluded therefore that this method, combined with daily inspection of the ostia and normal qualitative routine histologic examination of the biopsies, could be an excellent method for recognizing rejection crisis in its early stages. In the first transplantation group (group 3), spontaneous development of the grafts and of the animals was observed. No attempt was made to save the recipients by explanting the damaged grafts. Most animals in this group died of vascular complications, infection, or rejection crisis. In the second transplantation group (group 4), monitoring systems used in group 1–3 were tested for their practicability. Timely explantation that would enable the recipient to survive was attempted according to criteria based on information gatrered from groups 1–3. The results of the second transplantation group confirmed the validity of our monitoring system. Complications in the vascular axis of the graft or rejection crisis could be recognized early enough to allow timely removal of irreversibly damaged grafts, permitting the animals to survive. This safe monitoring system could reduce postoperative risk in patients who have undergone small-intestinal transplants so that it would no longer be greater than for other vascular abdominal surgery or for renal transplantation. It must, however, be stressed that this monitoring system, especially quantitative morphometric analysis, is a relatively time-consuming procedure which requires close cooperation between transplant surgeons and experienced pathologists. There is, for example, a 4- to 6-h time lapse between biopsy and the appearance of the first point on the curve of quantitative morphometric analysis. Despite this disadvantage, quantitative morphometric analysis allows for the establishment of objective quantitative histologic criteria of the rejection process that can be used early on. This can contribute to the safety of small-intestinal transplantation for recipients, a prerequisite for application in man.

References

Chalkley HW, Cornfield J, Park H (1949) A method for estimating volume/surface ratios. Science 110:295

Dunnhill MS, Whitehead R (1972) A method for the quantitation of small intestinal biopsy specimens. J Chir Path 25:243

Stauffer UG (1975) Transplantation of the small intestine. Prog Pediatr Surg 8, 1

Stauffer UG (1983) Die Dünndarm-Transplantation: Gegenwärtiger Stand und mögliche Zukunft. Z Kinderchir 38:286

Stauffer UG, Mona D, Shmerling DH (1975) Die Überwachung von Dünndarmtransplantaten durch fortlaufende Schleimhautsogbiopsien. Z Kinderchir 16:32

Stauffer UG, Becker M, Hirsig J, Meier HP, Kara O (1978a) The risk of small intestinal transplantation for the recipient: Experimental results in young minipigs. J Pediatr Surg 13:465

Stauffer UG, Becker M, Mona D, Kara O (1978b) Transplantation of the small intestine. Res Exp Med (Berl) 172:161

Weibel ER (1963) Principles and methods for the morphometric study of the lung and other organs. Lab Invest 12:131

*Monitoring of Small-Bowel Allograft Rejection: Maltose Absorption**

W. H. Schraut and K. K. W. Lee

Introduction

With the advent of effective control of the rejection process, believed to be possible with cyclosporine A, the clinical application of small-bowel transplantation may become a reality. An effective means of detecting rejection at its onset is therefore needed. Unlike renal transplants, in which serum creatinine levels can be followed, intestinal allografts offer no specific, easily measured parameters which can indicate the onset of rejection. Several approaches to the monitoring of small-bowel allografts have been taken; of these, surveillance by serial mucosal biopsy appears to be most accurate and has gained the widest acceptance (Stauffer et al. 1975; Madara and Kirkman 1985). It is difficult to obtain biopsies, however, if the graft is in intestinal continuity. Furthermore, several investigators have cautioned against biopsies as the sole means of surveillance because they noticed that the histologic alterations seen during rejection were sometimes variable in both distribution and intensity (Holmes et al. 1971; Raju et al. 1984; Rosemurgy and Schraut 1986). Therefore, random biopsies may not conclusively reflect the overall status of the allograft and should be supplemented by a graft function test.

In our search for a reliable, yet readily available method for the detection of incipient intestinal allograft rejection in the form of histologic evaluation and/or a function test, we studied the sequence of histologic rejection events and correlated the histologic findings with the results of a function test of our design, namely, a maltose absorption test (Billiar et al. 1984). Specifically, we sought to determine whether acute and chronic intestinal allograft rejection follow a clearly defined and predictable histologic sequence and whether the changes involve the graft uniformly or sporadically. In addition, we wanted to detect whether impairment of maltose absorption parallels or predates the clinical and histologic onset of rejection and, therefore, whether it might be suitable for monitoring purposes.

Materials and Methods

We used the rat model of accessory and of orthotopic small-bowel transplantation with the Lewis X Brown Norway F_1 (LBN-F_1) $\rightarrow$ Lewis (LEW) strain combination. In

* Supported by The National Institutes of Arthritis, Metabolism, and Digestive Diseases (Grant No. AM27332).

one group of animals ($n = 25$), the venous effluent of the allograft was drained into the inferior vena cava. In our experience (SCHRAUT et al. 1983; K. LEE and W. SCHRAUT, "Small-Bowel Transplantation in the Rat: Graft Survival with Heterotopic vs Orthotopic Position, this volume), this procedure is followed by acute rejection, i.e., graft necrosis, after 11.4 ± 0.4 days. In another group ($n = 14$), the effluent was drained into the portal vein; this allows delayed rejection as typified by graft fibrosis, which is complete after 19.8 ± 6.2 days. For the histologic studies, multiple full-thickness allograft biopsies were obtained from host animals at or near the time of their death and from graft recipients randomly killed at various intervals after transplantation. In rats with orthotopic grafts ($n = 6$), a jejunal full-thickness biopsy was performed at the time of the maltose test. Experimental groups and the type of studies performed are listed as follows:

Experimental group	Rats *(n)*
1. Accessory small-bowel allografts	
a) Followed to complete rejection	
Portocaval anastomosis	25
Portoportal anastomosis	14
b) Harvested at various intervals after transplantation	
Portocaval anastomosis	11
Portoportal anastomosis	9
c) Studied with the maltose absorption test	
Portocaval anastomosis	6
Portoportal anastomosis	6
2. Orthotopic small-bowel allografts	
a) Studied by biopsy and maltose absorption test	
Portocaval anastomosis	6

The maltose absorption test was performed on the 5th, 9th, 12th, and 15th days in 12 rats with accessory allografts and either portal or caval venous drainage. The six rats with orthotopic grafts underwent the absorption test on the 5th and the 8th–9th postoperative days. The technique for the maltose absorption test, as described previously by BILLIAR et al. (1984), involves instillation into the proximal stoma of accessory grafts (Fig. 1) or jejunum in orthotopic grafts of 0.5 mg maltose per gram rat body weight, dissolved in 2.5 cc normal saline. The serum glucose level is then determined at 15-min intervals until it returns to a previously measured baseline. Baseline and control studies have been performed previously in rats with accessory isografts (LEW → LEW; BILLIAR et al. 1984).

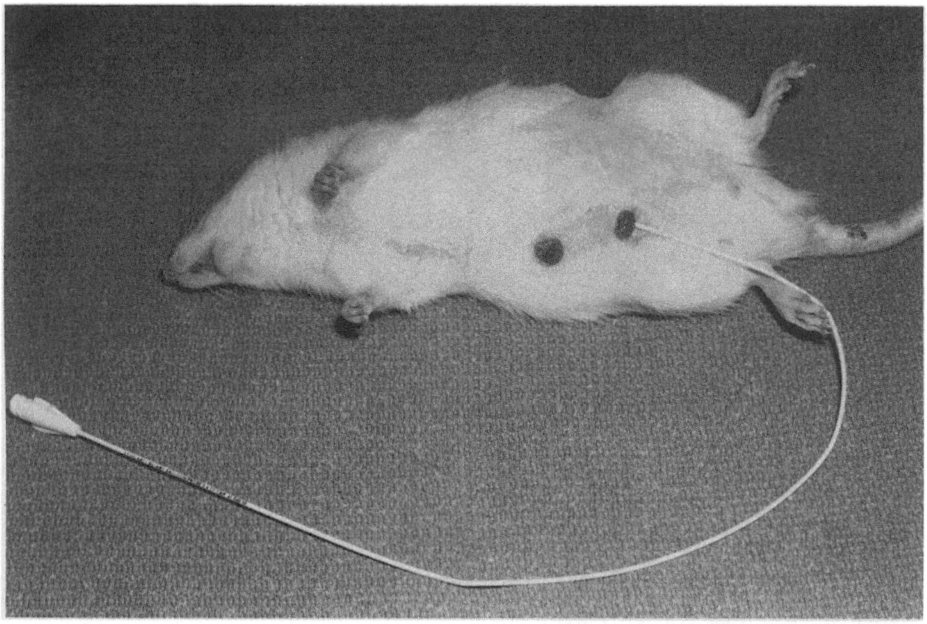

Fig. 1. The recipient of an accessory small-intestinal allograft has been prepared for the maltose absorption test, which is done under light ether anesthesia. The distal stoma *(right)* has been occluded with a biliary balloon catheter. The proximal stoma is next cannulated with a biliary irrigation catheter

Results

Histologic Studies

For the first 5 days after transplantation, all grafts were histologically identical to isografts and to the host's small intestine (Fig. 2A). For the grafts (accessory of orthotopic) undergoing acute rejection, the histologic sequence was as follows: by day 7, plasma cells and lymphocytes infiltrated the lamina propria; histologically, this was the obvious onset of rejection. Overall, the architecture of the allograft remained intact. By the 8th–9th day, the cellular infiltrate intensified and was then associated with villous blunting and epithelial sloughing (Fig. 2B). In the next 1–2 days, the rejection process seemed to accelerate, and by the 10th day, or often even sooner, complete mucosal destruction developed which was associated with heavy transmural cellular infiltration (Fig. 2C). This stage constituted irreversible graft rejection and destruction and led to death of the host.

Accessory allografts with portal drainage of the venous effluent were nearly always (11 of 14 animals) subject to a less rapid course of rejection. For the first 6 days, all of these grafts remained normal histologically. Lymphocytic infiltration of the otherwise morphologically intact allograft was the prominent feature up to the 9th postoperative day. As this cellular infiltation progressed, sporadic mucosal sloughing and villous blunting evolved with a noticeable increase in the thickness of the bowel wall. In this phase, sections with relatively well-preserved (but by no means normal) mucosal

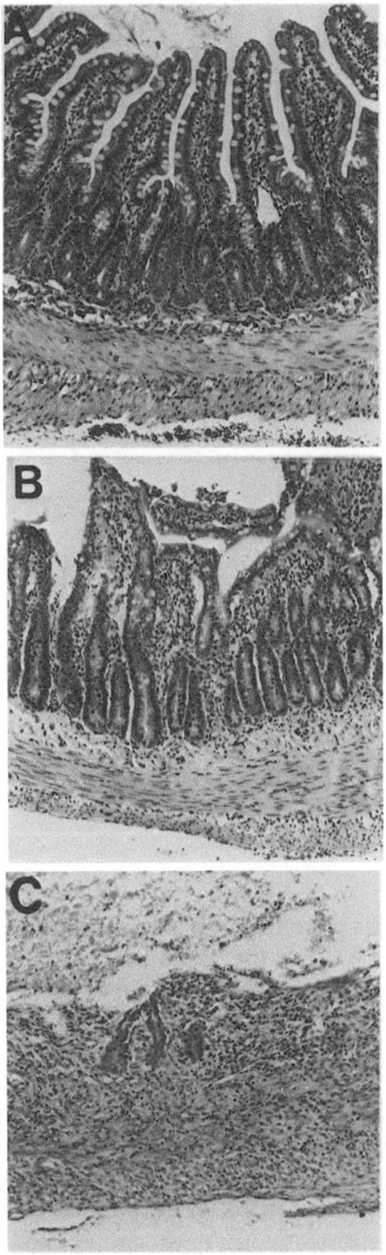

Fig. 2A–C. **A** Section from a heterotopic allograft harvested on the 5th postoperative day. The architecture of the intestine is histologically identical to that of the normal small bowel. **B** Heterotopic allograft (portocaval anastomosis) harvested on the 8th postoperative day. Marked cellular infiltration is associated with villus blunting and sporadic epithelial sloughing. **C** Histologic section from an acutely rejected allograft (10th postoperative day). There is near total mucosal destruction and heavy transmural cellular infiltration. (× 100)

architecture were interspersed with regions of severe destruction (Fig. 3). Aggressive immunosuppressive therapy, if it were available, might reverse some of these changes, but might result in fibrosis and would therefore lead to functional loss of the allograft even without rejection. This phase of rejection lasted through days 10–13, that is, 1–3 days longer than with allografts subject to acute rejection. Over the

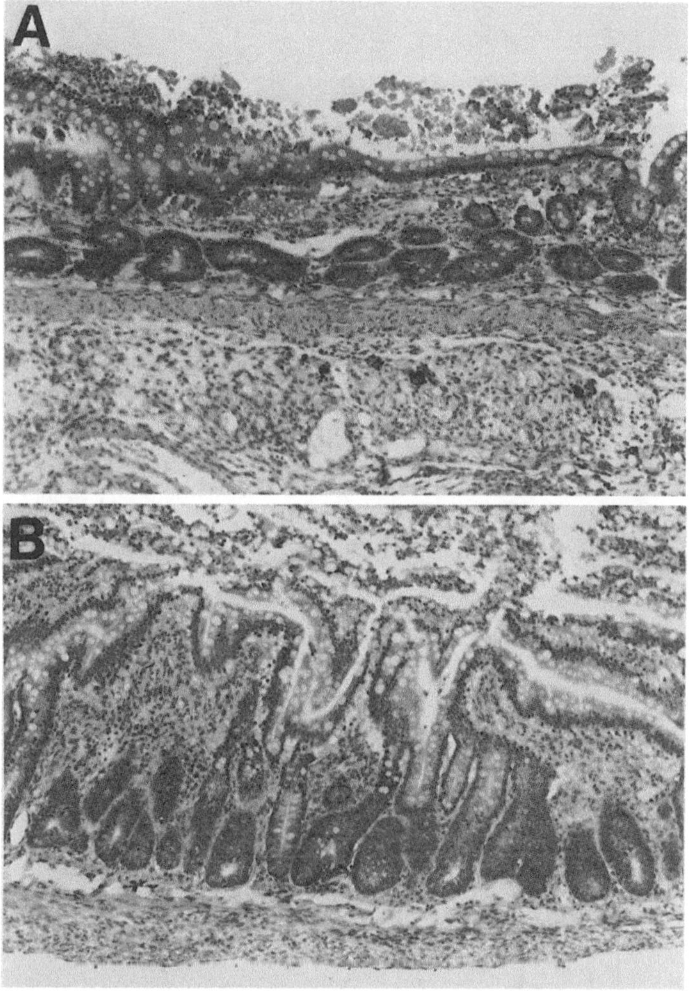

Fig. 3 A, B. Section from an intestinal allograft harvested on the 13th postoperative day (portoportal anastomosis). An area of complete loss of the mucosa is seen in **A.** A remnant of recognizable mucosa with prominent cellular infiltration and villus blunting was encountered in close proximity **(B).** (× 100)

ensuing days, destruction of the mucosa progressed rapidly and was associated with graft encapsulation and fibrosis (Fig. 4).

Maltose Absorption Test

The maltose absorption test undertaken on the 5th postoperative day in accessory grafts subject to acute rejection ($n = 6$) demonstrated a lesser rise in serum glucose than was seen in animals with isografts. The difference was statistically significant. A significantly reduced rise in the serum glucose level at 30 and 45 min was also seen on the 9th day. On the 12th postoperative day, the glucose curve was essentially flat in those animals (four of six rats) that survived (Fig. 5).

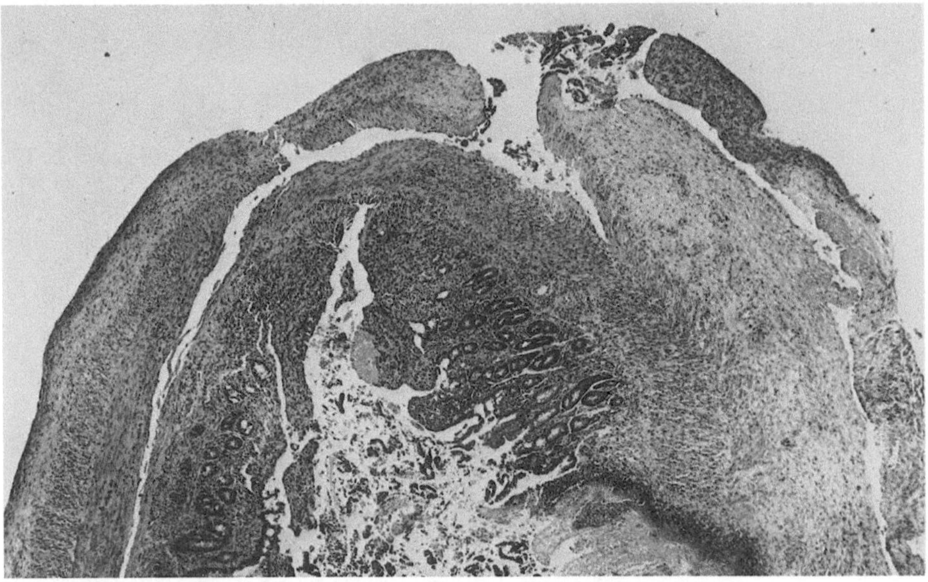

Fig. 4. Cross section of an accessory allograft subject to chronic rejection (29th postoperative day). Marked thickening of the bowel wall is associated with complete mucosal destruction. (× 25)

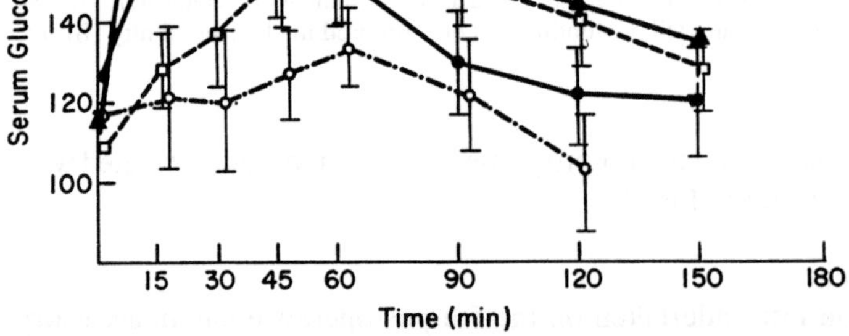

Fig. 5. Maltose absorption in heterotopic allografts with portocaval anastomosis. The curve with the *shaded triangles* (▲——▲) represents maltose absorption from accessory isografts (LEW → LEW, portocaval anastomosis) 4–6 weeks after transplantation. ●——●, 5th postoperative day; □ – – – □, 9th postoperative day; ○ –·–·– ○, 12th postoperative day. Reproduced from Rosemurgy and Schraut (1986)

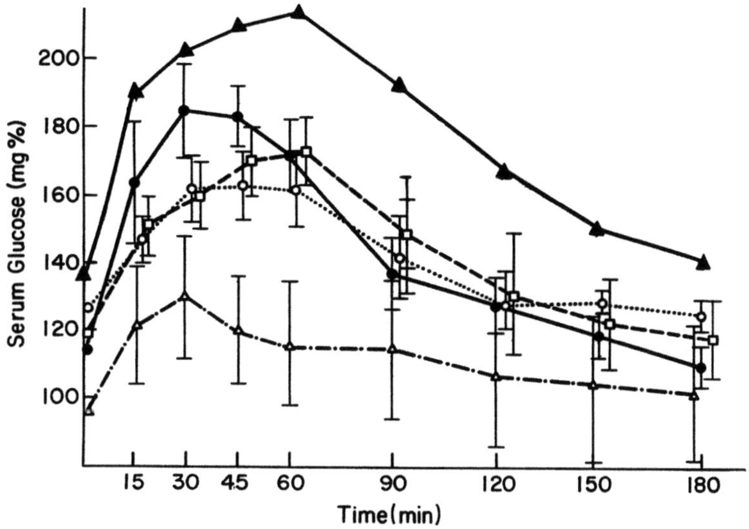

Fig. 6. Maltose absorption in heterotopic allografts with portoportal anastomosis. The curve with the *shaded* triangles (▲——▲) represents the maltose absorption from accessory isografts (LEW → LEW, porto-portal anastomosis) 4–6 weeks after transplantation ●——●, 5th postoperative day; ○····○, 9th postoperative day; □ - - - □, 12th postoperative day; △-·-·△, 15th postoperative day. Reproduced from Rosemurgy and Schraut (1986)

Accessory grafts that were subject to delayed rejection showed a similar progressive decline which began on the ninth postoperative day (Fig. 6). In this group, five of the six animals survived beyond 15 days, but, according to the maltose test, their accessory grafts were no longer functional by the 15th postoperative day. This indicates that the results of the absorption test parallels the histologic findings (Fig. 7).

Allografts in an orthotopic position showed a similar histologic and functional decline as rejection progressed (Fig. 7). However, there were two animals in which maltose absorption on the 8th postoperative day appeared to be less impaired than indicated by the histologic findings.

Discussion

This experimental study demonstrates that, during rejection, intestinal allografts undergo a sequence of histologic changes which is defined and predictable whether rejection is acute or delayed. Concerning reliance on light-microscope examination of biopsy specimens for monitoring of small-bowel allografts, several words of caution must be raised. Firstly, our findings are based on full-thickness cross sections which may not be readily obtained from an orthotopic graft. When we confined the histologic evaluation to the mucosal-submucosal level, which would simulate a superficial, "safe" suction biopsy, we repeatedly saw variability in the histologic indicators of the degree of rejection in different areas of each section and in different sections of any given specimen (Fig. 4). Although such variability was most often insufficient to cause us to classify any section erroneously in an incorrect stage of

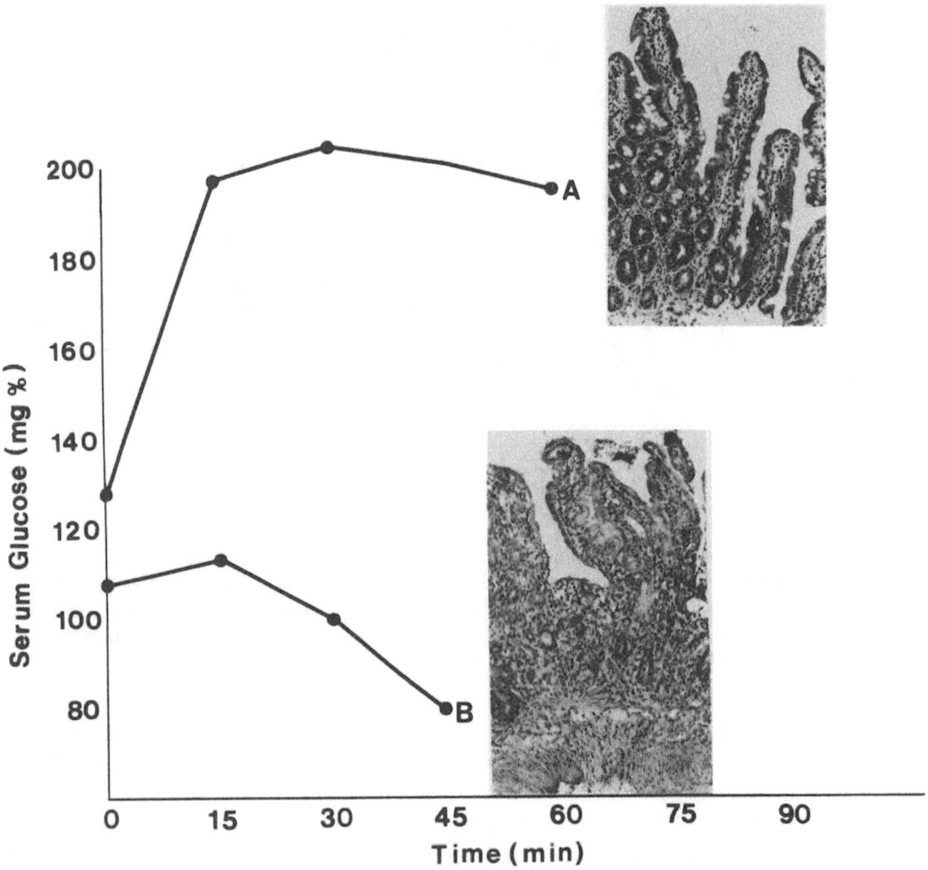

Fig. 7. Maltose absorption in an orthotopic allograft on the 5th *(A)* and 8th *(B)* postoperative days. Absorption is normal on the 5th and impaired on the 8th day. The simultaneous biopsy on the 5th day shows normal, intact intestinal architecture and, on the 8th day, cellular infiltration, with villus shortening and superficial erosion at the tips of the villi

rejection, such errors might be more likely in clinical small-bowel transplantation, where one would hesitate to do a deep biopsy for fear of causing a perforation.

Secondly, a disadvantage in relying on graft histology exclusively lies in the fact that orthotopic grafts are inaccessible to biopsy. One could circumvent this latter problem by creating a small-bowel pouch for biopsy, as suggested by Kunlin et al. (1971). Still another possibility for improving the diagnostic value of a biopsy would be to search for perivascular round-cell infiltrates of the villus arterioles (Madara and Kirkman 1985) or, following the suggestion of Stauffer et al. 1975), to perform morphometric measurements of the mucosa. The two latter techniques also appear to allow an earlier diagnosis of rejection than is possible with simple light-microscopic examination of random biopsies.

Given the limitations of monitoring by sequential graft biopsy, it would be preferable to use, for screening purposes, a function test that is easily done, can be repeated frequently, and is specific and sensitive. The present study indicates that the measurement of maltose absorption in the form of a glucose tolerance test can fulfill these requirements. In order to be absorbed, maltose must be split into its monosaccharide moiety, glucose, by the brush border enzyme maltase. Glucose is then absorbed actively into the mesenteric venous circulation. Both the peak and the shape of the serum glucose curve obtained with the maltose absorption test give information on the functional competence of the graft. Seemingly before the histologic alterations in the rejection process, or at least early in the course of rejection, the peak of the bell-shaped glucose curve is diminished and delayed. This course was, however, not seen uniformly in each animal, as was apparent in the series of experiments with the allograft in the orthotopic position in which we combined the maltose absorption test with a simultaneous jejunal biopsy. Maltose absorption appeared moderately impaired in several instances during the midcourse of rejection (8th–9th postoperative day), a time when histologic study indicated villus blunting, sporadic sloughing of the tips of the villi, and cellular infiltration of the submucosa (Fig. 7). This discrepancy between biopsy and function test may be explained by the fact that the disaccharidase maltase is present at very high concentration in the brush border. Therefore, impaired maltose absorption may not become evident unless there is widespread mucosal injury. It is also possible that, by chance, the random biopsy and histologic sections were taken from a jejunal area that was destroyed more severely than other regions of the graft. As rejection ensues and becomes clinically evident by stomal edema and by a hunched posture of the graft recipient, the curve flattens out. These changes are always paralleled by progressive destruction of the bowel architecture, which culminates in graft necrosis.

In summary, we find that the maltose absorption test provides a reliable and reproducible method for screening and monitoring of the functional integrity of small-bowel allografts. In future clinical applications, if functional impairment were detected by this function test, a confirmatory biopsy should be performed. Based on this combined information, the immunosuppressive regimen – of a type which still needs to be determined – would be adjusted. Functional and morphological evaluation must complement each other.

References

Billiar TR, Garberoglio C, Schraut WH (1984) Maltose absorption as an indicator of small-intestinal allograft rejection. J Surg Res 37:75–82

Holmes JT, Klein MS, Winawer SJ, Fortner JG (1971) Morphological studies of rejecion in canine jejunal allografts. Gastroenterology 61:693–706

Kunlin A, Gaston JP, Shiu MH, Winawer SJ, Fortner JG (1971) The isolated allograft pouch: A useful method for monitoring small bowel allografts. Surg Forum 22:237–239

Madara JL, Kirkman RL (1985) Structural and functional evolution of jejunal allograft rejection in rats and the ameliorating effects of cyclosporine therapy. J Clin Invest 75:502–512

Raju S, Didlake RH, Cayirli M, Turner MD, Grogan JB, Achord J (1984) Experimental small bowel transplantation utilizing cyclosporine. Transplantation 38:561–566

Rosemurgy AS, Schraut WH (1986) Small-bowel allografts: Sequence of histologic changes in acute and chronic rejection. Am J Surg (in press)

Schraut WH, Rosemurgy AS, Riddel RM (1983) Prolongation of intestinal allograft survival without immunosuppressive drug therapy. Transplantation of small bowel allografts. J Surg Res 34:597–607

Stauffer UG, Mona D, Shmerline DH (1975) Monitoring of small bowel transplants by sequential mucosal suction biopsies. Z Kinderchir Grenzgeb 16:32–37

Porcine Ileal Peptide: A Potential Marker for Rejection of Small-Intestine Allografts

A. BORGSTROM, M. WIDER, W.H. MARKS, and A. VINIK

Introduction

Successful transplantation of any organ requires a means by which to monitor rejection. This allows for attempts at reversing the rejection process while preserving graft function. Small-bowel transplantation may soon be used as a clinical tool, yet no reliable, noninvasive marker for rejection currently exists. A newly isolated protein from the gastrointestinal tract, porcine ileal peptide (PIP), may obviate this problem (WIDER et al. 1984). The purpose of our work was to determine the tissue distribution of this protein in order to determine its organ specificity.

Materials and Methods

Specimens

Tissue samples were taken from a 3-month-old pig (16 kg) under pentobarbital anesthesia. Sampled tissues were taken from salivary glands; esophagus; stomach; duodenum; upper and lower jejunum; upper, mid- and lower ileum; proximal, mid-, and distal colon. In addition, samples from heart, lung, diaphragm, liver, gallbladder, sciatic nerve, vagal nerve, skeletal muscle, pancreas, spleen, adrenal gland, kidney, ureter, urinary bladder, and skin were harvested. All samples were collected in phosphate-buffered, 10% formalin, and paraffin-embedded tissue sections were used for immunohistochemical staining.

Immunohistochemistry

Endogenous peroxidase was inhibited by incubation of the slides with equal parts of absolute methanol and 3% H_2O_2 for 10 min. This was followed by a 10-min incubation with normal goat serum diluted to 1:20 to reduce nonspecific background staining. All dilutions were made with a phosphate buffer (0.05 mol/liter) containing NaCl (0.15 mol/liter), bovine serum albumen (40 g/liter), and normal goat serum (1% v/v) at pH 7.4. A polyclonal monospecific rabbit anti-PIP serum was used. Antibody specificity was checked by immunoelectrophoresis in agarose and showed only a single precipitation line against both crude pig ileal extract and isolated PIP. The tissue sections were incubated for 2–3 h at room temperature with the above-mentioned rabbit anti-PIP serum diluted to 1:5000–1:40000. A biotinylated goat anti-rabbit IgG antiserum and a avidin-peroxidase complex, both obtained from Vector (Vectastain, Burlingame, California), were used according to the manufacturer's instructions. 3-3′-Diaminobenzidine tetrahydrochloride (0.4 g/liter in 0.05 mol/liter phosphate buffer, containing NaCl, 0.15 mol/liter and H_2O_2, 0.05% at pH 7.4) (Sigma Chemical Company, St. Louis, Missouri) was used for color complex development of the immune precipitate. The slides were then counterstained with hematoxylin (Gill No. 3, Sigma Chemical Co.).

Specificity of staining was determined by immune neutralization using fragment B, the largest fragment of PIP obtained following cyanogen bromide treatment of the

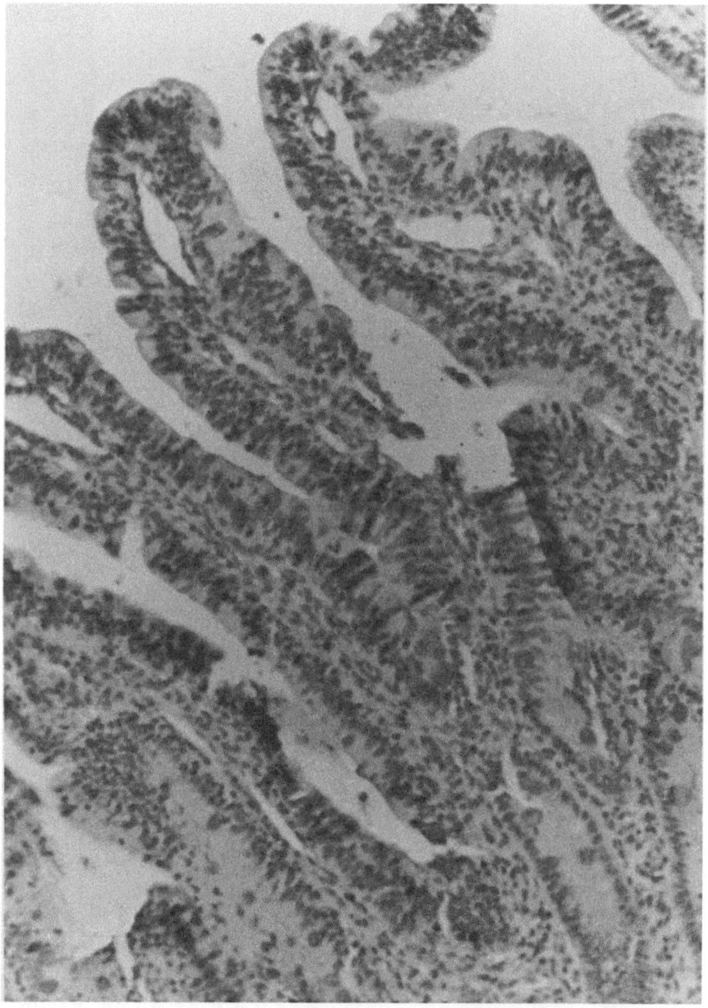

Fig. 1. Immunoreactive PIP in the proximal ileum. *Darkened area* is positive staining

native peptide (Wider and Duhaime 1985). The antiserum, diluted 1:10000, was incubated with fragment B in three different concentrations (5, 50, and 500 ng/ml) for 48 h at °C before application to the secions.

Results

In the gastrointestinal tract, immunoreactive PIP (IRPIP) was mainly found immunohistochemically in the distal small intestine. In the proximal ileum, IRPIP was confined to scattered single cells in the superficial mucosa (Fig. 1). In the distal ileum,

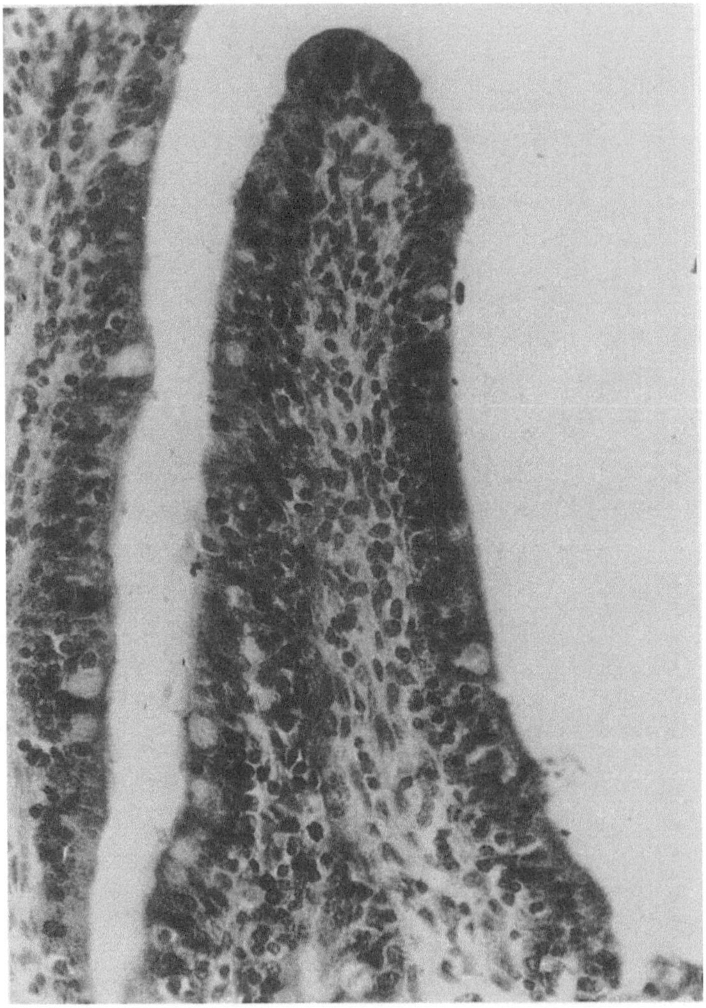

Fig. 2. Immunoreactive PIP in the distal ileum. *Darkened area* is positive staining

all superficial enterocytes except for goblet cells stained for IRPIP (Fig. 2). No cells in the deeper layers of the mucosa or in the crypts were stained.

No IRPIP was found in heart, lung, diaphragm, liver, gallbladder, sciatic nerve, vagal nerve, skeletal muscle, pancreas, spleen, adrenal gland, kidney, or skin using these antibody concentrations. In the urinary tract, however, IRPIP was seen in the mucosa of the ureter and the urinary bladder. In the bladder, staining was seen throughout the mucosa (Fig. 3) except for the most superficial cuticule. In the ureter, only occasional cells scattered in the deeper layers of the mucosa stained for IRPIP.

While the ileal mucosa stained intensely with antibody dilutions of 1:40000–1:20000, these antibody concentrations gave no or barely visible staining of the mucosa of the urinary tract. For intense staining in the urinary tract, higher antibody

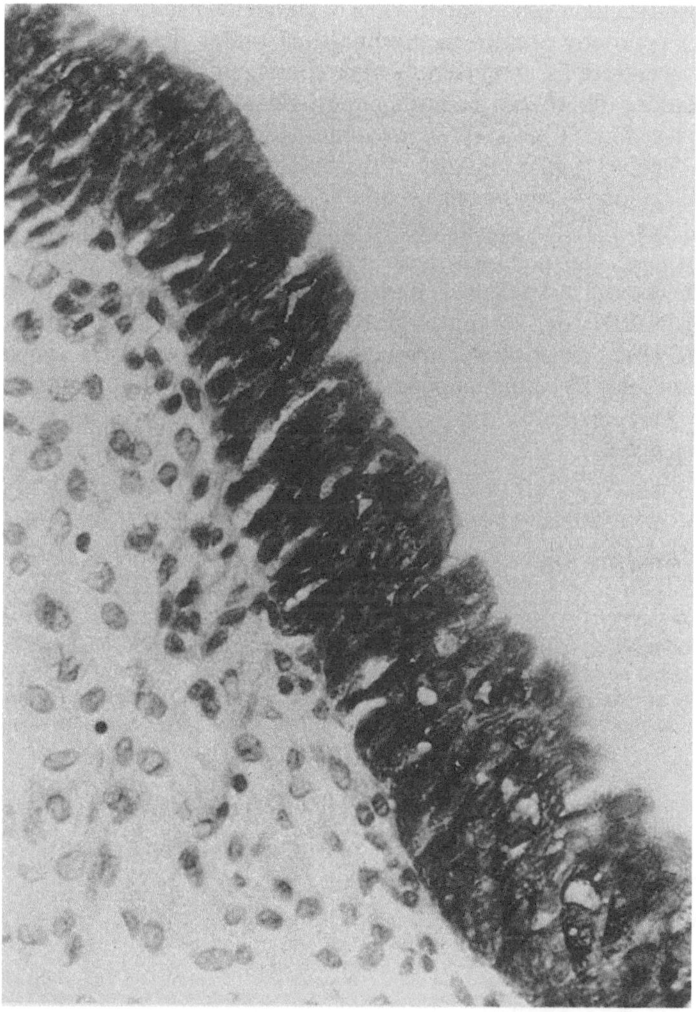

Fig. 3. Immunoreactive PIP in the urinary bladder. *Darkened area* is positive staining

concentrations of 1:10000–1:5000 had to be used. This could be done without the appearance of any visible background staining.

Preincubating the antibody diluted to 1:10000 with fragment B of PIP in a concentration of 5 ng/ml or more completely blocked staining of the urinary tract mucosa. Additions of 5 and 50 ng/ml of fragment B decreased staining of the ileal mucosa, while 500 ng/ml was needed to block completely all staining in the ileal mucosa.

Discussion

We have shown that immunoreactive PIP is uniquely distributed in the mucosa of the distal small intestine and to some extent in the urinary tract. The major concentration is apparently present in the intestinal rather than the bladder mucosa, as higher concentrations of antiserum were consistently necessary to demonstrate PIP in the bladder. However, the immunoperoxidase technique is not quantitative, and tissue extraction is necessary to prove this assumption.

The antigenic similarity of the bladder and intestinal staining is supported by the ability of the cyanogen bromide-generated fragment B to block staining in both tissues. PIP thus appears to be mainly localized in the distal few feet of ileum in the mucosa. The mucosa is in earliest jeopardy during rejection episodes. Disruption of the mucosa may result in either a transient increase of PIP in the peripheral circulation or in PIP's total disappearance. This may be anticipated, as we have demonstrated IRPIP in the peripheral circulation in a concentration of 6–12 ng/ml in our pilot studies for a IRPIP radioimmunoassay.

Therefore, PIP represents a potential organ-specific marker for small-bowel rejection.

References

Wider MD, Vinik AI, Heldsinger A (1984) Isolation and partial characterization of an enterooxyntin from porcine ileum. Endocrinology 115:1484–1491

Wider MD, Duhaime PMO (1985) Chromatographic and electrophoretic characterization of immunoreactive porcine ileal polypeptide in plasma. Endocrinology [Suppl] 116:A656

Session 9: Summary

A. Thiede

Postoperative clinical and immunologic monitoring is of particular importance in small-intestine transplantation. Fundamentally, we can say that in organ transplantation, it is useful to perform not only special analyses of the organ's functions, but also indirect or direct cytoimmunologic studies. Even more certainty can be attained with direct biopsies. Today, we are able to perform immunohistologic investigations on biopsy specimens and possibly to demonstrate the expression of antigenic determinants that are the initial prodromes of an impending rejection prior to any clinical manifestations, as Engemann (1985) has shown experimentally in rat liver transplantation.

In small-intestine transplantation, the direct biopsy is of transcendent importance as long as there is a stoma in the vulnerable postoperative phase – thus, the two-step technique is ideal for studying preclinical questions. With direct mucosa-submucosa biopsies, we can perform not only the investigations referred to above, but also make systematic macroscopic observations relating to blood circulation, and above all, perform quantitative morphometrical analyses of the form and volume of the villi and enzyme histochemical analyses of the microvilli (see contributions by Sandforth et al. and Stauffer). Postoperative monitoring is much more difficult after the second step of the operation, when the small-intestine graft is completely incorporated into the gastrointestinal passage, although this phase is immunologically much more stable. Repeated endoscopic biopsies are likely to cause unusual difficulties for technical reasons, so that we must depend on indirect hematologic and immunologic results and indirect absorption tests, such as the maltose absorption test for example (see Schraut and Lee). The reults of this test can probably be considered representative of the absorptive behavior of many substances during rejection reactions, since absorption studies have so far not shown any dissociation of the absorptive behavior of different substances during rejection reactions. We should also mention the demonstration of β_2-microglobulin in the serum, which is an easy test to perform for screening purposes and can be frequently repeated. This test also provides a considerable amount of information on the behavior of organ grafts. Whether the specific ileal peptide will turn out to be of particular significance as a potential rejection marker in small-intestine transplantation (see Borgstrom et al.) is a question that will have to be clarified by further experiments.

Reference

Engemann R (1985) Die orthotope Lebertransplantation: Funktionelle, morphologische und immunologische Untersuchung zur Toleranz allogener Rattenlebertransplantate. Habilitationsschrift, University of Kiel

Session 10

Indications for Small-Bowel Grafting in Children and Adults

Potential Recipients for Small-Bowel Transplantation in the United States and the United Kingdom

S. E. Talsma, W. H. Marks, C. Marks, and M. Brady

Introduction

The population which would benefit from small-bowel transplantation remains poorly defined. Both the United States and the United Kingdom have established registers of patients receiving home hyperalimentation. We chose to examine these records in an initial effort to identify the "at-need" population for this procedure. A further goal was to determine whether these registers contained sufficient information to act as a data base collection system for potential recipients of small-bowel transplants.

Materials and Methods

United States Registry of Patients on Home Total Parenteral Nutrition
(New York Academy of Medicine, New York, New York). The registry began in 1977, and data are available through 1983. Information is gathered by questionaires sent annually to participating institutions. The number of institutions reporting has increased from a low of 19 in 1977 to a current high of 93. Only the data from 1981–1983 were used in this review because the number of respondents was relatively constant (89, 90, 93 in the respective years). The United States data was limited, as individual patient records were not available for review owing to an agreement on the confidentiality of records with the participating institutions.

Information was obtained on the diagnoses initiating home total parenteral nutrition (HTPN), conditions resulting in the termination of HTPN, age and sex distribution of the patients, and cumulative statistics concerning length of time on HTPN and associated complications and cost of HTPN, where available.

United Kingdom Home Parenteral Nutrition Register
(University of Manchester, Salford, England). The register began in 1977, and data are available through April 1985. Information is gathered by annual questionaire. A total of 26 institutions report, with 14 hospitals accounting for 92.5% of the cases. Detailed patient information is available on all patients registered prior to 1983.

Information obtained from the British HTPN registry was similar to the data provided by its United States counterpart.

Independent Audit of Candidates

In the United States, medical records of patients identified by ICD-9-CM codes for short-bowel syndrome, acute vascular insufficiency of the intestine, volvulus, necrotizing enterocolitis, and unspecified intestinal malabsorption were reviewed at three tertiary care centers known to report to the U.S. HTPN registry. The goal was to determine if all potential candidates had been reported to the HTPN register in the years reviewed.

Results

United States HTPN Register

During the period studied, 1205 patients entered the registry. The diagnoses resulting in the initiation of HTPN are listed as follows:

1) Malignancy
2) Crohn's disease
3) Ulcerative colitis
4) Ischemic bowel disease
5) Motility disorders
6) Congenital bowel malformation
7) Pancreatic disease
8) Immune disorders
9) Trauma
10) Hyperemesis gravidarum
11) Cystic fibrosis
12) Bowel obstruction (nonmalignant)
13) Short-bowel syndrome
14) Persistent bowel fistulae
15) Other nonsurgical causes of malabsorption
16) Other/no information

Patients with motility disorders, trauma resulting in short-bowel syndrome, cystic fibrosis, and short bowel resulting from additional unrelated causes were likely candidates for small-bowel transplantation. In all, 177 patients were included in this category. The average age was 28.5 years, and 57% of patients were female.

United Kingdom HTPN Register

Data from 84 patients were entered. The diagnoses leading to the initiation of HTPN were similar to those in the United States. Of these 84 persons, 11 were identified as candidates for small-bowel transplantation. The average age was 31.9 years, and 57% were female.

Independent Audit of Candidates

Two infants were identified who had died in the hospital as a result of an inability to thrive on long-term hyperalimentation. These patients were not included in the registries. In the United Kingdom, there were seven cases (ages unknown) not registered.

Cost of HTPN

Data on cost were only available for 1982 in the United States data and not at all in the data provided by the United Kingdom (Table 1).

Table 1. HTPN-Related expenses in the United States

	Annual cost per patient (1982) in U.S. $
Pump	1155–2390
Supplies and solutions	36700–55380
Physician/clinic fees	277–385
Laboratory fees	824–987
Total mean cost per patient per year	40899–58819

Discussion

These data indicate that approximately 400 patients per year in the United States and 20 patients per year in the United Kingdom begin receiving HTPN. Many are not suitable candidates for small-bowel transplantation. We eliminated persons with malignancy or ischemic bowel disease due to atherosclerosis (assumed in patients over 50 years of age), as well as patients who were over 50 years of age. We also chose to eliminate patients with inflammatory bowel disease. These patients represent a large group of potential recipients. However, the disease has an unknown pathophysiology, may be systemic in nature, and has a tendency to recur, prompting us to exclude these patients as candidates at this time. Such a viewpoint may be unduly pessimistic and unnecessarily lower the number of potential recipients, just as 15 years ago patients with diabetic nephropathy would not have been considered renal transplant candidates.

Using these rough guidelines and the limited data bases available to us, we were able to identify 58 persons in the United States (1 per 5.2 million) and two persons in the United Kingdom (1 per 30 million) who became acceptable candidates each year. Although the numbers are small, the annual cost of maintaining these patients on HTPN is considerable, amounting to U.S. $ 3 million by 1982 prices for the United States patients alone. These figures include only basic costs for standard supplies and solutions and do not reflect hospital readmissions related to HTPN complications.

While all patients in the United Kingdom who would be acceptable candidates are apparently reported to their registry, it is important to note that, in the United States, we were able to identify at least two other candidates who were not reported to the registry over a 3-year period. In addition, only 93 United States medical centers were reporting, this in a country with at least 140 medical schools, each of which is associated with at least one tertiary care center. Therefore, it is likely that, at least in the United States data base, there are many more candidates available on an annual basis than are listed.

Finally, while the United States register was established largely to act as a listing and data retrieval system for small-bowel transplant candidates, the system currently available does not lend itself to rigorous statistical analysis, and the numbers generated are estimates by necessity. Much of the information is unavailable owing to the failure to differentiate between transplant and nontransplant candidates. Nonetheless, the United States register has been helpful as a first step in estimating the magnitude of the problem and will be helpful in the design of a more specific and useful small-bowel transplant candidate listing and data base system for the future. It is also clear that, especially in the United States, a more complete system is necessary in order to identify the potential recipients who do not currently have access to the register.

Indications for Small-Bowel Transplantation in Children

W. MENGEL and TH. SCHANG

It is not an easy task to comment on small-bowel transplantation in newborns and infants, when experimental work will be applied clinically in the next future. Nevertheless, small-bowel transplantation as seen from the point of view of a pediatric surgeon will be discussed here.

In children, short-bowel syndrome resulting from irreversible damage of extensive parts of small-intestine is not very often caused by disorders of vascular supply, such as thrombosis of the superior mesenteric vein. More frequently, various malformations and diseases affecting mostly newborns raise the question of whether small-bowel transplantation can be considered a therapy of choice or not for this group of patients.

Among the indications for small-bowel transplantation, we must mention atresia of the small bowel, either involving the entire organ or occurring in multiple segments, volvulus in malrotation, followed by small-bowel necrosis, gastroschisis, necrotizing enterocolitis (NEC), and ganglionosis of the entire intestine. The situation after continued partial resecions for NEC should also be listed here. Accidental damage of the superior mesenteric vessels in surgery for very large retroperitoneal tumors is a very specific cause of short-bowel syndrome that need only be mentioned for the sake of completeness.

According to STAUFFER (1977; 1983), a small bowel of 15–20 cm in length seems to be a critical threshold for sufficient enteric resorption. Total parenteral nutrition has been the only chance of survival until now, if the length of small bowel is less than 15 cm. Hickmann and Broviac catheters of Silastic available today make it possible to manage parenteral nutrition for months and even years, given correct handling of the catheters and avoidance of septic infections, which have been limiting factors in the past. Today, the problem of maintaining a parenteral line has thus been solved even if repeated changes of catheters are necessary, as we know from experience with bone marrow transplantation.

Patients can be placed in one of two groups according to whether they have more or less than the critical length of 15 cm of small bowel. Children having less than 15 cm of functional small intestine are likely to require long-term parenteral hyperalimentation. Based on experiences, small-bowel transplantation is the only change of survival for these children because it is not possible for them to develop enough resorptive surface, even by hypertrophy.

Submitting to a request for case reports, departments of pediatric surgery all over the Federal Republic of Germany sent reports concerning cases in the last 10 years in which there might have been indications for small-bowel transplantation. The evaluation of these reports has disclosed several remarkable findings. Although this survey cannot claim completeness, 19 departments of pediatric surgery reported data

Table 1. Case reports of short-bowel syndrome (1975–1985)

Patient	Year	Age	Clinical description	Result
1	1975	Newborn	Multiple intestinal atresia, 9 cm small bowel, multiple anastomoses	Died
2	1975	Newborn	Multiple intestinal atresia, 12 cm small bowel, multiple anastomoses	Died
3	1976	Newborn	Gastroschisis, intestinal atresia beginning in the duodenum, pars IV	Died after 100 days
4	1978	Newborn	Multiple intestinal atresia, 12 cm small bowel	Died
5	1979	Newborn	Gastroschisis, intestinal atresia, no small bowel left, 15 cm large bowel	Died
6	1979	3 years	NEC after chemotherapy for Wilms' tumor	Died
7	1983	Newborn	Gastroschisis, multiple intestinal atresia, 17 cm small bowel	Died after 6 months
8	1985	2 years	Thrombosis of superior mesenteric vein, duodenum pars I and II remaining	Parenteral nutrition since 2/85

on patients suffering from small-bowel syndrome who had undergone surgery in the last 10 years. The cases reported by one of these clinics are summarized in Table 1 and make clear, as do all the other case reports, that most pediatric surgeons are challenged by the problem of developing an adequate therapy for children who have less than 20 cm of small intestine. Though a calculation based on the reported cases may be very speculative, one might guess that, by extrapolating from the 64 cases in the last 10 years reported by 19 departments out of the 34 queried, there are at least 15–20 new cases of short-bowel syndrome every year in the 47 departments of the Federal Republic of Germany. For these children, a therapeutic solution must be found.

The number of children having more than 20 cm of small bowel seems to be similar. These children require parenteral nutrition and enteric administration of hydrolized proteins causing hypertrophy of the remaining mucosa, which is the preferred therapy today. There is no doubt that there is an indication for small-bowel transplantation in true short-bowel syndrome because, if the child survives, lifelong parenteral nutrition would be the only alternative, and this cannot really be the therapy of choice for functional and ethical reasons. In contrast, there is a relative indication for transplantation.

The experience of several surgeons shows that many children do not gain weight and suffer from generally impaired development, even though they have more than 20–30 cm of small intestine. Presumably in these cases, we are dealing with the following problem: Because of efforts to leave as much of the damaged intestine as possible, for instance in NEC, some damaged tissue remains in situ which is incapable of rebuilding functioning mucosa. Thus, a functional short-bowel syndrome is created.

With the possibility that successful clinical small-bowel transplantation will probably be available in the near future, the question arises of whether a more radical primary resection would be of value in these cases. This technique would leave less, but only healthy small intestine, thus avoiding reoperations. Of course, successful transplantation is the prerequisite for discussions of relative indications.

Pediatric surgeons have different points of view concerning indications for small-bowel transplantation, and one might have the impression that the majority do not really see any indication for it at all. This attitude might derive from the fact that everybody has experience of single cases only that do not leave a lasting impression. However, when all reported cases of children suffering from short-bowel syndrome are put together, the following situation is apparent: After repeated operations and tremendous efforts to allow these children to survive, where they must undergo a painful martyrdom lasting a few days for some children and up to 16 months for others, almost all of them succumb to death in the end. Successful small-bowel transplantation could save 15–20 children per year suffering from short-bowel syndrome.

References

Stauffer UG (1977) The present state of small bowel transplantation in animal research and in man. Z Kinderchir 22:241

Stauffer UG (1983) Die Dünndarm-Transplantation: Gegenwärtiger Stand und mögliche Zukunft. Z Kinderchir 38:286

Session 10: Summary

U. G. STAUFFER

In this last session of the symposium, which was devoted to the current status of small-bowel transplantation in man, we heard that there would probably be between 100 and 400 candidates for small-intestinal transplantation in the United States, 30–50 in the United Kingdom, and 30–40 in Germany. Four patients have already been placed on a transplantation list in Zürich. The first small-intestinal transplantation in man since 1972 was carried out by the Toronto team of Dr. COHEN this year. Five more attempts to perform small-intestinal transplantation in man have been approved for his group by the counselling ethical committee in Toronto. Fifteen patients, mainly children, are awaiting small-intestinal transplantation in Paris.

It must stressed, however, that we all realize that small-intestinal transplantation is still an experimental therapy. In spite of all our efforts so far, there are still many unsolved or only partially solved problems. I would like to mention some of these: First, it is important to realize that there are no regular series over years of truly long-term survivors of small-intestinal transplantations, even for animal experiments. Long-term survivors are still the exception rather than the rule. Furthermore, the results obtained so far in experiments in small animals, mainly in rats, are of course not directly applicable to large animals and certainly not to man. Regarding clinical application, we learned from the recent Toronto case that identical blood groups between donor and recipient are absolutely mandatory, as is of course a negative cross-match. However, at least now that cyclosporine A has been introduced, HLA typing no longer seems to be of prime importance. Cyclosporine A seems to be an excellent immunosuppressive drug, and there was some agreement that a serum level of 300 ng/L would probably be adequate, at least in animals. However, here again, this has not yet been confirmed for humans. There is also no clear agreement as to whether cyclosporine A should be combined with corticosteroids or not, or how long cyclosporine A should be given after transplantation. Nor is there a definite answer yet as to which route (intravenous or oral) should be preferred in the long run. Therefore, we still need further pharmacodynamic studies, mainly concerning intestinal absorption in normal intestine and in the transplanted intestine over longer periods of time.

As for transplantation techniques, most of us prefer initially to transplant the intestine using Thiry-Vella loops with double enterostomies, at least for the first 3–4 weeks. However, we still have some doubts as to whether there is a significant difference between orthotopic and heterotopic transplants. The enterostomies allow for early recognition of vascular complications during the initial hours or days after transplantation. It also seems that biopsies and histologic studies with special techniques (for instance, quantitative morphometric analysis) provide the safest monitoring systems, allowing recognition of an incipient rejection crisis early enough to start intensive immunosuppressive therapy or, in the event of graft failure, to explant the graft without danger to the recipient. If intestinal continuity is restored between the residual bowel and the transplant after a period of several weeks or months, most transplant surgeons agree that a biopsy pouch should be left for further monitoring, but there is no complete consensus on this point. The length of the bowel to be transplanted is also still being debated. Because of the immense numbers of immunocompetent cells involved, graft-versus-host-reaction may play a role at least in total allotransplantation in spite of the use cyclosporine A. This may have an influence on the function of these transplants over longer periods of time. On the other hand, we know that in transplants of up to 150 cm a graft-versus-host-reaction does not occur. Shorter intestinal segments should therefore be preferred for small-intestinal transplantation. However, we do not know how long this segment should be in order to assure normal intestinal function over months or years. Given that a rejection crisis can be brought under control, we still also lack information on whether transplant function can recover completely or only partially. With a few exceptions, studies on the function of intestinal allografts have covered only shorter periods of time. In intact small-intestinal allografts, we know that there is a normal function capacity for amino acids, proteins, and glucose, but that there is a delay in fat absorption. The latter is probably due to the time needed for reconstruction of the lymph vessels, which usually takes between 6 and 10 weeks. We also know that intestinal enzymes, for instance disaccharidases, are at normal levels in the well-functioning transplant. This appears very encouraging, but here again, the function of the transplanted intestinal segments could deteriorate over months or years, and therefore, more detailed resorption studies performed on successful intestinal transplants over months or years are imperative.

In considering all these unsolved or only partially solved problems, it became clear during the session that the majority of the audience think that it would be ethically debatable or even wrong to accept living donors. However, in practice, the short ischemia time of 5–6 h is an important consideration in harvesting the transplant, as was mentioned by several speakers.

The only alternative therapy to small-intestinal transplantation is home parenteral nutrition, and it seems that this is still the treatment of choice for most adults today. On the other hand, there is also considerable morbidity and mortality in adults on home parenteral nutrition, and for some patients, this treatment is not feasible or is eventually rejected by the patient himself, as in Dr. COHEN's recent case. For these selected patients, small-intestinal transplantation is a possible alternative today. However, such candidates for small-intestinal transplantation have to be fully informed about the present state of knowledge concerning this technique, including the fact that we still lack long-term human survivors. On the other hand, it can also be mentioned that small-intestinal transplantation is a relatively safer procedure today, which can be undertaken without undue risk to the recipient because we are able to recognize rejection crisis and other complications on the axis of the graft early enough. This is, of course, the prime prerequisite for small-intestinal transplantation in humans.

In contrast to the situation for adults, home parenteral nutrition in the pediatric age group is much more difficult. Complication rates are higher, and the value of continuous total parenteral nutrition over periods of more than 6 months or even years is questionable and ethically debatable, especially with infants and very young children. Small-intestinal transplantation therefore seems to be indicated for this group. Possible candidates would be infants and children who have a total loss of small-intestinal function or extreme short-bowel syndrome and in whom intestinal rehabilitation has failed after 6–8 months of total parenteral nutrition. These are currently the criteria for the patients on the transplantation list in Zürich and Paris. I expect, therefore, that in the next years we will hear mainly about small-intestinal transplantations in infants and children. In the near future, adults will probably receive transplants only in those selected cases where home parenteral nutrition is not feasible for one reason or another. This may change with further experience in basic and clinical research. An international registry should be instituted to record every attempt to perform small-intestinal transplantation, and the details of every case should be reported and described, as Dr. Cohen did in his presentation.

I thank all the speakers and panelists for their contributions and hope that this symposium will be a landmark that will represent another important step forward toward the clinical applications of small-intestinal transplantation in humans. In the name of all the participants, I would also like to thank the organizers for their hospitality and the opportunity to share and discuss together all aspects of the experimental and clinical fundamentals of small-bowel transplantation. I also hope that we will be able to meet again in a few years to discuss first of all further progress in basic research directed toward the remaining unsolved problems touched on here and, secondly, the results of a small initial series of at least partially successful small-intestinal transplantation in humans.

Subject Index

MIX
Papier aus verantwortungsvollen Quellen
Paper from responsible sources
FSC® C105338

If you have any concerns about our products,
you can contact us on
ProductSafety@springernature.com

In case Publisher is established outside the EU,
the EU authorized representative is:
Springer Nature Customer Service Center GmbH
Europaplatz 3, 69115 Heidelberg, Germany

Printed by Libri Plureos GmbH
in Hamburg, Germany